T0262725

Encyclopedia of DNA Repair and Human Health

Volume III

Encyclopedia of DNA Repair and Human Health
Volume III

Edited by **Nas Wilson**

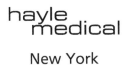

hayle
medical

New York

Published by Hayle Medical,
30 West, 37th Street, Suite 612,
New York, NY 10018, USA
www.haylemedical.com

Encyclopedia of DNA Repair and Human Health
Volume III
Edited by Nas Wilson

International Standard Book Number: 978-1-63241-002-3 (Hardback)

Contents

Preface

This book provides comprehensive information regarding DNA repair and human health. Over the past decades, significant developments have been made in cellular DNA repair pathways. Simultaneously, a wealth of elucidative knowledge of human diseases has been compiled. Now, the fundamental research of the mechanisms of DNA repair is integrating with clinical research, placing the action of the DNA repair pathways in light of the whole organism. Such integrative approach allows understanding of the disease mechanisms and is useful in enhancing diagnostics and prevention, as well as designing improved therapies. This book throws light on the primary role of DNA repair in human health and well-being by discussing repair and aging, damage and disease, and inflammation in relation to DNA.

The researches compiled throughout the book are authentic and of high quality, combining several disciplines and from very diverse regions from around the world. Drawing on the contributions of many researchers from diverse countries, the book's objective is to provide the readers with the latest achievements in the area of research. This book will surely be a source of knowledge to all interested and researching the field.

In the end, I would like to express my deep sense of gratitude to all the authors for meeting the set deadlines in completing and submitting their research chapters. I would also like to thank the publisher for the support offered to us throughout the course of the book. Finally, I extend my sincere thanks to my family for being a constant source of inspiration and encouragement.

Editor

Part 1

DNA Repair and Aging

Transcriptional Functions of DNA Repair Proteins Involved in Premature Aging

Robin Assfalg and Sebastian Iben
Department of Dermatology and Allergic Diseases
University of Ulm
Germany

1. Introduction

Premature aging diseases or progerias are rare genetical disorders displaying symptoms of the aging body early in life or even in childhood. They are called segmental because they show some, but not all features of aging. There is the progeria of the adult, Werner syndrome and, more severe because limiting lifespan to the first or second decade, the progerias of the childhood, Cockayne syndrome, trichothiodystrophy and Hutchinson-Gilford syndrome. With the exception of Hutchinson-Gilford syndrome, the progerias are caused by recessive mutations. Cockayne syndrome and trichothiodystrophy are polygenic disorders- the recessive mutation in five respective three different genes can cause the same devastating phenotype. All genes of a polygenic disorder may function in a critical redundant pathway . The identification of these pathways is topic of intensive labour in different laboratories for more than one reason. First, the identification of the molecular defects will help us to treat these diseases. Second, as these diseases mimic the normal aging process, understanding these diseases will strengthen our understanding of aging in general. Third, as these disorders display accelerated aging, the underlying pathways may be critical for the rate of aging and may help us to slow aging respectively allow us to affect healthy aging. Aging is believed to be due to the accumulation of molecular and macromolecular damage (Kirkwood, 2010), thus accelerated aging might be caused by a higher damage rate or by an impairment of counteracting pathways as repair mechanisms. The later assumption is generally believed to be the explanation for the accelerated aging seen in progerias, defects in macromolecular repair pathways, especially in DNA-repair pathways are generally considered as being causal for accelerated aging. Although there is ample evidence that aging is accompanied by macromolecular damage and DNA damage in particular, the causal connection between DNA damage and tissue or organismal aging is far from understood. Here the investigation of progerias is able to fuel our understanding of the mechanisms of aging as most of the involved genes play roles in different DNA repair pathways. But it is not so simple because all the progeria genes display multiple functions in the cells and are also involved in the regulation of gene expression by acting as basal transcription factors or as chromatin modifying enzymes. The discovery of the transcriptional function of DNA repair factors was accompanied by the hypothesis that accelerated aging could also be caused by alterations in gene expression mechanisms (Drapkin et al, 1994, Guzder et al, 1994). Since then the "transcriptional" versus the "DNA repair" hypothesis were intensively discussed and today there is a lot of evidence for the involvement of both pathways in the pathogenesis of premature aging (Chalut et al,1994, Winkler and Hoeijmakers,1998, Bergmann and Egly 2001, deBoer et al 2002). Transcription of DNA by the RNA polymerases serves as a DNA damage sensor and recruits DNA repair proteins to sites of DNA damage. Moreover, hitherto as pure DNA repair factors recognized proteins turned out to be involved in chromatin remodeling and epigenetic modulation of gene expression of undamaged DNA (Schmitz et al, 2009, LeMay et al, 2010). Thus repair of DNA and gene expression at the level of transcription are intimately structurally and functionally linked. Here we review the current knowledge about transcriptional functions of DNA repair proteins involved in the pathogenesis of progerias.

2. Premature aging syndromes

2.1 Werner syndrome

Werner syndrome (WS) or the progeria of the adult, is an autosomal recessive genetic instability and cancer predisposition syndrome that mimics premature aging. WS patients lack the pubertal growth spurt and develop bilateral cataracts, premature graying and loss of hair and scleroderma-like skin changes already beginning in the second decade of life. Patients have an elevated risk of age-associated diseases as atherosclerotic cardiovascular disease, diabetes mellitus, osteoporosis and cancer. Life expectancy is shortened to 47 years.

The WS gene WRN encodes a member of the RecQ helicase protein family and posseses an additional 3´-5´exonuclease domain. WRN is involved in different DNA metabolizing pathways as DNA repair and replication, telomere maintenance and transcription (Rossi et al, 2010, Chu and Hickson, 2009, Ding and Shen 2008). WRN deficient cells display a telomere lagging strand replication defect and karyotypic instability associated with short telomers (Crabbe et al, 2004, Crabbe et al, 2007). Moreover, premature aging in mice deficient for WRN is dependent on telomere shortening in the telomerase RNA subunit TERC deficient background (Chang et al, 2004). These double knockout mice also show a hallmark of cells derived from Werner syndrome patients- premature senescence. Whereas fibroblasts from normal donors enter the stage of irreversible division stop, replicative senescence, after 60 population doublings, cells from Werner syndrome patients enter senescence after 15-20 population doublings (Faragher et al, 1993). Thus it seems that the role of the WRN protein at the telomeres might be critical to protect us from premature aging. Nonetheless, there are host of questions arising. It is not clear if replicative senescence is responsive for aging pathologies, although markers of replicative senescence accumulate in aged skin of baboons (Herbig et al 2006). Studies on telomere length dynamics in Werner syndrome cells revealed that telomeres did not erode faster than in normal cells (Baird et al, 2004). Expression of telomerase in Werner syndrome cells can overcome premature senescence (Wyllie et al, 2000, Choi et al, 2001), but inhibition of the stress-activated kinase p38 by the compound PD203580 also extended the replicative lifespan of WS cells to that observed in normal fibroblasts (Davis et al 2005). These observations substanstiate that our knowledge about the pathophysiology of Werner syndrome is still limited and that alternative concepts also deserve attention.

The first indication of the involvement of RecQ helicases in gene expression came from studies of the yeast WRN homolog sgs1. As in WS, the *sgs1* deletion decreases the average life span of cells and accelerates aging (Sinclair et al, 1997). Conditional mutation of *sgs1* in a yeast strain lacking the helicase *srs2* is followed by a drastical inhibition of DNA replication and RNA polymerase I transcription. The authors concluded that the replication defect could contribute to the genomic instability of WS, whereas impaired ribosomal RNA chain elongation may render RNA polymerase I prone to pausing that could trigger the formation of double strand breaks. Repair by nonhomologous end-joining could result in the accumulation of deletions in the genomic rDNA and contribute to premature aging in WS (Lee et al, 1999). Shiratori and co-workers showed that in human WS cells RNA polymerase I transcription is reduced and can be restored by wildtype WRN. Moreover, nucleolar localization of WRN is dependent on ongoing RNA polymerase I transcription. WRN can be co-immunoprecipitated with RNA polymerase I. In humans, the decreased transcriptional rate of rRNA could be the primary molecular defect causing the premature aging phenotype in WS patients, the authors speculated (Shiratori et al, 2002). Another study with human WS cells described, that the stimulation of RNA polymerase I transcription by some growth factors is impaired in WS cells. Moreover, WRN acts as a transcription factor and stimulates the step of promoter clearance of RNA polymerase I transcription. Chromatin-immunoprecipitations revealed that WRN binds to quiescent and unmethylated rDNA, implicating a role of WRN in epigenetic regulation of RNA polymerase I transcription. Taken together, this study implicated that WRN acts as a growth factor dependent transcription factor of RNA polymerase I and may prevent inactivation of rDNA genes in the absence of growth factors (Lutomska et al, 2008). These mechanisms may contribute to the lack of the pubertal growth spurt, impaired wound healing and premature aging in WS patients.

Beside RNA polymerase I transcription several publications show that WRN influences gene expression by RNA polymerase II. One study from 1999 describes a significant reduction of RNA polymerase II transcription in WS cells. This is reflected in *in vitro* transcription and can be rescued by addition of wildtype but not mutant WRN. Moreover a 27aa repeated sequence in the WRN gene was identied as a strong transcriptional activator domain. The transcription defect in WS cells may be global or may affect certain genes or categories of genes within the genome (Balajee et al, 1999). The later hypothesis is supported by a report showing that the transcriptional activator function of p53 is stimulated by WRN (Blander et al, 1999). Gene expression profiling comparing cells from young donors and cells from old donors with WS cells unravelled that mutation of WRN affects the expression of certain genes within the genome. Moreover transcription alterations in WS were strikingly similar to those in normal aging (Kyng et al, 2003). These findings validated WS as a model disease for aging research and established, that WRN influences the expression of certain genes within the genome. To investigate if the observed changes in the transcriptome are due to the direct loss of WRN or are secondary consequences of genomic instability, Turaga et al used short-term siRNA based knockdown of WRN. This was sufficient to trigger an expression profile resembling fibroblasts established from old donor patients and identified genes involved in 14 distinct biological pathways to be affected by loss of WRN. It is conceivable that WRN might associate with chromatin and affect the activity of classical transcription factors (Turaga et al, 2009). A recent report also used microarray expression analysis to investigate if RecQ helicases and WRN in particular regulate genes enriched in G-quadruplex DNA, a family of non-canonical nucleic acids structures formed by certain G-rich sequences. RecQ helicases can unwind these structures *in vitro* and *in vivo*. In fact the authors found significant associations between loci that are regulated in WS and loci containing potential G-quadruplex forming sequences. These findings indicate that WRN can regulate transcription globally by targeting G-quadruplex DNA (Johnson et al, 2010).

Taken together there is ample evidence that the WRN protein influences transcription by RNA polymerase I and II and is involved in gene regulation of certain genes that are also regulated throughout the normal aging process and in the globally regulation of genes with G-quadruplex forming sequences.

2.2 Cockayne syndrome

Cockayne syndrome is an autosomal recessive neurodegenerative disorder characterized by progressive growth failure, retinal degeneration, cataracts, sensorineural deafness, mental retardation, and photosensitivity (Nance and Berry, 1992, Laugel et al, 2009). Cataracts, loss of retinal cells, neurological degeneration and cachexia are prominent premature aging symptoms of this disorder followed by infant death. Cockayne syndrome is caused by mutations in *CSA* and *CSB* genes and rare combinations with the cancer prone skin disease xeroderma pigmentosum and complementation groups *XPB*, *XPD* and *XPG* have been described. All five genes are involved in repair of helix-distorting lesions of DNA by the nucleotide excision repair pathway (NER). Damage recognition mechanisms differ in the subpathways transcription-coupled repair (TCR) in which CSA and CSB are involved and global genomic repair (GGR). Both pathways of damage recognition flow into a common DNA repair mechanism. Premature aging in Cockayne syndrome is commonly attributed to defective transcription coupled repair (Hoeijmakers, 2009), although this view raises a plethora of questions. There are multiple mutations in NER proteins described (XPA, XPB, XPD, XPF, XPG) that completely impair both branches of this DNA repair pathway, but are not followed by premature aging but cause the severe cancer prone skin disease xeroderma pigmentosum. Xeroderma pigmentosum patients, when shed from UV-light do not develop the premature aging traits of Cockayne syndrome although the same type of DNA lesions remain unrepaired and should accumulate and disturb cellular fidelity. Thus transcription coupled repair might also be responsive for the repair of hitherto undefined DNA lesions that compromise transcription (Laugel et al, 2009). It is conceivable that all five genes that, when mutated cause Cockayne syndrome, are involved in a critical redundant function that protects us from accelerated aging. This function is not identified yet. Transcription-coupled repair is responsible for the recruitment of the repair machinery to the transcribed strand of active genes. It has been shown, that nearly all factors involved in transcription coupled repair are coincidental participating in basal transcription mechanisms thus raising the possibility that premature aging might be due to aberrant transcription. This hypothesis is discussed since two decades without a definitive answer. Here, we would like to review the current knowledge about the transcriptional functions of the five proteins involved in the pathogenesis of Cockayne syndrome.

2.2.1 Cockayne syndrome protein A (CSA)

As the *CSA* gene was identified, the interaction of the corresponding protein with CSB and the TFIIH subunit p44 were described. TFIIH, beside being essential for Nucleotide Excision Repair (NER) of UV damaged DNA, is a general transcription factor of RNA polymerase II (see below). Thus the authors proposed a transcriptional function of CSA (Henning et al, 1995). In vitro transcription studies with a template bearing oxidative lesions showed a reduced RNA polymerase II transcription in nuclear extracts of CSA cells, that could be rescued by the overexpression of CSA indicating a transcriptional function of CSA (Dianov et al, 1997). However, microinjection of CSA antibodies in cells reduced the repair capacity of the cells, but did not influence the rate of transcription by RNA polymerase II (van Gool et al, 1997). Since then additional evidence for a direct involvement of CSA in transcription was not found.

2.2.2 Cockayne syndrome protein B (CSB)

Mutations in the *ERCC6/CSB* gene are responsible for 62% of Cockayne syndrome cases (Laugel et al, 2009). The *ERCC6* gene product belongs to the family of SWI/SNF chromatin remodeling enzymes (Troelstra et al, 1992). ATP-dependent chromatin remodeling enzymes coordinate changes in chromatin structure to help regulate transcription. This structure of CSB implies a regulatory role in transcription. The first study investigating a transcriptional role of CSB used in vivo labeling and permeabilisation of cells to show that CSB mutant cells exhibit a severely reduced RNA polymerase II transcription that could be restored by addition of CSB. As transcription of chromatin from permeabilized cells represent the elongation activity of RNA polymerase II, the authors proposed a role of CSB in transcription elongation (Balajee et al, 1997). Using microinjection of antibodies against CSB, van Gool et al did not detect an inhibition of transcription by all three RNA polymerases measured by labelled thymidine incorporation However, CSB cofractionates with RNA polymerase II over chromatographic columns and RNA polymerase II can be coimmunoprecipitated with CSB (van Gool et al, 1997). As these complexes do not contain initiation factors of RNA polymerase II, the authors speculated that CSB might be involved in a non-essential step of transcription elongation. Another study confirmed the interaction of RNA polymerase II with CSB and could convincingly show, that CSB stimulates elongation by RNA polymerase II in vitro (Selby and Sancar, 1997). If this function of CSB is relevant for transcription elongation in vivo, the study by van Gool et al should have detected a reduction of transcription by microinjection of CSB antibodies. The recruitment of CSB to RNA polymerase II elongation complexes in vitro was also demonstrated by other investigators (Tantin et al, 1997) but the in vivo relevance of this interaction was not studied. CSB mutant cells were found to exhibit metaphase fragility of highly transcribed genes of RNA polymerase II and III that are coding for structural RNAs. The authors proposed that CSB might play a role in transcription elongation of these genes and lack of CSB would be followed by stalled polymerases inducing metaphase fragility (Yu et al, 2000). ATP-dependent chromatin remodeling activity of CSB was substantiated in another study, thus implicating that CSB may play a role in facilitating transcription by RNA polymerase II through pause sites on natural chromatin templates in vivo by modulating nucleosome structure on DNA. It is possible that defective chromatin rearrangements during DNA repair or transcription may contribute to the severe clinical symptoms of CS patients (Citterio et al, 2000). A study performed in Saccharomyces cerevisiae provided in vivo evidence for a role of *rad26*, the counterpart of the *CSB* gene, in transcription elongation by RNA polymerase II. Under conditions requiring rapid synthesis of new mRNAs, growth is considerably reduced in cells lacking *rad26*. These findings implicate a role for CSB in transcription elongation, and they strongly suggest that impaired transcription elongation is the underlying cause of the developmental problems in CS patients (Lee et al, 2001).

The same authors showed that the CSB homolog *rad26* plays a role in promoting transcription by RNA polymerase II through bases damaged by the alkylating agent MMS. Transcription through these bases is severely inhibited in *rad26Δ* cells lacking both the NER (nucleotide excision repair) and BER (base excision repair) pathways required for the removal of these lesions (Lee et al, 2002). This report demonstrates a transcriptional function of CSB independent from DNA repair and, moreover, fit to the observation, that nuclear extracts from CS cells of three complementation groups exhibit reduced RNA polymerase II in vitro transcription only on oxidised template (Dianov et al, 1997).

Microarray analysis of gene expression profiles did not identify significant differences in gene expression between CSB deficient and transfected cells indicating that CSB does not function as a gene specific transcription factor (Selzer et al, 2002). Bradsher et al reported a novel aspect of CSB as a component of RNA polymerase I transcription in the nucleolus. CSB was localized to nucleoli and isolated in a complex with RNA polymerase I, transcription initation factors of RNA polymerase I, TFIIH and XPG. CS mutations in TFIIH subunits rendered this complex instable and stability of this transcription competent complex was speculated to contribute to Cockayne syndrome phenotype. RNA polymerase I transcription was reduced in CSB mutant cells and restored by transfection of CSB (Bradsher et al, 2002). This report is inasmuch interesting as it describes a functional complex of 4 from 5 proteins that, when mutated cause Cockayne syndrome, indicating that rDNA transcription by RNA polymerase I might be the redundant function of the CS proteins whose failure causes premature aging.

Microarray analysis after oxidative stress revealed that there is a bundle of genes that is differently regulated after H_2O_2 treatment of CSB deficient and CSB competent cells. If the identified genes are directly regulated by CSB was not further specified (Kyng et al, 2003).

Confocal microscopy and quantitative digital image analysis of different photobleaching (FRAP) procedures showed transient interactions of CSB with the transcription machinery, which are prolonged when RNA polymerases are arrested at sites of DNA damage. Active RNA polymerase II could be immunopurified with CSB, but no transcription factors were found to be associated (van dem Boom et al, 2003). The CSB function in transcription was to this timepoint always linked to transcription elongation. A novel study discovered functions of CSB upstream of transcription initiation. The authors unveiled the crucial role played by CSB in the transcription initiation of a certain set of protein coding genes after UV irradiation. CSB cells cannot transcribe even nondamaged genes if the cells were previously UV irradiated. The recruitment of TBP, which is supposed to initiate transcription, was severely decreased; also, the recruitment of TFIIB was almost absent. Furthermore, histone H4 acetylation does not occur properly, highlighting a defect in one of the earlier events of the transcriptional process. The fact that CSB associates mainly with the unphosphorylated RNA pol IIA and the serine 5 phosphorylated RNA pol IIO, strongly supports a role for CSB during the first phases of the transcription reaction (Proietti-Di-Santis et al, 2006). Although earlier microarray analysis did not yield gene expression differences in CS-cells (Selzer et al,2002), refined methodology using microarrays in combination with a unique method for comparative expression analysis found many genes regulated by CSB. Remarkably, many of the genes regulated by CSB are also affected by inhibitors of histone deacetylase and DNA methylation, as well as by defects in poly(ADP-ribose)-polymerase function and RNA polymerase II elongation. This data indicate a general role for CSB protein in maintenance and remodeling of chromatin structure and suggest that CS is a disease of transcriptional deregulation caused by misexpression of growth-suppressive, inflammatory, and proapoptotic pathways (Newman et al , 2006). In vitro transcription analysis using a reconstituted transcription system showed, that bypass of different oxidative lesions in the template requires elongation factors like CSB, thus again evaluating the initial observation by Dianov et al, that CSB deficient cells exhibit reduced RNA polymerase II transcription on oxidised template (Charlet-Berguerant et al, 2006).

Extending the findings of Newman et al, that CSB influences chromatin remodeling to transcription of RNA polymerase I, Yuan et al demonstrated in an intricate analysis that transcription activation of RNA polymerase I is dependent on CSB. CSB is recruited to active rDNA repeats by TTF-I bound to the promoter-proximal terminator T_0. Depletion of CSB by siRNA impairs the formation Pol I preinitiation complexes and inhibits rDNA transcription. CSB recruits G9a that methylates histone H3 on lysine 9 (H3K9) in the pre-rRNA coding region. The results demonstrate that the functional cooperation between CSB and G9a is important for efficient pre-rRNA synthesis (Yuan et al, 2007). This study integrates findings of several above mentioned publications. A gene specific regulatory function upstream of transcription initiation was mechanistically deciphered and a chromatin organisation mode of CSB was described in detail.

Analysis of in vitro transcription by RNA polymerase I revealed that CSB plays a role as an elongation factor in rDNA transcription and that truncated CSB still localizes to the rDNA repeats in vivo. Truncated CSB actively represses in vitro transcription of RNA polymerase I thus providing an explanation for the observation that a null mutation in CSB is not necessarily followed by CS (Horibata et al, 2004) whereas truncating mutations are devastating (Lebedev et al, 2008).

CSB is also a critical mediator of the hypoxic response and influences binding of the general transcription factors and RNA polymerase II in a gene-specific manner in response to hypoxia as demonstrated by chromatin-immunoprecipitation analysis. CSB binds to p53 and might also influence its transcriptional activity, the authors speculated (Filippi et al, 2008). Thus it becomes evident that CSB is not only an elongation factor of RNA polymerase II but exhibits gene regulatory functions in a gene-specific manner.

The reviewed studies clearly show that CSB is an elongation factor of transcription by RNA polymerase I and II and that CSB facilitates transcription through damaged bases. Additional, CSB functions upstream of initiation by RNA polymerase I and II by recruiting chromatin modifying cofactors or by remodeling chromatin itself in a gene specific manner.

2.2.3 TFIIH

TFIIH is a multisubunit complex composed of ten subunits. It habors three enzymatic activities, two ATP dependent helicases of opposite orientation, XPB and XPD and the cyclin dependent kinase cdk7. Mutations in the XPB and XPD helicases are followed by the skin cancer prone xeroderma pigmentosum syndrome but also by the premature aging syndromes Cockayne and trichothiodystrophy. Mutations in the recently discovered tenth subunit p8/TTDA destabilize TFIIH and is followed by trichothiodystrophy. Xeroderma pigmentosum is characterized by a 1000fold elevated skin cancer risk, the german term "Mondscheinkinder" translated "moonshine-children" denominates the fact that the failure of Nucleotide excision repair (NER) renders the skin of affected children so sensitive to UV-induced DNA damage and consecutive development of skin destructive cancers that they need to be shed totally from UV-light by special clothing. Then they develop normally. The ATPase of XPB and XPD helicase activity of TFIIH are necessary for the unwinding of the damaged DNA strand that can then be cleaved and resynthesized. Thus highly mutagenic DNA lesions persist in the genome when the helicase functions of TFIIH are reduced or inactivated by mutations. The second main function of TFIIH is as a general transcription factor of RNA polymerase II. General or basal transcription factors are needed at every protein coding gene for bending of the promoter, positioning of the polymerase or promoter opening as through the ATPase activity of the XPB subunit of TFIIH (Kim et al, 2000,

Douziech et al, 2000). TFIIH has also been reported to play a postinitiation role in transcription by RNA polymerase I, the key step of ribosomal biogenesis, that accounts for up to 60% of ongoing transcription in a growing cell (Iben et al, 2002).

Xeroderma pigmentosum is due to unrepaired DNA damage, whereas premature aging in Cockayne syndrome and trichothiodystrophy might be caused by transcriptional deficiencies. Several studies addressed this hypothesis and an unequivocal answer to the question "is it repair or transcription?" has not been delivered yet.

Trichothiodystrophy mice with a mutation in XPD reflect to a remarkable extent the human disorder, including brittle hair, developmental abnormalities, reduced life span, UV sensitivity, and skin abnormalities. The cutaneous symptoms are associated with reduced transcription of a skin-specific gene strongly supporting the concept of TTD as a human disease due to inborn defects in basal transcription. To explain the characteristic hair and skin abnormalities of TTD, TTD-type *XPD* mutations may alter the XPD conformation and in this way affect the stability of the TFIIH complex. Under normal conditions, de novo synthesis of TFIIH is thought to compensate for the reduced half-life. However, in terminal differentiating tissues where de novo synthesis gradually declines, the mutated TFIIH might get exhausted before the transcriptional program has been completed (de Boer et al, 1998). These authors describe that late in the differentiation pathway and thus gene-specific transcription is severely disturbed in trichothiodystrophy in contrast to general transcription deficiencies (whole genome).

A study comparing XP versus TTD mutations in the helicase XPD showed the following: all XPD mutations, regardless of causing Xeroderma pigmentosum or trichothiodystrophy are detrimental for XPD helicase activity, thus explaining the NER defect. TFIIH from TTD patients, but not from XP patients, exhibits a significant in vitro basal transcription defect in addition to a reduced intracellular concentration. Moreover, when XPD mutations prevent interaction with the p44 subunit of TFIIH, transactivation directed by certain nuclear receptors is inhibited, regardless of TTD versus XP phenotype, thus explaining the overlapping symptoms (Dubaele et al, 2003). TTD can also be caused by mutations in the TTDA subunit of TFIIH. Although this subunit is dispensable for the transcriptional activity of TFIIH in RNA polymerase II transcription, it nonetheless stabilizes TFIIH allowing expression of late acting genes and thus performs a specific gene expression activity (Hashimoto and Egly, 2009 and references therein).

Asking if TTD might be a transcription syndrome, the authors of the next study used microarrays to detect transcriptional differences between TTD and XP cells from the XP-D complementation group. They compared gene expression profiles in cultured fibroblasts from normal, XP and TTD donors and concluded that there are minimal differences in gene expression in proliferating fibroblasts from TTD, XP-D and normal donors (Offmann et al, 2008) thus arguing against transcriptional deficiencies being causal for trichothiodystrophy.

Mutations in XPB and XPD subunits of TFIIH can also cause a combination of xeroderma pigmentosum and Cockayne syndrome. As the failure of the DNA repair function of TFIIH explains the cancer susceptibility of xeroderma pigmentosum, additional functions of TFIIH might be responsible for the premature aging phenotype of Cockayne syndrome.

An optimized cell-free in vitro RNA polymerase II transcription assay was used to analyze transcription activity of XP-B and XP-D as well as XPB/CS and XPD/CS. Although the growth rate was normal, the XP-B and XP-D cells contained reduced amounts of TFIIH. Extracts prepared from XP-B and XP-D lymphoblastoid cells exhibited similar transcription activity from the adenovirus major late promoter when compared to that in extracts from normal cells. Thus, the authors concluded that the XP-B and XP-D lymphoblastoid cells do not have impaired RNA transcription activity. They considered the possible consequences of the reduced cellular content of TFIIH for the clinical symptoms in XP-B or XP-D patients, and discuss a 'conditional phenotype' that may involve an impairment of cellular function only under certain growth conditions (Satoh and Hanawald, 1997).

Subsequent another study investigated mutant TFIIH in a reconstituted RNA polymerase II transcription assay. Mutations in XP-B/Cockayne syndrome patients decrease the transcriptional activity of the corresponding TFIIH by preventing promoter opening of RNA polymerase II. The XP-B patient with the most severe symptoms was the patient with the lowest TFIIH transcription activity *in vitro*. These finding points out that the severity of the clinical symptoms observed within the XP-B patients is a function of the TFIIH activity in transcription rather than in NER. Both XPB mutations result in an almost total inhibition (~ 95%) of NER. Western blot analysis and enzymatic assays indicate that XPD mutations affect the stoichometric composition of TFIIH due to a weakness in the interaction between XPD-CAK complex and the core TFIIH, resulting in a partial reduction of transcription activity. The authors concluded that XP-B and XP-D patients are more likely to suffer from transcription repair syndromes rather than DNA repair disorders (Coin et al, 1999). This report identified failures of mutant TFIIH acting on the adenovirus-major-late promoter representative for all RNA polymerase II genes. Thus it describes a general deficiency in gene expression rather than a gene specific effect expected to be causative for Cockayne syndrome. TFIIH does influence gene-specific transcription by the interaction with transcriptional regulators or by phosphorylation of transcription factors like nuclear receptors (reviewed in Zurita and Merino, 2003).

2.2.4 XPG in transcription

XPG also called ERCC5 is a endonuclease that excises the 3`end of an unwinded damaged DNA single strand in nucleotide excision repair (NER). Endonuclease inactivating mutations are followed by xeroderma pigmentosum, whereas truncating mutations in XPG are followed by a severe form of Cockayne syndrome. The authors hypothesised that XPG exhibits a second function critical for the development of Cockayne syndrome (Nouspikel et al, 1997). That XPG as well as its yeast counterpart RAD2 are biochemically isolatable in a complex with TFIIH and interact with multiple subunits of this DNA repair/basal transcription factor was early recognized (Iyer et al,1996, Habraken et al, 1996). Genetic studies in yeast cells, knocking out the yeast counterparts of XPG and CSB, Rad2 and Rad26, unravelled an involvement of both proteins in transcription by RNA polymerase II.

The authors provide evidence for the involvement of *RAD2* in Pol II-dependent transcription. Interestingly, they found that both transcription and growth are more severely inhibited in the *rad2Δ rad26Δ* double mutant than in the *rad2Δ* and *rad26Δ* single mutants. These results indicate that *RAD2* and *RAD26* provide alternate means for efficient transcription, and further, they implicate transcriptional defects as the underlying cause of growth impairment that occurs in the *rad2Δ*, *rad26Δ*, and *rad2Δ rad26Δ* mutant strains under conditions that would require the synthesis of new mRNAs. From these studies, they infer that CS is likely a transcription syndrome and that growth and developmental defects in CS could result from defects in transcription (Lee et al, 2002). In a report studying the involvement of CSB in RNA polymerase I transcription, functional XPG was identified in a complex with CSB, TFIIH, RNA polymerase I initiation factor TIF-IB and RNA polymerase I indicating that XPG might play a role in ribosomal transcription by RNA polymerase I

(Bradsher et al, 2002). Thorel and coworkers described a mild case of Cockayne syndrome characterised by a XPG with nuclease activity that lost the interaction domain with TFIIH. This interaction might be critical for the development of the disease (Thorel et al, 2004).

Another level of complexity was added by the description of an epigenetic function of XPG. DNA methylation is an epigenetic modification that is essential for gene silencing and genome stability in many organisms. The authors show that Gadd45a (growth arrest and DNA-damage-inducible protein 45 alpha), a nuclear protein involved in maintenance of genomic stability, DNA repair and suppression of cell growth, has a key role in active DNA demethylation. Active demethylation occurs by DNA repair and Gadd45a interacts with and requires the DNA repair endonuclease XPG. They concluded that Gadd45a relieves epigenetic gene silencing by promoting DNA repair, which erases methylation marks (Barreto et al, 2007).

XPG forms a stable complex with TFIIH, which is active in transcription and NER. Mutations in XPG found in XP-G/CS patient cells that prevent the association with TFIIH also resulted in the dissociation of CAK and XPD from the core TFIIH. As a consequence, the phosphorylation and transactivation of nuclear receptors were disturbed in XP-G/CS as well as xpg(-/-) MEF cells and could be restored by expression of wild-type XPG. These results provide an insight into the role of XPG in the stabilization of TFIIH and the regulation of gene expression and provide an explanation of some of the clinical features of XP-G/CS. (Ito et al, 2007). This is the first report indicating that XPG serves a gene-specific regulatory function in transcription. An involvement of XPG in the regulation of RNA polymerase I transcription described a mechanism that seems to be conserved between RNA polymerase I and II. In both cases, Gadd45a recruits the NER proteins including XPG to demethylate and activate epigenetic silenced promoter regions The results reveal a mechanism that recruits the DNA repair machinery to the promoter of active genes, keeping them in a hypomethylated state (Barreto et al, 2007; Schmitz et al, 2009). An intimate functional link between Nucleotide excision repair (NER) and transcription by RNA polymerase II was unravelled in the groundbreaking study by Egly and co-workers.

Upon gene activation, they found that RNA polymerase II transcription machinery assembles sequentially with the nucleotide excision repair (NER) factors at the promoter. This recruitment occurs in absence of exogenous genotoxic attack, is sensitive to transcription inhibitors, and depends on the XPC protein. The presence of these repair proteins at the promoter of activated genes is necessary in order to achieve optimal DNA demethylation and histone posttranslational modifications (H3K4/H3K9 methylation, H3K9/14 acetylation) and thus efficient RNA synthesis. Deficiencies in some NER factors impede the recruitment of others and affect nuclear receptor transactivation. This data suggest that there is a functional difference between the presence of the NER factors at the promoters (which requires XPC) and the NER factors at the distal regions of the gene (which requires CSB). While the latter may be a repair function, the former is a function with respect to transcription (LeMay et al, 2010).

2.3 Hutchinson-Gilford progeria syndrome

Hutchinson-Gilford progeria syndrome (HGPS) is a very rare genetic disorder with an estimated incidence rate of 1 in 8 million. Taken in consideration misdiagnosed or unreported cases, the true figure might be closer to 1 in 4 million (Pollex et al, 2004). HGPS was first described by Dr. Jonathan Hutchinson in 1886 and Dr. Hastings Gilford in 1897 and ever since just over 100 cases of HGPS have been reported. Like all progeria HGPS is characterised by segmental premature aging. Children with this disease appear normal at birth but manifestations of HGPS appear at the age between 12-24 months. Characteristic features include delayed dentition, micrognathia, loss of subcutaneous fat, growth retardation, midface hypoplasia, alopecia, atherosclerosis and generalised osteodysplasia with osteolysis and pathologic fractures (www.progeriaresearch.org). The median age at death is about 13 years, and at least 90% of all patients die from progressive atherosclerosis of the coronary and cerebrovascular arteries (Baker et al. 1981).

HGPS is caused by mutations in *LMNA* which encodes lamins A and C. Most patients (80%) reveal a de novo heterozygous point mutation (G608G: GGC$\rightarrow$ GGT) in exon 11 of *LMNA* gene. (Eriksson et al, 2003; De Sandre-Giovannoli et al, 2003). Lamins A and C are type V intermediate filaments which are major components of the nuclear lamina, a protein scaffold at the inner nuclear membrane, which also extends as a network throughout the nucleus.

However, the *LMNA* G608G mutation responsible for most cases of HGPS does not cause an amino acid change, but activates a cryptic splice site leading to a truncated variant of lamin A (progerin) with an in-frame deletion of 50 amino acids near the carboxy terminus (Eriksson et al, 2003; De Sandre-Giovannoli et al, 2003). Due to the loss of 50 amino acids, progerin is lacking an important endoprotease cleavage site required for excision of the farnesylcystein methyl ester. Thus, the HGPS mutation causes the accumulation of permanently farnesylated progerin in the cell nucleus.

One of the most apparent outcomes of the accumulation of progerin is the morphological change of nuclei. HGPS is characterised by significant changes in nuclear size and shape, including lobulation of the nuclear envelope, wrinkle formation, thickening of the the nuclear lamina and clustering of nuclear pores (Goldman et al, 2004.; Eriksson et al, 2003; De Sandre-Giovannoli et al, 2003; Scaffidi et al, 2005;Lammerding et al, 2005).

Another aspect widely discussed in literature is the potential regulatory role of progerin in gene expression as lamins are also interacting with chromatin. Chromatin in *Zmpste24-/-* MEFs, which are also accumulating farnesylated prelamin A (progerin), aggregates at discrete regions in a balloon shape and further analysis showed a variety of chromosomal abnormalities (aneuploidy, ring structures, chromosome instability and DNA breaks) (Liu et al, 2005). Further studies revealed that HGPS cells show significant changes in epinetic control of heterochromatin (Goldman et al, 2004; Shumaker et al, 2006). Heterochromatin markers such as histone H3 trimethylated on lysine 27 (H3K27me3), for facultative heterochromatin, as well as H3 trimethylated on lysine 9 (H3K9me3), for pericentric constitutive heterochromatin, are lost in HGPS cells (Shumakers et al, 2006). These changes could be directly link to progerin expression and are detectable even before changes in shapes of nuclei occur, suggesting that progerin changes gene regulation and silencing even at low levels.

It is suggested that lamin A has diverse roles in DNA metabolism, including DNA replication and transcription and also gene expression. Genome expression profiling of HGPS revealed differentially expressed genes in HGPS fibroblasts compared to age matched control cell lines, which play a role in a variety of biological processes. The most prominent categories encode transcription factors and extracellular matrix proteins, many of which are known to function in the tissues severely affected in HGPS. The most affected gene was *MEOX/GAX*, a homeobox gene that functions as a negative regulator of mesodermal tissue proliferation (Csoka et al, 2004). Microarray analysis from another study showed significant changes in 352 genes of which 306 were down regulated and 46 up regulated in HGPS cells. Functional analysis indicated that most of the genes are important for lipid metabolism, cell growth and differentiation, cell cycle, DNA replication and repair as well as cardiovascular system development (Marji et al, 2010). The only altered expressed gene encoding a protein known to directly interact with A-type lamins has been *Rb1*. Rb plays an important role in cell cycle control and also regulates differentiation. The level of Rb expression at the mRNA and protein level was down regulated in cells derived from HGPS patients and also downstream targets of *Rb1* were affected (Marji et al, 2010). There is also evidence for a significant reduction of hyperphosphorylated Rb in HGPS fibroblasts (Dechat et al, 2007). Based on these observations, decreased Rb expression and reduction of hyperphosphorylated Rb in HGPS cells may lead to deregulation of proliferation (Marji et al, 2010). Similar observation have been reported in cells derived from Lmna -/- mice implicating that absence or mutation of lamin A lead to unstable Rb and a altered lamin A/C-Rb signaling in HGPS cells (Johnson et al, 2004).

Transcription is also in part regulated by the nuclear scaffold which regulates the association and organisation of genes and transcription factors. Certain observations implicate that active transcription complexes are bound to the nuclear lamina and transcription factors as well as active genes are reported to be enriched in nuclear matrix preparations (Jackson et al, 1985; Stein et al, 1995). The contribution of nuclear lamins in transcription has been suggested by different studies. Loss of function mutation of lamin (Dm$_0$) in *Drosophila* disrupts the directed outgrowth of cytoplasmic extensions from terminal cells of the tracheal system, and oocytes from germ line mutants show improper localization of mRNA in the cytoplasm (Guillemin et al., 2001). These results confirm the requirement of nuclear lamin for cytoplasmic as well as nuclear organization. Lamin associated protein 2B (LAP 2B) is a lamin binding protein and has been shown to mediate transcriptional repression (Mancini et al, 1994). Another study revealed that during vertebrate development, changes in the expression of lamins correlates with the beginning of transcription and cell differentiation (Moir et al, 1995). Additionally, disruption of normal lamin organization in active embryonic nuclei from *Xenopus* leads to inhibition of RNA polymerase II activity. The authors suggested that lamins may act as a scaffold upon which the basal transcription factors required for RNA polymerase II transcription are organized (Spann et al, 2002). A recent study by Osorio et al. also demonstrate reduction of RNA polymerase I transcription in Zmpst24 deficient mice. This decrease is due to hypermethylation and hypoacetylation of rDNA leading to a more compact, silent and dysfunctional rDNA gene activity (Osorio et al, 2010). It is also reported that DNA replication can be regulated by the lamina scaffold. Nuclei from *Xenopus* eggs lost their ability to synthesise DNA after immunodepletion of lamins (Newport et al, 1990). Furthermore, mutation in lamina in *Xenopus* blocks DNA replication at the transition from the initiation to the elongation phase of DNA replication (Moir et al, 2000).

3. Conclusion

Transcriptional alterations as the driving force behind premature aging- the implications are vast. The dispute of the competing hypothesis if its primarily unrepaired, accumulating DNA damage or if there is a kind of genetic program that drives premature and normal aging is not solved yet. As both pathways, the DNA damage response and transcriptional regulation are intimately connected by bi- or multifunctional proteins, the separation of progerias in DNA-repair or transcriptional syndromes might turn out to be artificial. The gene expression profiles, the transcriptomes of the aging body might be initiated by DNA damage but executed by specific transcription factors that respond to DNA damage. Mutations in these specific transcription factors could initiate a gene expression profile that resembles the normal answer to accumulating DNA damage. To prove these hypothesis there is a lot of exciting work ahead.

4. Acknowlegdement

We thank Sylvia Koch and Omar Garcia Gonzalez for stimulating discussions and Meinhard Wlaschek and Karin Scharffetter-Kochanek for continuos support. R.A. and S.I. are supported by a Grant of the German Research Society (DFG), Klinische Forschergruppe KFO142.

5. References

Baird, D.M., Davis, T., Rowson, J., Jones, C.J. and Kipling, D. (2004) Normal telomere erosion rates at the single cell level in Werner syndrome fibroblast cells. *Hum Mol Genet*, 13, 1515-1524.

Baker, P.B., Baba, N. and Boesel, C.P. (1981) Cardiovascular abnormalities in progeria. Case report and review of the literature. *Arch Pathol Lab Med*, 105, 384-386.

Barreto, G., Schafer, A., Marhold, J., Stach, D., Swaminathan, S.K., Handa, V., Doderlein, G., Maltry, N., Wu, W., Lyko, F. and Niehrs, C. (2007) Gadd45a promotes epigenetic gene activation by repair-mediated DNA demethylation. *Nature*, 445, 671-675.

Bergmann, E. and Egly, J.M. (2001) Trichothiodystrophy, a transcription syndrome. *Trends Genet*, 17, 279-286.

Blander, G., Kipnis, J., Leal, J.F., Yu, C.E., Schellenberg, G.D. and Oren, M. (1999) Physical and functional interaction between p53 and the Werner's syndrome protein. *J Biol Chem*, 274, 29463-29469.

Chalut, C., Moncollin, V. and Egly, J.M. (1994) Transcription by RNA polymerase II: a process linked to DNA repair. *Bioessays*, 16, 651-655.

Chang, S., Multani, A.S., Cabrera, N.G., Naylor, M.L., Laud, P., Lombard, D., Pathak, S., Guarente, L. and DePinho, R.A. (2004) Essential role of limiting telomeres in the pathogenesis of Werner syndrome. *Nat Genet*, 36, 877-882.

Charlet-Berguerand, N., Feuerhahn, S., Kong, S.E., Ziserman, H., Conaway, J.W., Conaway, R. and Egly, J.M. (2006) RNA polymerase II bypass of oxidative DNA damage is regulated by transcription elongation factors. *Embo J*, 25, 5481-5491.

Chu, W.K. and Hickson, I.D. (2009) RecQ helicases: multifunctional genome caretakers. *Nat Rev Cancer*, 9, 644-654.

Coin, F., Bergmann, E., Tremeau-Bravard, A. and Egly, J.M. (1999) Mutations in XPB and XPD helicases found in xeroderma pigmentosum patients impair the transcription function of TFIIH. *Embo J*, 18, 1357-1366.

Crabbe, L., Jauch, A., Naeger, C.M., Holtgreve-Grez, H. and Karlseder, J. (2007) Telomere dysfunction as a cause of genomic instability in Werner syndrome. *Proc Natl Acad Sci U S A*, 104, 2205-2210.

Crabbe, L., Verdun, R.E., Haggblom, C.I. and Karlseder, J. (2004) Defective telomere lagging strand synthesis in cells lacking WRN helicase activity. *Science*, 306, 1951-1953.

Csoka, A.B., English, S.B., Simkevich, C.P., Ginzinger, D.G., Butte, A.J., Schatten, G.P., Rothman, F.G. and Sedivy, J.M. (2004) Genome-scale expression profiling of

Hutchinson-Gilford progeria syndrome reveals widespread transcriptional misregulation leading to mesodermal/mesenchymal defects and accelerated atherosclerosis. *Aging Cell*, 3, 235-243.

de Boer, J., Andressoo, J.O., de Wit, J., Huijmans, J., Beems, R.B., van Steeg, H., Weeda, G., van der Horst, G.T., van Leeuwen, W., Themmen, A.P., Meradji, M. and Hoeijmakers, J.H. (2002) Premature aging in mice deficient in DNA repair and transcription. *Science*, 296, 1276-1279.

De Sandre-Giovannoli, A., Bernard, R., Cau, P., Navarro, C., Amiel, J., Boccaccio, I., Lyonnet, S., Stewart, C.L., Munnich, A., Le Merrer, M. and Levy, N. (2003) Lamin a truncation in Hutchinson-Gilford progeria. *Science*, 300, 2055.

Dechat, T., Shimi, T., Adam, S.A., Rusinol, A.E., Andres, D.A., Spielmann, H.P., Sinensky, M.S. and Goldman, R.D. (2007) Alterations in mitosis and cell cycle progression caused by a mutant lamin A known to accelerate human aging. *Proc Natl Acad Sci U S A*, 104, 4955-4960.

Dianov, G.L., Houle, J.F., Iyer, N., Bohr, V.A. and Friedberg, E.C. (1997) Reduced RNA polymerase II transcription in extracts of cockayne syndrome and xeroderma pigmentosum/Cockayne syndrome cells. *Nucleic Acids Res*, 25, 3636-3642.

Douziech, M., Coin, F., Chipoulet, J.M., Arai, Y., Ohkuma, Y., Egly, J.M. and Coulombe, B. (2000) Mechanism of promoter melting by the xeroderma pigmentosum complementation group B helicase of transcription factor IIH revealed by protein-DNA photo-cross-linking. *Mol Cell Biol*, 20, 8168-8177.

Drapkin, R., Reardon, J.T., Ansari, A., Huang, J.C., Zawel, L., Ahn, K., Sancar, A. and Reinberg, D. (1994) Dual role of TFIIH in DNA excision repair and in transcription by RNA polymerase II. *Nature*, 368, 769-772.

Eriksson, M., Brown, W.T., Gordon, L.B., Glynn, M.W., Singer, J., Scott, L., Erdos, M.R., Robbins, C.M., Moses, T.Y., Berglund, P., Dutra, A., Pak, E., Durkin, S., Csoka, A.B., Boehnke, M., Glover, T.W. and Collins, F.S. (2003) Recurrent de novo point mutations in lamin A cause Hutchinson-Gilford progeria syndrome. *Nature*, 423, 293-298.

Faragher, R.G., Kill, I.R., Hunter, J.A., Pope, F.M., Tannock, C. and Shall, S. (1993) The gene responsible for Werner syndrome may be a cell division "counting" gene. *Proc Natl Acad Sci U S A*, 90, 12030-12034.

Filippi, S., Latini, P., Frontini, M., Palitti, F., Egly, J.M. and Proietti-De-Santis, L. (2008) CSB protein is (a direct target of HIF-1 and) a critical mediator of the hypoxic response. *Embo J*, 27, 2545-2556.

Goldman, R.D., Shumaker, D.K., Erdos, M.R., Eriksson, M., Goldman, A.E., Gordon, L.B., Gruenbaum, Y., Khuon, S., Mendez, M., Varga, R. and Collins, F.S. (2004) Accumulation of mutant lamin A causes progressive changes in nuclear architecture in Hutchinson-Gilford progeria syndrome. *Proc Natl Acad Sci U S A*, 101, 8963-8968.

Guillemin, K., Williams, T. and Krasnow, M.A. (2001) A nuclear lamin is required for cytoplasmic organization and egg polarity in Drosophila. *Nat Cell Biol*, 3, 848-851.

Guzder, S.N., Sung, P., Bailly, V., Prakash, L. and Prakash, S. (1994) RAD25 is a DNA helicase required for DNA repair and RNA polymerase II transcription. *Nature*, 369, 578-581.

Habraken, Y., Sung, P., Prakash, S. and Prakash, L. (1996) Transcription factor TFIIH and DNA endonuclease Rad2 constitute yeast nucleotide excision repair factor 3: implications for nucleotide excision repair and Cockayne syndrome. *Proc Natl Acad Sci U S A*, 93, 10718-10722.

Hashimoto, S. and Egly, J.M. (2009) Trichothiodystrophy view from the molecular basis of DNA repair/transcription factor TFIIH. *Hum Mol Genet*, 18, R224-230.

Henning, K.A., Li, L., Iyer, N., McDaniel, L.D., Reagan, M.S., Legerski, R., Schultz, R.A., Stefanini, M., Lehmann, A.R., Mayne, L.V. and Friedberg, E.C. (1995) The Cockayne syndrome group A gene encodes a WD repeat protein that interacts with CSB protein and a subunit of RNA polymerase II TFIIH. *Cell*, 82, 555-564.

Herbig, U., Ferreira, M., Condel, L., Carey, D. and Sedivy, J.M. (2006) Cellular senescence in aging primates. *Science*, 311, 1257.

Hoeijmakers, J.H. (2009) DNA damage, aging, and cancer. *N Engl J Med*, 361, 1475-1485.

Horibata, K., Iwamoto, Y., Kuraoka, I., Jaspers, N.G., Kurimasa, A., Oshimura, M., Ichihashi, M. and Tanaka, K. (2004) Complete absence of Cockayne syndrome group B gene product gives rise to UV-sensitive syndrome but not Cockayne syndrome. *Proc Natl Acad Sci U S A*, 101, 15410-15415.

Iben, S., Tschochner, H., Bier, M., Hoogstraten, D., Hozak, P., Egly, J.M. and Grummt, I. (2002) TFIIH plays an essential role in RNA polymerase I transcription. *Cell*, 109, 297-306.

Ito, S., Kuraoka, I., Chymkowitch, P., Compe, E., Takedachi, A., Ishigami, C., Coin, F., Egly, J.M. and Tanaka, K. (2007) XPG stabilizes TFIIH, allowing transactivation of nuclear receptors: implications for Cockayne syndrome in XP-G/CS patients. *Mol Cell*, 26, 231-243.

Iyer, N., Reagan, M.S., Wu, K.J., Canagarajah, B. and Friedberg, E.C. (1996) Interactions involving the human RNA polymerase II transcription/nucleotide excision repair complex TFIIH, the nucleotide excision repair protein XPG, and Cockayne syndrome group B (CSB) protein. *Biochemistry*, 35, 2157-2167.

Jackson, D.A. and Cook, P.R. (1985) Transcription occurs at a nucleoskeleton. *Embo J*, 4, 919-925.

Johnson, B.R., Nitta, R.T., Frock, R.L., Mounkes, L., Barbie, D.A., Stewart, C.L., Harlow, E. and Kennedy, B.K. (2004) A-type lamins regulate retinoblastoma protein function by promoting subnuclear localization and preventing proteasomal degradation. *Proc Natl Acad Sci U S A*, 101, 9677-9682.

Johnson, J.E., Cao, K., Ryvkin, P., Wang, L.S. and Johnson, F.B. Altered gene expression in the Werner and Bloom syndromes is associated with sequences having G-quadruplex forming potential. *Nucleic Acids Res*, 38, 1114-1122.

Kim, T.K., Ebright, R.H. and Reinberg, D. (2000) Mechanism of ATP-dependent promoter melting by transcription factor IIH. *Science*, 288, 1418-1422.

Kirkwood, T.B. Global aging and the brain. *Nutr Rev*, 68 Suppl 2, S65-69.

Kyng, K.J., May, A., Brosh, R.M., Jr., Cheng, W.H., Chen, C., Becker, K.G. and Bohr, V.A. (2003) The transcriptional response after oxidative stress is defective in Cockayne syndrome group B cells. *Oncogene*, 22, 1135-1149.

Lammerding, J., Hsiao, J., Schulze, P.C., Kozlov, S., Stewart, C.L. and Lee, R.T. (2005) Abnormal nuclear shape and impaired mechanotransduction in emerin-deficient cells. *J Cell Biol*, 170, 781-791.

Laugel, V., et al., (2009) Mutation update for the CSB/ERCC6 and CSA/ERCC8 genes involved in Cockayne syndrome. *Hum Mutat*, 31, 113-126.

Le May, N., Mota-Fernandes, D., Velez-Cruz, R., Iltis, I., Biard, D. and Egly, J.M. NER factors are recruited to active promoters and facilitate chromatin modification for transcription in the absence of exogenous genotoxic attack. *Mol Cell*, 38, 54-66.

Le May, N., Mota-Fernandes, D., Velez-Cruz, R., Iltis, I., Biard, D. and Egly, J.M. NER factors are recruited to active promoters and facilitate chromatin modification for transcription in the absence of exogenous genotoxic attack. *Mol Cell*, 38, 54-66.

Lebedev, A., Scharffetter-Kochanek, K. and Iben, S. (2008) Truncated Cockayne syndrome B protein represses elongation by RNA polymerase I. *J Mol Biol*, 382, 266-274.

Lee, S.K., Johnson, R.E., Yu, S.L., Prakash, L. and Prakash, S. (1999) Requirement of yeast SGS1 and SRS2 genes for replication and transcription. *Science*, 286, 2339-2342.

Lee, S.K., Yu, S.L., Prakash, L. and Prakash, S. (2001) Requirement for yeast RAD26, a homolog of the human CSB gene, in elongation by RNA polymerase II. *Mol Cell Biol*, 21, 8651-8656.

Lee, S.K., Yu, S.L., Prakash, L. and Prakash, S. (2002) Requirement of yeast RAD2, a homolog of human XPG gene, for efficient RNA polymerase II transcription. implications for Cockayne syndrome. *Cell*, 109, 823-834.

Lee, S.K., Yu, S.L., Prakash, L. and Prakash, S. (2002) Yeast RAD26, a homolog of the human CSB gene, functions independently of nucleotide excision repair and base excision repair in promoting transcription through damaged bases. *Mol Cell Biol*, 22, 4383-4389.

Liu, B., Wang, J., Chan, K.M., Tjia, W.M., Deng, W., Guan, X., Huang, J.D., Li, K.M., Chau, P.Y., Chen, D.J., Pei, D., Pendas, A.M., Cadinanos, J., Lopez-Otin, C., Tse, H.F., Hutchison, C., Chen, J., Cao, Y., Cheah, K.S., Tryggvason, K. and Zhou, Z. (2005) Genomic instability in laminopathy-based premature aging. *Nat Med*, 11, 780-785.

Lutomska, A., Lebedev, A., Scharffetter-Kochanek, K. and Iben, S. (2008) The transcriptional response to distinct growth factors is impaired in Werner syndrome cells. *Exp Gerontol*, 43, 820-826.

Mancini, M.A., Shan, B., Nickerson, J.A., Penman, S. and Lee, W.H. (1994) The retinoblastoma gene product is a cell cycle-dependent, nuclear matrix-associated protein. *Proc Natl Acad Sci U S A*, 91, 418-422.

Marji, J., O'Donoghue, S.I., McClintock, D., Satagopam, V.P., Schneider, R., Ratner, D., Worman, H.J., Gordon, L.B. and Djabali, K. Defective lamin A-Rb signaling in Hutchinson-Gilford Progeria Syndrome and reversal by farnesyltransferase inhibition. *PLoS One*, 5, e11132.

Moir, R.D., Spann, T.P. and Goldman, R.D. (1995) The dynamic properties and possible functions of nuclear lamins. *Int Rev Cytol*, 162B, 141-182.

Moir, R.D., Spann, T.P., Herrmann, H. and Goldman, R.D. (2000) Disruption of nuclear lamin organization blocks the elongation phase of DNA replication. *J Cell Biol*, 149, 1179-1192.

Nance, M.A. and Berry, S.A. (1992) Cockayne syndrome: review of 140 cases. *Am J Med Genet*, 42, 68-84.

Newman, J.C., Bailey, A.D. and Weiner, A.M. (2006) Cockayne syndrome group B protein (CSB) plays a general role in chromatin maintenance and remodeling. *Proc Natl Acad Sci U S A*, 103, 9613-9618.

Newport, J.W., Wilson, K.L. and Dunphy, W.G. (1990) A lamin-independent pathway for nuclear envelope assembly. *J Cell Biol*, 111, 2247-2259.

Nouspikel, T., Lalle, P., Leadon, S.A., Cooper, P.K. and Clarkson, S.G. (1997) A common mutational pattern in Cockayne syndrome patients from xeroderma pigmentosum group G: implications for a second XPG function. *Proc Natl Acad Sci U S A*, 94, 3116-3121.

Osorio, F.G., Varela, I., Lara, E., Puente, X.S., Espada, J., Santoro, R., Freije, J.M., Fraga, M.F. and Lopez-Otin, C. Nuclear envelope alterations generate an aging-like epigenetic pattern in mice deficient in Zmpste24 metalloprotease. *Aging Cell*, 9, 947-957.

Pollex, R.L. and Hegele, R.A. (2004) Hutchinson-Gilford progeria syndrome. *Clin Genet*, 66, 375-381.

Proietti-De-Santis, L., Drane, P. and Egly, J.M. (2006) Cockayne syndrome B protein regulates the transcriptional program after UV irradiation. *Embo J*, 25, 1915-1923.

Rossi, M.L., Ghosh, A.K. and Bohr, V.A. Roles of Werner syndrome protein in protection of genome integrity. *DNA Repair (Amst)*, 9, 331-344.

Satoh, M.S. and Hanawalt, P.C. (1997) Competent transcription initiation by RNA polymerase II in cell-free extracts from xeroderma pigmentosum groups B and D in an optimized RNA transcription assay. *Biochim Biophys Acta*, 1354, 241-251.

Scaffidi, P., Gordon, L. and Misteli, T. (2005) The cell nucleus and aging: tantalizing clues and hopeful promises. *PLoS Biol*, 3, e395.

Schmitz, K.M., Schmitt, N., Hoffmann-Rohrer, U., Schafer, A., Grummt, I. and Mayer, C. (2009) TAF12 recruits Gadd45a and the nucleotide excision repair complex to the promoter of rRNA genes leading to active DNA demethylation. *Mol Cell*, 33, 344-353.

Schmitz, K.M., Schmitt, N., Hoffmann-Rohrer, U., Schafer, A., Grummt, I. and Mayer, C. (2009) TAF12 recruits Gadd45a and the nucleotide excision repair complex to the promoter of rRNA genes leading to active DNA demethylation. *Mol Cell*, 33, 344-353.

Selby, C.P. and Sancar, A. (1997) Cockayne syndrome group B protein enhances elongation by RNA polymerase II. *Proc Natl Acad Sci U S A*, 94, 11205-11209.

Shiratori, M., Suzuki, T., Itoh, C., Goto, M., Furuichi, Y. and Matsumoto, T. (2002) WRN helicase accelerates the transcription of ribosomal RNA as a component of an RNA polymerase I-associated complex. *Oncogene*, 21, 2447-2454.

Shumaker, D.K., Dechat, T., Kohlmaier, A., Adam, S.A., Bozovsky, M.R., Erdos, M.R., Eriksson, M., Goldman, A.E., Khuon, S., Collins, F.S., Jenuwein, T. and Goldman, R.D. (2006) Mutant nuclear lamin A leads to progressive alterations of epigenetic control in premature aging. *Proc Natl Acad Sci U S A*, 103, 8703-8708.

Sinclair, D.A., Mills, K. and Guarente, L. (1997) Accelerated aging and nucleolar fragmentation in yeast sgs1 mutants. *Science*, 277, 1313-1316.

Spann, T.P., Goldman, A.E., Wang, C., Huang, S. and Goldman, R.D. (2002) Alteration of nuclear lamin organization inhibits RNA polymerase II-dependent transcription. *J Cell Biol*, 156, 603-608.

Stein, G.S., van Wijnen, A.J., Stein, J., Lian, J.B. and Montecino, M. (1995) Contributions of nuclear architecture to transcriptional control. *Int Rev Cytol*, 162A, 251-278.

Tantin, D., Kansal, A. and Carey, M. (1997) Recruitment of the putative transcription-repair coupling factor CSB/ERCC6 to RNA polymerase II elongation complexes. *Mol Cell Biol*, 17, 6803-6814.

Thorel, F., Constantinou, A., Dunand-Sauthier, I., Nouspikel, T., Lalle, P., Raams, A., Jaspers, N.G., Vermeulen, W., Shivji, M.K., Wood, R.D. and Clarkson, S.G. (2004) Definition of a short region of XPG necessary for TFIIH interaction and stable recruitment to sites of UV damage. *Mol Cell Biol*, 24, 10670-10680.

Troelstra, C., van Gool, A., de Wit, J., Vermeulen, W., Bootsma, D. and Hoeijmakers, J.H. (1992) ERCC6, a member of a subfamily of putative helicases, is involved in Cockayne's syndrome and preferential repair of active genes. *Cell*, 71, 939-953.

Turaga, R.V., Paquet, E.R., Sild, M., Vignard, J., Garand, C., Johnson, F.B., Masson, J.Y. and Lebel, M. (2009) The Werner syndrome protein affects the expression of genes involved in adipogenesis and inflammation in addition to cell cycle and DNA damage responses. *Cell Cycle*, 8, 2080-2092.

van Gool, A.J., Citterio, E., Rademakers, S., van Os, R., Vermeulen, W., Constantinou, A., Egly, J.M., Bootsma, D. and Hoeijmakers, J.H. (1997) The Cockayne syndrome B protein, involved in transcription-coupled DNA repair, resides in an RNA polymerase II-containing complex. *Embo J*, 16, 5955-5965.

Winkler, G.S. and Hoeijmakers, J.H. (1998) From a DNA helicase to brittle hair. *Nat Genet*, 20, 106-107.

Yu, A., Fan, H.Y., Liao, D., Bailey, A.D. and Weiner, A.M. (2000) Activation of p53 or loss of the Cockayne syndrome group B repair protein causes metaphase fragility of human U1, U2, and 5S genes. *Mol Cell*, 5, 801-810.

Yuan, X., Feng, W., Imhof, A., Grummt, I. and Zhou, Y. (2007) Activation of RNA polymerase I transcription by cockayne syndrome group B protein and histone methyltransferase G9a. *Mol Cell*, 27, 585-595.

Zurita, M. and Merino, C. (2003) The transcriptional complexity of the TFIIH complex. *Trends Genet*, 19, 578-584.

2

Involvement of Histone PTMs in DNA Repair Processes in Relation to Age-Associated Neurodegenerative Disease

Chunmei Wang, Erxu Pi, Qinglei Zhan and Sai-ming Ngai
School of Life Sciences, State Key laboratory of Agrobiotechnology
The Chinese University of Hong Kong
China

1. Introduction

Neurodegenerative diseases, such as Alzheimer's disease (AD), Parkinson's disease (PD) and Huntington's disease (HD), are becoming common in the world with increasing number of aged people in the population. Many investigations have been performed in an attempt to elucidate the mechanisms of neurodegenerative diseases. However, no single etiopathological factor was found to be responsible for such diseases, and therefore no effective therapeutic strategy could be designed.

Aging is regarded as the greatest risk factor for the development of neurodegenerative diseases. Upon aging, reactive oxygen species (ROS) accumulation induces damage to DNA as well as protein and lipid, thus resulting in a progressive loss in the functional efficiency of the brain. Recently, it has been demonstrated that hundreds of proteins including KIN-19, a homolog of mammalian casein kinase 1 isoform alpha (CK1a), become more insoluble with age in *Caenorhabditis elegans* and its over-expression could enhance polyglutamine-repeat pathology (David et al., 2010). Such discovery indicated that aging process itself could be a causative factor for protein aggregation. Increasing aggregation of proteins, such as amyloid beta peptide, could also promote the generation of ROS, DNA damage and thus accelerate neurodegenerative events (Butterfield, 2002). In addition, redox-active metals Cu and Fe could also generate ROS. Normal aging resulted in an elevation of Cu and Fe in the brain, and further interruption of metal homeostasis was noted in AD (Tabner et al., 2010).

Oxidative DNA lesions, such as 8-oxoguanine (8-oxoG) and 8-hydroxyguanosine (8-OHG), were increased dramatically in patients with PD (Nakabeppu et al., 2007; Lovell et al., 1999). Statistically significant elevation of 8-hydroxy-2'-deoxyguanosine (8-OHdG) was detected on DNA of AD subjects, even at the early stage of AD (Lovell et al., 1999; Markesbery & Lovell, 2006). At the same time, DNA repair deficiency in aged or neurodegenerative brain was observed. Both base excision repair (BER) and non-homologous end joining (NHEJ) pathway were deficient in AD subjects (Shackelford, 2006; Weissman et al., 2007). The animals with deficiencies in DNA repair exhibited neurological abnormalities or severe postnatal neurodegeneration and shortened life span (Laposa & Cleaver, 2001; Best, 2009; Dollé et al., 2006), that proved the role of DNA repair deficiency in neurodegeneration. DNA damage combined with inefficient repair mechanism could induce the apoptosis of brain cells, as well as transcriptional inhibition of the vulnerable genes involved in learning, memory and neuronal survival (Hetman et al., 2010). All these contribute to the pathogenesis of age related neurodegenerative diseases.

Now, histone posttranslational modifications (PTMs) have become an emerging discipline of research, exploring various physiological and pathological processes. Histone PTMs take part in diverse biological processes by inducing chromatin remodelling and regulating gene expression. Increasing evidence suggests that altered patterns of histone PTMs are central to many human diseases. The involvement of histone PTMs in normal nervous system development has been demonstrated and the aberrant PTMs patterns were detected in neurodegenerative disorders (Büttner et al., 2010; Mattson, 2001; Wang et al., 2010; Penner et al., 2010).

It has been widely accepted that histone modifications play important roles in response to DNA damage and in DNA repair (Méndez-Acuña et al., 2010). In the cellular repair machinery, these modified histone sites not only signal the presence of damage, but also provide a landing platform for necessary repair/signaling proteins. Moreover, different PTMs could work together during DNA damage response (Van Attikum & Gasser, 2009). Here, we summarize the abnormal histone PTMs patterns in nuclear DNA damage response (DDR). The role of abnormally expressed histone PTMs in age-associated neurodegenerative disease and their mechanisms are also proposed.

2. Histone PTMs in DNA damage and repair

The core unit of chromatin is the nucleosome which consists of 147 bp of DNA wrapped around histone octamer containing two of each of the core histone proteins H2A, H2B, H3 and H4. The residues at the histone N-terminal tails and globular domains are subjected to PTMs. There are at least nine different types of covalent modifications found in histone proteins, including acetylation, methylation, phosphorylation, deimination, ubiquitination, sumoylation, ADP-ribosylation, proline isomerization and O-linked β-N-acetylglucosamination. Méndez-Acuña has summarized four types of these histone PTMs related to DNA damage response (Méndez-Acuña et al., 2010). Here, we will focus on histone PTMs which are related to DNA damage response during aging and neurodegeneration.

2.1 Phosphorylation

Histone H2A has four variants including H2A1, H2A2, H2AX, and H2AZ. Among them, H2AX is the histone guardian of the genome (Fernandez-Capetillo et al., 2004b). H2AX-/- mice showed the phenomena of radiation sensitivity, growth retardation and immune deficiency (Celeste et al., 2002). Phosphorylation of histone H2AX at serine 139, named gamma-H2AX, is the most characterized PTM at DNA double strand breaks (DSBs). It is catalyzed by the kinases of the PI3-family (ATM, ATR and DNA-PK), especially by ATM (Kinner et al., 2008). It appeared rapidly after the exposure to ionizing radiation and half-maximal amounts were reached by 1 min and maximal amounts by 10 min (Rogakou et al., 1998). Therefore, gamma-H2AX is the first step in recruiting and localizing DNA repair proteins after damage. Presently, gamma-H2AX is regarded as a novel biomarker for DNA breaks and for early stage of apoptosis. Moreover, its expression in a wide range of eukaryotic organisms has indicated its conserved function (Foster & Downs, 2005).

Gamma-H2AX was suggested as a molecular marker of aging and diseases (Mah et al., 2010). The level of H2AX in astrocytes and neurons was found to significantly decrease with the age of participants (Simpson et al., 2010). Meanwhile, the incidence of endogenous gamma-H2AX foci was increased with age (Sedelnikova et al., 2008). The number of gamma H2AX-immunopositive nuclei was significantly increased in the astrocytes of both gray and white matter, and consistently in the cornus ammonus (CA) regions of the hippocampus of AD patients compared to those of control cases (Myung et al., 2008). However, the rate of recruitment of DSB repair proteins to gamma-H2AX foci was correlated inversely with age for both normal and premature aging disease donors (Sedelnikova et al., 2008).

Nuclear localization of DNA repair enzyme DNA-PK and of damaged base 8-OHdG reflect different aspects of the cell response to DNA damage. DNA-PK is required for the NHEJ pathway of DNA repair, whereas, 8-OHdG indicates DNA lesion caused by oxidative damage. Simpson and his colleagues found that the localization of H2AX and DNA-PK demonstrated a good correlation, whereas 8-OHdG localization expression demonstrated a weak correlation with DNA-PK and no significant correlation with H2AX (Simpson et al., 2010). This indicates that H2AX preferentially detects DSBs and is involved in NHEJ repair.

Besides gamma-H2AX, other histone serine phosphorylation events also take place during DDR. Yeast H2A is phosphorylated at serine 122 (threonine 119 in higher eukaryotes) upon DNA damage. Such serine residue was essential for cell survival in the presence of DNA damaging agents (Harvey et al., 2005). The phosphorylation at serine 14 of histone H2B (H2BS14ph) and the phosphorylation at serine 1 of histone H4 (H4S1ph) also occurred in response to DNA damage, and H4S1ph has been shown to be required for an efficient DSB repair by NHEJ (Fernandez-Capetillo et al., 2004a; Cheung et al., 2005). However, the expression of all these PTM sites in aged or neurodegenerative brain has not been reported yet.

Recently, histone phosphorylation at tyrosine was found to be involved in aging, such as phosphorylation of histone H2AX on tyrosine 142 (H2AXY142ph) and histone H3 on tyrosine 99 (H2AXY99ph) (Singh & Gunjan, 2011). Histone H2AXY142 was phosphorylated by the WICH complex and dephosphorylated by the EYA1/3 phosphatases, determining the relative recruitment of either DNA repair or pro-apoptotic factors to DNA damage sites (Stucki, 2009). In contrast to H2AX serine 139 phosphorylation, tyrosine 142 appeared to be constitutively phosphorylated in undamaged cells, but was gradually dephosphorylated in chromatin bearing unrepaired DSBs (Stucki, 2009).

2.2 Methylation

Along the histone polypeptide chain, one, two, or three methyl groups could be added onto the lysine residues by histone methyltransferases (HMT) and could also be removed by histone demethyltransferase (HDMT). Histone methylation is generally associated with transcriptional repression with the exception that several methylation sites are involved in transcriptional activation.

Tri-methylated histone H3 at position lysine 4 (H3K4me3), an important modification associated with transcriptional regulation, showed different epigenome in neuron cells comparing with non-neuronal cells (Cheung et al., 2010). During aging, a significant decrease in H3K4me3 was observed at migrated neural progenitor double cortin gene promoters, indicating the possibility of H3K4me3 in the mechanism of aging-dependent hippocampal dysfunction (Kuzumaki et al., 2010). Other investigation also found that H3K4me3 was related to DDR and could be detected at newly created DSB. In budding yeast cells, H3K4me3 was important for a proper response to DNA damaging agents, and the cells that cannot methylate H3K4 displayed a defect in DSB repair by NHEJ (Faucher & Wellinger, 2010). During meiosis, H3K4me3 was critical for the formation of the programmed DSB that initiated homologous recombination (Kniewel & Keeney, 2009).

Histone H3 is constitutively methylated at lysine 79 (H3K79me) in both mammalian and yeast cells. In yeast, H3K79 methylation played an important role in the activation of the G1 and intra S-phase DNA damage checkpoint (Wysocki et al., 2005). It was also detected in the brains of senescence-accelerated prone 8 mice and increased with aging (Wang et al., 2010). Lysine 79 locates in a loop connecting the first and the second α helixes in H3 structure (Luger et al., 1997). This region is exposed and adjacent to the interface between H3/H4 tetramer and H2A/H2B dimer, which could influence the access of molecules to the interface. Therefore, the added methyl group on H3K79 might alter the properties of the nucleosome and play an important role in regulating the access of other DNA binding factors to chromatin (Feng et al., 2002). However, the expression level of H3K79 methylation was found unchanged in response to DNA damage. Therefore, methylated H3K79 site might change the higher-order chromatin structure and expose the binding site to DNA damage and repair factors, e.g. the exposure of 53BP1 binding site (Huyen et al., 2004). In addition, H3K79me worked together with phosphorylated H2A serine 129 for the recruitment of budding yeast homolog Rad9 to the DNA damage sites (Huyen et al., 2004; Toh et al. 2006).

Previous investigation has shown that methylated histone H4 at lysine 20 (H4K20me) increased in kidneys and liver of the old-aged rat (Sarg et al., 2002). Except for transcriptional regulation, H4K20me is another reported methylation site that related to DDR. DNA breakage might cause exposure of methylated H4K20 previously buried within the chromosome. At the same time, the level of H4K20 methylation increased locally upon the induction of DSBs by the enzyme named histone methyltransferase MMSET (also known as NSD2 or WHSC1) in mammals (Pei et al., 2011).

2.3 Acetylation

During neurodegeneration, the degree of acetylation balance in brain was greatly impaired (Saha & Pahan, 2006). The inhibition of histone deacetylation induced the sprouting of dendrites, an increased number of synapses, learning behavior reinstatement and long-term memories in bi-transgenic CK-p25 Tg mice (Fischer et al., 2007). All these changes are mainly caused by transcriptional regulation of histone acetylation and/or deacetylation. Actually, DNA damage response regulated by histone acetylation and deacetylation state is also important in neurodegenerative diseases. Moreover, histone deacetylases (HDAC) 1- and 2-depleted cells were hypersensitive to DNA-damaging agents and showed defective DSB repair, particularly NHEJ repair pathway (Miller et al., 2010).

It was found that the acetylation of histone H3 lysine 56 (H3K56ac) was involved in DDR. Mutation of K56 site made the cells sensitive to genotoxic agents (Masumoto et al., 2005). After DNA damage, H3K56ac co-localized with gama-H2AX and other proteins, involved in DNA damage signaling pathways, such as phospho-ATM, CHK2, and p53, at the sites of DNA repair (Vempati et al., 2010). Furthermore, GCN5, histone acetyltransferase (HAT) for H3K56 was shown to have an important role in maintaining genome stability (Burgess & Zhang, 2010). Knocking down of GCN5 resulted in impaired recruitment of NER factors to sites of damage and inefficient DNA repair (Guo et al., 2011). Histone deacetylases HDAC1 and HDAC2 could be rapidly recruited to DNA-damage sites and promote hypoacetylation of H3K56. However, HDAC1/2 depletion or inhibition did not affect the amount of DNA damage produced by DSB-inducing agents but impaired DNA repair particularly through NHEJ (Miller et al., 2010)

Histone H4 is acetylated at lysine 16 (H4K16ac) by a human MOF gene encoded protein. Reduced level of H4K16ac correlated with a defective DDR and DSB repair after exposure to ionizing radiation (IR). MOF depletion greatly decreased DSB repair by both NHEJ and homologous recombination (HR) (Sharma et al., 2010). Its specific deacetylase Sir2 was recruited to the HO lesion during HR repair process in budding yeast cells (Tamburini & Tyler, 2005). In response to DNA damage, SIRT1, a mammalian homologue of yeast Sir2, re-localized to DNA breaks to promote repair, resulting in transcriptional changes that parallel those in the aging mouse brain (Oberdoerffer et al., 2008).

Acetylation of H2AX on lysine 36 (H2AXK36Ac) also plays a key role in DSB repair pathway. This modification site is constitutively acetylated by the CBP/p300 acetyltransferase. Though its level was not increased by DNA damage, this modification was required for cells to survive in IR exposure. However, H2AXK36Ac did not affect phosphorylation of H2AX or the formation of DNA damage foci, indicating that H2AXK36Ac was a novel, constitutive histone modification regulating radiation sensitivity independently of H2AX phosphorylation (Jiang et al., 2010).

2.4 Ubiquitination

Increased level of monoubiquitinated histone H2A and decreased level of monoubiquitinated H2B were found to be involved in transcriptional repression during HD, and these two ubiquitylation states inhibited methylation of histone H3K9 and histone H3K4, respectively (Kim et al., 2008). Interestingly, histone acetylation could affect monoubiquitination of histone H2A (Sadri-Vakili et al., 2007), whereas monoubiquitinated histone H2B controlled histone methylation (Sun and Allis, 2002). Thus, histone monoubiquitylation provided a potential bridge between histone acetylation and methylation, which leaded to the change of gene expression in neurodegenerative diseases (Kim et al., 2008).

Same as other modifications, histone ubiquitination is also involved in DNA damage response. Monoubiquitination of histone H2B, known for its involvement in transcription, was also important for a proper response of budding yeast cells to DNA damaging agents (Faucher & Wellinger, 2010). In human cells, DSBs induced monoubiquitination of histone H2B on lysine 120, and this monoubiquitination was required for timely repair of DSBs (Moyal et al., 2011).

2.5 Poly ADP-ribosylation

Poly ADP-ribosylation of histones is carried out by poly ADP-ribose polymerases (PARPs). Poly ADP-ribosylated histones could stimulate local chromatin relaxation to facilitate the repair process (Monks et al., 2006). Poly (ADP-ribose) polymerase-1 (PARP-1) is a nuclear enzyme that contributed to both neuronal death and survival under stress conditions (Kauppinen & Swanson, 2007). PARPs were activated in AD in response to oxidative damage to DNA (Love et al., 1999). PARP-1 activation enhanced core histone acetylation, and the acetylated histone H4 facilitated ADP-ribosylation of histones (Cohen-Armon et al., 2007; Boulikas, 1990). 3-aminobenzamide was found to inhibit poly (ADP-ribose) polymerase as well as histone H3 phosphorylation (Tikoo et al., 2001). Therefore, histone H3 phosphorylation was often coupled to poly-(ADP-ribosylation) during ROS-induced cell death. However, the appearance of histone ADP-ribosylation preceded histone H3 phosphorylation after DNA damage (Monks et al., 2006).

3. How are PTMs involved in DNA damage response and repair?

Several histone modifications are associated with DNA damage and repair by directly regulating activation or repression of DNA repair genes. For example, the expression of manganese-dependent superoxide dismutase (Mn-SOD) was regulated by the acetylation of histones H3 and H4 at Mn-SOD proximal promoter (Maehara et al., 2002). In addition, decreased level of dimethyl H3K4 and acetylated H3K9 also regulated the expression of SOD2 gene (Hitchler et al., 2008). SODs are a group of critical enzymes in counteracting the superoxide toxicity. Altered expression and activity of SOD are all associated with oxidative DNA damage. It was found that *SOD1* mutation could cause familial amyotrophic lateral sclerosis (ALS) (Li et al., 2010). High level of MnSOD was detected in hippocampus of AD patients (Marcus et al., 2005).

On the other hand, these PTM signals are directly read to initiate DNA repair process. 53BP1 is found as one key point protein connecting the PTM signals with other repair molecules. It is a conserved checkpoint protein with properties of a DSB sensor. DNA damage-induced PTMs could change higher-order structure of chromatin and then expose the 53BP1-binding site. In response to DNA damage, 53BP1 is recruited to DSBs sites by binding to gamma-H2AX. A region of 53BP1 upstream of tandem tudor domains bound gamma-H2AX in vitro (Ward et al., 2003). Moreover, 53BP1 was recruited to the sites of DSBs by binding of its tandem tudor domain to methylated histones, such as H4K20me1/2, H3K79me1/2 (Huyen et al., 2004; Pei et al., 2011).

However, the binding of 53BP1 to DNA damage sites is not the first step in DDR. The upstream molecules could regulate such binding activity, such as mediator of DNA damage checkpoint protein 1 (MDC1) and E3 ubiquitin-protein ligase RNF8. MDC1 is a cell cycle checkpoint protein, activated in response to DNA damage. Through its BRCT motifs, MDC1 interacted with gamma-H2AX at sites near DDR within minutes after exposure to ionizing radiation, which facilitated the recruitment of ATM kinase to DNA damage foci (Stewart et al., 2003). Then RNF8 was rapidly assembled at DSBs via interaction of its FHA domain with the phosphorylated adaptor protein MDC1 (Mailand et al., 2007). After that, ubiquitinated H2A and H2AX by RNF8 made the translocation of 53BP1 to the sites of DNA damage (Yan & Jetten, 2008). At the same time, phosphorylated histone methyltransferase MMSET (at Ser 102 site) was also recruited with the interaction to MDC1 BRCT domain, which induced H4K20 methylation around DSBs and also facilitates 53BP1 recruitment (Pei et al., 2011).

What about the mechanism of histone acetylation in DDR? Evidence has indicated that acetylated histones and histone acetyltransferases were involved in DDR by recruiting DNA repair proteins as well as chromatin remodeling factors to DSB sites (Tamburini & Tyler, 2005; Ogiwara et al., 2011). For example, the recruitment of CBP and p300 to the DSB sites induced the acetylation of lysine 18 within histone H3, and lysines 5, 8, 12, and 16 within histone H4, which facilitated the recruitment of KU70 and KU80 for NHEJ. At the same time, BRM, a catalytic subunit of the SWI/SNF complex, was also recruited at DSB sites to establish a relaxed chromatin environment for DNA damage repair. During homologous recombinational repair, histone acetyltransferases GCN5 and Esa1 and histone deacetylases Rpd3, Sir2 and Hst1 were recruited to the HO lesion (Tamburini & Tyler, 2005). Dynamic changes in histone acetylation were detectable at DSB sites, which might represent important signal for cells indicating that chromosomal repair was complete and might be required to turn off the DNA damage or chromatin structure checkpoint (Tamburini & Tyler, 2005).

Recently, researchers explained the mechanism of ubiquitination of histone H2A at lysine 119 (H2AK119ub) in DDR (Ginjala et al., 2011). ATM, phosphorylated H2AX and RNF8 firstly recruited polycomb protein BMI1 to sites of DNA damage. BMI1 then catalyzed ubiquitination of histone H2AK119 and activated homologous recombination.

Kauppinen and Swanson have described the possible mechanism of poly ADP-ribosylation in DDR (Kauppinen & Swanson, 2007). Poly ADP-ribosylation of histones induced local relaxation of the chromatin structure, which in turn facilitated access of repair proteins to damaged DNA. In addition, the binding of PARP induced the synthesis of a poly ADP-ribose chain (PAR), which worked as a signal for the other DNA repair enzymes, such as DNA ligase III (LigIII) and DNA polymerase beta (polβ), which were necessary for BER process. Regretfully, over-activation of PARP might induce a progressive ATP depletion and finally result in cell death.

4. Specificity of DNA damage and repair in age-associated neurodegenerative diseases

DNA damage could be caused by both exogenous and endogenous damaging agents. However, some external agents, such as UV light, are unlikely to affect neuronal cells because they are never exposed to sunlight. Endogenous DNA damaging agents, such as ROSs, is the predominant DNA damaging agent in age-associated neurodegenerative diseases. The DNA damage and repair occurring in neurodegenerative diseases have been summarized in a number of reviews (Fishel et al., 2007; Martin, 2008). The main forms of damage detected in AD brains as well as in other neurodegenerative diseases are DNA single-strand breaks (SSBs) and DSBs, which are intermediates in repair of oxidative DNA damage. SSBs are primarily removed by BER pathway and nucleotide excision repair (NER) pathway. Neuronal cells also have the capacity to repair DNA lesions by direct repair and mismatch repair (MMR) and have the ability to repair DSBs through homologous recombination (HR) and NHEJ mode. However, the cohesive end joining activity decreased with age of the animal (Vyjayanti & Rao, 2006).

Interestingly, different types of DNA damage had different distribution patterns in neurodegenerative brain, and different cells showed various fates (Barzilai et al., 2008). Most of DNA damage was found in the hippocampus and cortex during aging, which was consistent with the decline in memory and cognitive capacity as the early features of neurodegenerative disease. Astrocytes and neurons, but not microglia, were associated with the presence of DNA damage-associated molecules (H2AX, DNA-PK and 8-OHdG). PARP protein recognizes SSBs sites. Most of the cells containing poly (ADP-ribose), end-product of PARP, were neurons, such as small pyramidal neurons in cortex and some astrocytes, but not microglia (Love et al., 1999). Interestingly, accumulation of poly (ADP-ribose) was not detectable in the cells containing tangles and relatively low accumulation occurred within plaques, which were caused by tau or amyloid beta protein (Love et al., 1999). This might imply that the damage form caused by tau or amyloid beta protein might be DSBs rather than SSBs.

The destiny of different brain cells in response to the same type of DNA damage was diverse, which leaded researchers to propose that brain cells had different thresholds to

DNA damage (Barzilai et al., 2008). Certain types of neurons, such as hippocampal, pyramidal and granule cells as well as cerebellar granule cells, suffer from an age-associated accumulation of DNA damage but do not reduce in number during aging. Other types of neurons, such as cerebellar Purkinje cells, reduce cell number during aging, but remaining cells show no age-associated accumulation of DNA damage.

In conclusion, DDR differs between various neuronal cells. Therefore certain histone PTM types and their role in repair pathways might be specific to certain age-associated neurodegenerative diseases. However, we should note that some conclusions on histone PTMs involving in DDR came from the investigations on budding yeast cells or non- human mammalian cells. Therefore, further work focusing on human neuronal cells is needed.

5. PTMs in cell cycle re-entry

It is commonly believed that neurons are postmitotic cells, which remains in G0 phase of the cell cycle indefinitely. Actually, neurons in the adult human brain are able to re-enter the cell-division cycle. Schwartz and colleagues have demonstrated cell cycle re-entry phenomenon in neurons (Schwartz et al., 2007). They found that subtoxic concentrations of H_2O_2 induced the formation of repairable DSBs associated with the activation of cyclin D1, G1 cell cycle component, and the phosphorylation of retinoblastoma tumor suppressor protein (pRB) at serine 795, a marker of G0-G1 transition, was also significantly elevated. In addition, DNA helicase subunit minichromosome maintenance (Mcm) protein 2, which is strongly down regulated in quiescent, terminally differentiated or senescent cells, was higher in H_2O_2 -treated cells. Nuclear antigen Ki-67 positive neurons, a marker of cells in G1, S, G2 and mitosis, were also increased after treatment. Except for the expression of several cell cycle proteins (Nagy et al., 1997), H3 phosphorylation at serine 10, as a marker for mitosis and transcriptional activation, was also significantly increased in the cytoplasm of neurons in the hippocampus of AD cases (Ogawa et al., 2003).

It seemed that neuronal cells also need to re-enter the cell cycle to activate DNA repair and/or contribute to apoptosis, which shared the same function with proliferating cells (Kruman, 2004). The transition from G0 to G1 was required for NHEJ repair in neurons (Tomashevski et al., 2010). In the brains of AD patients, the cell cycle of neurons could progress as far as the G2 phase, which was also required for repairing DNA lesions (Obulesu & Rao, 2010).

Dynamic change of histone PTMs during cell cycle has been analyzed in HeLa cells (Bonenfant et al., 2007). For example, phosphorylated histone H3 at serine 10 and threonine 3 was only detected in G2/M phase and acetylation on histone H2A and H2B was reduced in G2/M phase, while histone H3K79me showed no change during the cell cycle. Such studies provide us with valuable information for understanding the roles of histone PTMs in cell cycle regulation. However, several recent investigations have reported the roles of histone PTMs in cell cycle re-entry under DNA damage stress (see above), which may be more important in terminally differentiated neurons and likely represent a new research area in the future.

6. Conclusions

Oxidative stress-induced DNA damage has been proposed as pathological mechanism contributing to age-associated neurodegenerative diseases. The modified histone sites not only signal the presence of damage, but also provide a landing platform for necessary repair/signaling proteins in cellular repair machinery. Moreover, histone residues covalently modified alone or in combination could provide distinct docking sites for multiple nuclear proteins, and thus regulate the expression of genes in response to oxidative stress or other extracellular signals. Therefore, both direct and indirect participation of histone PTMs in DNA damage recognition and repair might play a critical role in the pathological process of age-related neurodegenerative diseases.

Except for nuclear DNA damage, mitochondrial DNA (mtDNA) damage is also proposed to play a critical role in aging and in the pathogenesis of several neurological disorders (Yang et al., 2008). According to previous studies, no histone proteins were found in mitochondria. DNA damage detection and DNA repair processes that involve histone PTMs might not be suitable for mtDNA damage. However, Katherine and her group recently found the positive signal of histone H3 in mitochondrial extracts from Brassica oleracea by western blot (Katherine et al., 2010). Regretfully, the function of mitochondrial H3 has not been demonstrated by experimental data. More evidence in other species had not been reported. The question whether there is a relationship between PTMs and mtDNA damage or not needs more hard experimental work to be answered.

In summary, studies of the mechanisms involving histone PTMs will enrich our basic knowledge of the role of histone PTMs in DNA damage response and thus will benefit the strategies for clinical interventions in age-related neurodegenerative diseases in the future.

7. Abbreviations

8-oxoG, 8-oxoguanine; 8-OHG, 8-hydroxyguanosine; 8-OHdG, 8-hydroxy-2'-deoxyguanosine; BER, base excision repair; DDR, DNA damage response; DSBs, DNA double strand breaks; HMT, histone methyltransferases; HDMT, histone demethyltransferase; HDAC, histone deacetylases; HAT, histone acetyltransferase; HR, homologous recombination; IR, ionizing radiation; NER, nucleotide excision repair; NHEJ, non-homologous end joining; PARPs, poly ADP-ribose polymeras; PTMs, histone post translational modifications; ROS, reactive oxygen species; SSBs, single-strand breaks.

8. References

Barzilai, A., Biton, S. & Shiloh, Y. (2008). The role of the DNA damage response in neuronal development, organization and maintenance. *DNA Repair (Amst)*, 7(7), 1010-27.

Best, BP. (2009). Nuclear DNA damage as a direct cause of aging. *Rejuvenation Res*, 12(3), 199-208.

Bonenfant, D., Towbin, H., Coulot, M., Schindler, P., Mueller, DR. & van Oostrum, J. (2007). Analysis of dynamic changes in post-translational modifications of human histones during cell cycle by mass spectrometry. *Mol Cell Proteomics*, 6(11), 1917-32.

Boulikas, T. (1990). Poly (ADP-ribosylated) histones in chromatin replication. *J Biol Chem*. 265(24), 14638-47.

Butterfield, DA. (2002). Amyloid beta-peptide (1-42)-induced oxidative stress and neurotoxicity: implications for neurodegeneration in Alzheimer's disease brain. *Free Radic Res*, 36(12), 1307-13.

Büttner, N., Johnsen, SA., Kügler, S. & Vogel, T. (2010). Af9/Mllt3 interferes with Tbr1 expression through epigenetic modification of histone H3K79 during development of the cerebral cortex. *Proc Natl Acad Sci U S A*, 107(15), 7042-7.

Celeste, A., Petersen, S., Romanienko, PJ., Fernandez-Capetillo, O., Chen, HT., Sedelnikova, OA., Reina-San-Martin, B., Coppola, V., Meffre, E., Difilippantonio, MJ., Redon, C., Pilch, DR., Olaru, A., Eckhaus, M., Camerini-Otero, RD., Tessarollo, L., Livak, F., Manova, K., Bonner, WM., Nussenzweig, MC. & Nussenzweig, A. (2002). Genomic instability in mice lacking histone H2AX. *Science*, 296(5569), 922-7.

Cheung, I., Shulha, HP., Jiang, Y., Matevossian, A., Wang, J., Weng, Z. & Akbarian, S. (2010). Developmental regulation and individual differences of neuronal H3K4me3 epigenomes in the prefrontal cortex. *Proc Natl Acad Sci U S A*, 107(19), 8824-9.

Cheung, WL., Turner, FB., Krishnamoorthy, T., Wolner, B., Ahn, SH., Foley, M., Dorsey, JA., Peterson, CL., Berger, SL. & Allis, CD. (2005). Phosphorylation of histone H4 serine 1 during DNA damage requires casein kinase II in S. cerevisiae. *Curr Biol*, 15(7), 656-60.

Cohen-Armon, M., Visochek, L., Rozensal, D., Kalal, A., Geistrikh, I., Klein, R., Bendetz-Nezer, S., Yao, Z. & Seger, R. (2007). DNA-independent PARP-1 activation by phosphorylated ERK2 increases Elk1 activity: a link to histone acetylation. *Mol Cell*, 25(2), 297-308.

David, DC., Ollikainen, N., Trinidad, JC., Cary, MP., Burlingame, AL. & Kenyon, C. (2010). Widespread protein aggregation as an inherent part of aging in C. elegans. *PLoS Biol*, 8(8), e1000450.

Dollé, ME., Busuttil, RA., Garcia, AM., Wijnhoven, S., van Drunen, E., Niedernhofer, LJ., van der Horst, G., Hoeijmakers, JH., van Steeg, H. & Vijg, J. (2006). Increased genomic instability is not a prerequisite for shortened lifespan in DNA repair deficient mice. *Mutat Res*, 596(1-2), 22-35.

Faucher, D. & Wellinger, RJ. (2010). Methylated H3K4, a transcription-associated histone modification, is involved in the DNA damage response pathway. *PLoS Genet*, 6(8), pii: e1001082.

Feng, Q., Wang, H., Ng, HH., Erdjument-Bromage, H., Tempst, P., Struhl, K. & Zhang, Y. (2002). Methylation of H3-Lysine 79 Is Mediated by a New Family of HMTases without a SET Domain. *Current Biology*, 12(12), 1052–8.

Fernandez-Capetillo, O., Allis, CD. & Nussenzweig, A. (2004a). Phosphorylation of histone H2B at DNA double-strand breaks. *J Exp Med*, 199(12), 1671-7.

Fernandez-Capetillo, O., Lee, A., Nussenzweig, M. & Nussenzweig, A. (2004b). H2AX: the histone guardian of the genome. *DNA Repair (Amst)*, 3(8-9), 959-67.

Fischer, A., Sananbenesi, F., Wang, X., Dobbin, M. &Tsai LH. (2007). Recovery of learning and memory is associated with chromatin remodelling. *Nature*, 447 (7141), 178-182.

Fishel, ML., Vasko, MR. & Kelley, MR. (2007). DNA repair in neurons: so if they don't divide what's to repair? *Mutat Res*, 614(1-2), 24-36.

Foster, ER. & Downs, JA. (2005). Histone H2A phosphorylation in DNA double-strand break repair. *FEBS J*, 272(13), 3231-40.

Ginjala, V., Nacerddine, K., Kulkarni, A., Oza, J., Hill, SJ., Yao, M., Citterio, E., van Lohuizen, M. & Ganesan, S. (2011). BMI1 is recruited to DNA breaks and contributes to DNA damage induced H2A ubiquitination and repair. *Mol Cell Biol*, Doi: 10.1128/MCB.00981-10.

Harvey, AC., Jackson, SP. & Downs, JA. (2005). Saccharomyces cerevisiae histone H2A Ser122 facilitates DNA repair. *Genetics*, 170(2), 543-53.

Hetman, M., Vashishta, A. & Rempala, G. (2010). Neurotoxic mechanisms of DNA damage: focus on transcriptional inhibition. *J Neurochem*, 114(6), 1537-49.

Hitchler, MJ., Oberley, LW. & Domann, FE. (2008). Epigenetic silencing of SOD2 by histone modifications in human breast cancer cells. *Free Radic Biol Med*, 45(11), 1573-80.

Huyen, Y., Zgheib, O., Ditullio, RA Jr., Gorgoulis, VG., Zacharatos, P., Petty, TJ., Sheston, EA., Mellert, HS., Stavridi, ES. & Halazonetis, TD. (2004). Methylated lysine 79 of histone H3 targets 53BP1 to DNA double-strand breaks. *Nature*, 432(7015), 406-11.

Jiang, X., Xu, Y., & Price, BD. (2010). Acetylation of H2AX on lysine 36 plays a key role in the DNA double-strand break repair pathway. *FEBS Lett*, 584(13), 2926-30.

Katherine, B., Zanin, M., Donohue, JM., & Everitt, BA. (2010). Evidence that core histone H3 is targeted to the mitochondria in Brassica oleracea. *Cell Biol Int*, 34(10), 997-1003.

Kauppinen, TM. & Swanson, RA. (2007). The role of poly (ADP-ribose) polymerase-1 in CNS disease. *Neuroscience*, 145(4), 1267-72.

Kim, MO., Chawla, P., Overland, RP., Xia, E., Sadri-Vakili, G. & Cha, JH. (2008). Altered histone monoubiquitylation mediated by mutant huntingtin induces transcriptional dysregulation. *J Neurosci*, 28(15), 3947-57.

Kinner, A., Wu, W., Staudt, C. & Iliakis, G. (2008). Gamma-H2AX in recognition and signaling of DNA double-strand breaks in the context of chromatin. *Nucleic Acids Res*, 36(17), 5678-94.

Kniewel, R. & Keeney, S. (2009). Histone methylation sets the stage for meiotic DNA breaks. *EMBO J*, 28(2), 81-3.

Kruman, II. (2004). Why do neurons enter the cell cycle? *Cell Cycle*, 3(6), 769-73.

Kuzumaki, N., Ikegami, D., Tamura, R., Sasaki, T., Niikura, K., Narita, M., Miyashita, K., Imai, S., Takeshima, H., Ando, T., Igarashi, K., Kanno, J., Ushijima, T., Suzuki, T., & Narita, M. (2010). Hippocampal epigenetic modification at the doublecortin gene is involved in the impairment of neurogenesis with aging. *Synapse*, 64(8), 611-6.

Laposa, RR. & Cleaver, JE. (2001). DNA repair on the brain. *Proc Natl Acad Sci U S A*, 98(23), 12860-2.

Li, Q., Vande Velde, C., Israelson, A., Xie, J., Bailey, AO., Dong, MQ., Chun, SJ., Roy, T., Winer, L., Yates, JR., Capaldi, RA., Cleveland, DW. & Miller, TM. (2010). ALS-linked mutant superoxide dismutase 1 (SOD1) alters mitochondrial protein composition and decreases protein import. *Proc Natl Acad Sci U S A*,107(49), 21146-51.

Love, S., Barber, R. & Wilcock, GK. (1999). Increased poly(ADP-ribosyl)ation of nuclear proteins in Alzheimer's disease. *Brain*, 122 (Pt 2), 247-53.

Lovell, MA., Gabbita, SP. & Markesbery, WR. (1999). Increased DNA oxidation and decreased levels of repair products in Alzheimer's disease ventricular CSF. *J Neurochem*, 72(2), 771-6.

Luger, K., Mäder, AW., Richmond, RK., Sargent, DF. & Richmond, TJ. (1997). Crystal structure of the nucleosome core particle at 2.8 A resolution. *Nature*, 389(6648), 251–260.

Maehara, K., Uekawa, N. & Isobe K. (2002). Effects of histone acetylation on transcriptional regulation of manganese superoxide dismutase gene. *Biochem Biophys Res Commun*, 295(1), 187-92.

Mah, LJ., El-Osta, A. & Karagiannis, TC. (2010). GammaH2AX as a molecular marker of aging and disease. *Epigenetics*, 5(2), 129-36.

Mailand, N., Bekker-Jensen, S., Faustrup, H., Melander, F., Bartek, J., Lukas, C., Lukas, J., Marcus, DL., Strafaci, JA. & Freedman, ML. (2006). Differential neuronal expression of manganese superoxide dismutase in Alzheimer's disease. *Med Sci Monit*, 12(1), BR8-14.

Mailand, N., Bekker-Jensen, S., Faustrup, H., Melander, F., Bartek, J., Lukas, C. & Lukas, J. (2007). RNF8 ubiquitylates histones at DNA double-strand breaks and promotes assembly of repair proteins. *Cell*, 131(5), 887-900.

Markesbery, WR. & Lovell, MA. (2006). DNA oxidation in Alzheimer's disease. Antioxid *Redox Signal*, 8(11-12), 2039-45.

Martin, LJ. (2008). DNA damage and repair: relevance to mechanisms of neurodegeneration. *J Neuropathol Exp Neurol*, 67(5), 377-87.

Mattson, MP. (2003). Methylation and acetylation in nervous system development and neurodegenerative disorders. *Ageing Res Rev*, 2(3), 329-42.

Méndez-Acuña, L., Di Tomaso, MV., Palitti, F. & Martínez-López, W. (2010) Histone post-translational modifications in DNA damage response. *Cytogenet Genome Res*, 128(1-3), 28-36.

Monks, TJ., Xie, R., Tikoo, K. & Lau, SS. (2006). Ros-induced histone modifications and their role in cell survival and cell death. *Drug Metab Rev*, 38(4), 755-67.

Moyal, L., Lerenthal, Y., Gana-Weisz, M., Mass, G., So, S., Wang, SY., Eppink, B., Chung, YM., Shalev, G., Shema, E., Shkedy, D., Smorodinsky, NI., van Vliet, N., Kuster, B., Mann, M., Ciechanover, A., Dahm-Daphi, J., Kanaar, R., Hu, MC., Chen, DJ., Oren, M. & Shiloh, Y. (2011) Requirement of ATM-dependent monoubiquitylation of histone H2B for timely repair of DNA double-strand breaks. *Mol Cell*, 41(5), 529-42.

Myung, NH., Zhu, X., Kruman, II., Castellani, RJ., Petersen, RB., Siedlak, SL., Perry, G., Smith, MA. & Lee, HG. (2008). Evidence of DNA damage in Alzheimer disease: phosphorylation of histone H2AX in astrocytes. *Age (Dordr)*, 30(4), 209-15.

Nakabeppu, Y., Tsuchimoto, D., Yamaguchi, H. & Sakumi, K. (2007). Oxidative damage in nucleic acids and Parkinson's disease. *J Neurosci Res*, 85(5), 919-34.

Oberdoerffer, P., Michan, S., McVay, M., Mostoslavsky, R., Vann, J., Park, SK., Hartlerode, A., Stegmuller, J., Hafner, A., Loerch, P., Wright, SM., Mills, KD., Bonni, A., Yankner, BA., Scully, R., Prolla, TA., Alt, FW. & Sinclair, DA. (2008). SIRT1 redistribution on chromatin promotes genomic stability but alters gene expression during aging. *Cell*, 135(5), 907-18.

Obulesu, M. & Rao, DM. (2010). DNA damage and impairment of DNA repair in Alzheimer's disease. *Int J Neurosci*, 120(6), 397-403.

Ogawa, O., Zhu, X., Lee, HG., Raina, A., Obrenovich, ME., Bowser, R., Ghanbari, HA., Castellani, RJ., Perry, G. & Smith, MA. (2003). Ectopic localization of phosphorylated histone H3 in Alzheimer's disease: a mitotic catastrophe? *Acta Neuropathol*, 105(5), 524-8.

Ogiwara, H., Ui, A., Otsuka, A., Satoh, H., Yokomi, I., Nakajima, S., Yasui, A., Yokota, J. & Kohno, T. (2011). Histone acetylation by CBP and p300 at double-strand break sites facilitates SWI/SNF chromatin remodeling and the recruitment of non-homologous end joining factors. *Oncogene*, Doi:10.1038/onc.2010.592.

Pei, H., Zhang, L., Luo, K., Qin, Y., Chesi, M., Fei, F., Bergsagel, PL., Wang, L., You, Z. & Lou, Z. (2011). MMSET regulates histone H4K20 methylation and 53BP1 accumulation at DNA damage sites. *Nature*, 470(7332), 124-8.

Penner, MR., Roth, TL., Barnes, CA. & Sweatt. JD. (2010). An epigenetic hypothesis of aging-related cognitive dysfunction. *Front Aging Neurosci*, Doi: 10.3389/fnagi.2010.00009.

Rogakou, EP., Pilch, DR., Orr, AH., Ivanova, VS. & Bonner, WM. (1998). DNA double-stranded breaks induce histone H2AX phosphorylation on serine 139. *J Biol Chem*, 273(10), 5858-68.

Sadri-Vakili, G., Bouzou, B., Benn, CL., Kim, MO., Chawla, P., Overland, RP., Glajch, KE., Xia, E., Qiu, Z., Hersch, SM., Clark, TW., Yohrling, GJ. & Cha, JH. (2007) Histones associated with downregulated genes are hypo-acetylated in Huntington's disease models. *Hum Mol Genet*, 16(11), 1293-306.

Saha, RN. & Pahan, K. (2006). HATs and HDACs in neurodegeneration: a tale of disconcerted acetylation homeostasis. *Cell Death Differ*, 13(4), 539-50.

Sarg, B., Koutzamani, E., Helliger, W., Rundquist, I. & Lindner, HH. (2002) Postsynthetic trimethylation of histone H4 at lysine 20 in mammalian tissues is associated with aging. *J Biol Chem*, 277(42), 39195-201.

Schwartz, EI., Smilenov, LB., Price, MA., Osredkar, T., Baker, RA., Ghosh, S., Shi, FD., Vollmer, TL., Lencinas, A., Stearns, DM., Gorospe, M. & Kruman, II. (2007). Cell cycle activation in postmitotic neurons is essential for DNA repair. *Cell Cycle*, 6(3), 318-29.

Sedelnikova, OA., Horikawa, I., Redon, C., Nakamura, A., Zimonjic, DB., Popescu, NC. & Bonner, WM. (2008). Delayed kinetics of DNA double-strand break processing in normal and pathological aging. *Aging Cell*, 7(1), 89-100.

Shackelford, DA. (2006). DNA end joining activity is reduced in Alzheimer's disease. *Neurobiol Aging*, 27(4), 596-605.

Sharma, GG., So, S., Gupta, A., Kumar, R., Cayrou, C., Avvakumov, N., Bhadra, U., Pandita, RK., Porteus, MH., Chen, DJ., Cote, J. & Pandita, TK. (2010). MOF and histone H4 acetylation at lysine 16 are critical for DNA damage response and double-strand break repair. *Mol Cell Biol*, 30(14), 3582-95.

Simpson, JE., Ince, PG., Haynes, LJ., Theaker, R., Gelsthorpe, C., Baxter, L., Forster, G., Lace, GL., Shaw, PJ., Matthews, FE., Savva, GM., Brayne, C. & Wharton, SB. (2010). MRC cognitive function and ageing neuropathology study group. population variation in oxidative stress and astrocyte DNA damage in relation to Alzheimer-type pathology in the ageing brain. *Neuropathol Appl Neurobiol*, 36(1), 25-40.

Singh, RK. & Gunjan, A. (2011). Histone tyrosine phosphorylation comes of age. *Epigenetics*, 6(2), 153-60.

Stewart, GS., Wang, B., Bignell, CR., Taylor, AM. & Elledge, SJ. (2003). MDC1 is a mediator of the mammalian DNA damage checkpoint. *Nature*, 421(6926), 961-6.

Stucki, M. (2009). Histone H2A.X Tyr142 phosphorylation: a novel sWItCH for apoptosis? *DNA Repair (Amst)*, 8(7), 873-6.

Sun, ZW. & Allis, CD. (2002). Ubiquitination of histone H2B regulates H3 methylation and gene silencing in yeast. *Nature*, 418(6893), 104-8.

Tabner, BJ., Mayes, J. & Allsop, D. (2010). Hypothesis: soluble aβ oligomers in association with redox-active metal ions are the optimal generators of reactive oxygen species in Alzheimer's disease. *Int J Alzheimers Dis*, 2011, 546380.

Tamburini, BA. & Tyler, JK. (2005). Localized histone acetylation and deacetylation triggered by the homologous recombination pathway of double-strand DNA repair. *Mol Cell Biol*, 25(12), 4903-13.

Tikoo, K., Lau, SS. & Monks, TJ. (2001). Histone H3 phosphorylation is coupled to poly-(ADP-ribosylation) during reactive oxygen species-induced cell death in renal proximal tubular epithelial cells. *Mol Pharmacol*, 60(2), 394-402.

Toh, GW., O'Shaughnessy, AM., Jimeno, S., Dobbie, IM., Grenon, M., Maffini, S., O'Rorke, A. & Lowndes, NF. (2006). Histone H2A phosphorylation and H3 methylation are required for a novel Rad9 DSB repair function following checkpoint activation. *DNA Repair (Amst)*, 5(6), 693-703.

Tomashevski, A., Webster, DR., Grammas, P., Gorospe, M. & Kruman, II. (2010). Cyclin-C-dependent cell-cycle entry is required for activation of non-homologous end joining DNA repair in postmitotic neurons. *Cell Death Differ*, 17(7), 1189-98.

Van Attikum, H. & Gasser, SM. (2009). Crosstalk between histone modifications during the DNA damage response. *Trends Cell Biol*, 19(5), 207-17.

Vyjayanti, VN. & Rao, KS. (2006). DNA double strand break repair in brain: reduced NHEJ activity in aging rat neurons. *Neurosci Lett*, 393(1): 18-22.

Wang, CM., Tsai, SN., Yew, TW., Kwan, YW. & Ngai, SM. (2010). Identification of histone methylation multiplicities patterns in the brain of senescence-accelerated prone mouse 8. *Biogerontology*, 11(1), 87-102.

Ward, IM., Minn, K., Jorda, KG. & Chen, J. (2003). Accumulation of checkpoint protein 53BP1 at DNA breaks involves its binding to phosphorylated histone H2AX. *J Biol Chem*, 278(22): 19579-82.

Weissman, L., Jo, DG., Sørensen, MM., de Souza-Pinto, NC., Markesbery, WR., Mattson, MP. & Bohr, VA. (2007). Defective DNA base excision repair in brain from individuals with Alzheimer's disease and amnestic mild cognitive impairment. *Nucleic Acids*, 35(16), 5545-55.

Wysocki, R., Javaheri, A., Allard, S., Sha, F., Côté, J. & Kron, SJ. (2005). Role of Dot1-dependent histone H3 methylation in G1 and S phase DNA damage checkpoint functions of Rad9. *Mol Cell Biol*, 25(19), 8430-43.

Yan, J. & Jetten, AM. (2008). RAP80 and RNF8, key players in the recruitment of repair proteins to DNA damage sites. *Cancer Lett*, 271(2), 179-90.

Yang, JL., Weissman, L., Bohr, VA. & Mattson, MP. (2008). Mitochondrial DNA damage and repair in neurodegenerative disorders. *DNA Repair (Amst)*, 7(7), 1110-20.

Part 2

DNA Damage and Disease

3

Relationship Between DNA Damage and Energy Metabolism: Evidence from DNA Repair Deficiency Syndromes

Sarah Vose and James Mitchell
Harvard School of Public Health
Department of Genetics and Complex Diseases, Boston, MA
USA

1. Introduction

It is estimated that the human genome incurs on the order of $1,000$-$1,000,000$ DNA lesions/cell/day (Lodish 2000). A majority of these are thought to be due to endogenous sources, including reactive oxygen and nitrogen species (ROS, RNS) that can oxidize cellular macromolecules including lipid, protein and nucleic acid. These free radicals can be generated for specific purposes by cellular enzymes; for example, nitric oxide synthases generate NO in endothelial cells for signaling purposes, while NADPH oxidase and myeloperoxidase generate ROS in granulocytes to kill invading pathogens. However, ROS can also occur as a byproduct of cellular energy metabolism (Beckman and Ames 1998). Most cells use mitochondrial respiration as a means of energy production. The process of moving electrons across the mitochondrial membrane can at some frequency result in their transfer to molecular oxygen and the generation of superoxide and hydrogen peroxide, which together can generate the highly reactive hydroxyl radical and damage nearby molecules, including DNA.

The frequency of superoxide formation is influenced by many factors, including the rate of electron transport and the capacity of the mitochondria to couple the proton gradient created across the inner membrane to ATP production, or to dissipate it in the form of heat through the use of uncoupling proteins. High rates of electron transport and efficient ATP production or uncoupling are consistent with reduced ROS generation, while low rates of transport or inefficient ATP production (for example when ATP/ADP ratios are already high) are consistent with increased ROS generation. Different substrates may also influence mitochondrial ROS production. Oxidation of ketone bodies, for example, may generate more ROS than oxidation of acetyl CoA from glucose (Tieu et al. 2003). Substrate utilization further depends on cell type and nutritional status. For example, neurons prefer to oxidize glucose, but can also use ketone bodies derived from fat oxidation in the liver. Skeletal muscle can use either fat or glucose, depending on availability, but tends to use one at the exclusion of the other (Randle et al. 1963). In cooperation with mitochondria, peroxisomes also play a major role in energy metabolism by oxidizing long-chain fatty acids. Peroxisomes can further participate in ketogenesis, amino acid oxidation and the oxidative phase of the pentose phosphate pathway depending on substrate availability. Like mitochondria, they are a major source of ROS and RNS generating enzymes, and thus a potential source of oxidative macromolecular damage by leakage of ROS/RNS across the organelle membrane. Mitochondria and peroxisomes also produce abundant amounts of antioxidants enzymes such as superoxide dismutase and catalase to neutralize ROS. Thus, mitochondria and peroxisomes can both contribute to ROS as well as play a role in ROS detoxification.

In order to generate energy efficiently, cells oxidize carbon units derived from glucose, amino acids or fatty acids in mitochondria. The use of these substrates is governed by nutritional status and is further subject to hormonal control. Insulin and glucagon are major regulators of organismal substrate utilization. In the fed state, elevated blood glucose promotes insulin secretion by the pancreas and transport of glucose into insulin-responsive tissues including liver, muscle and fat. In the liver, glucose is stored as glycogen or used as a substrate for *de novo* lipogenesis. Insulin signaling also inhibits release of free fatty acids from white adipose tissue and promotes *de novo* lipogenesis and dietary lipid repackaging in the liver for storage in white adipose tissue. After a meal, glucose levels fall and counter-regulatory hormones such as glucagon reverse the actions of insulin and glucose by promoting hepatic glycogenolysis and gluconeogenesis for glucose-dependent tissues such as red blood cells and neurons, and release of fatty acids from the white adipose tissue for oxidation in other organs. Defects in insulin signaling caused by overeating are associated with a spectrum of pathologies including diabetes, obesity and atherosclerosis collectively known as the metabolic syndrome. Although the underlying mechanisms are not entirely clear, it is associated with chronic inflammation and oxidative stress (Hotamisligil 2006). In stark contrast to metabolic syndrome is the spectrum of phenotypes associated with dietary restriction (DR, also known as calorie restriction), defined as reduced food intake without malnutrition. Originally described in rodents to reduce the incidence of cancer and extend lifespan (McCay, Crowel, and Maynard 1935), DR has proven efficacy at increasing lifespan, stress resistance and metabolic fitness in a wide range of experimental organisms. In mammals, the DR state is characterized by reduced serum glucose, reduced growth factors and growth factor signaling, improved insulin sensitivity, increased resistance to oxidative stress and reduced adiposity (Fontana and Klein 2007). While the molecular mechanisms underlying the benefits of DR remain unclear, reduced steady state levels of macromolecular oxidative damage suggest reduced ROS production and/or increased antioxidant defenses play a role.

When DNA damage occurs, there are a number of overlapping repair pathways that recognize and remove the damage, as well as a battery of signaling pathways that influence immediate decisions on cell fate and longer-term adaptations to stress. DNA damage repair pathways are distinguished in large part by the lesions that they recognize. Oxidative base lesions are typically recognized by the base excision repair (BER) pathway, while bulky helix distorting lesions are typically removed by the nucleotide excision repair (NER) pathway. Although the latter is chiefly responsible for removal of UV lesions from sunlight, endogenous oxidative lesions are also partially dependent on NER pathways (Brooks et al. 2000). Oxidative stress can also cause breaks in the sugar-phosphate backbone, resulting in single strand breaks that can interrupt transcription or replication. When the density of such breaks is high, they can occur nearby on opposite strands and result in double strand breaks. Such lesions can be repaired by homologous recombination in the presence of a sister chromatid (for example during S phase of the cell cycle) or by non-homologous recombination during other phases of the cell cycle when the sister chromatid is not readily available to serve as a template for repair. The so-called DNA damage response (DDR) is not a single response but a network of signaling and repair pathways activated by genotoxic stress. Upon DNA damage such as a double strand break or a collapsed replication fork, the serine/threonine kinases ATM or ATR, respectively, initiate a cascade of cellular responses resulting in cell cycle arrest and recruitment of repair factors. One of the targets of ATM and ATR is the tumor suppressor p53, which is stabilized by phosphorylation and activates transcription of genes involved in cell fate, including apoptosis or senescence. Other proteins such as poly ADP ribose polymerase (PARP) are activated by DNA damage and can have indirect effects on cell fate decisions by depleting ATP and NAD+.

Given the connection between production of ROS by cellular metabolism and DNA damage, one might predict coordinate regulation of the cellular response to DNA damage and growth and metabolism on the cellular and organismal levels. In this chapter, we will discuss existing evidence of such a connection. First, we will consider metabolic changes associated with defects in NER disorders and their resemblance to the adaptive response to DR, particularly in mouse models of these diseases. Next, we will consider metabolic changes in a variety of other DNA damage repair and signaling disorders, ranging from DR-like phenotypes to metabolic disorder. We will conclude by reviewing the evidence linking DNA damage repair and signaling pathways directly and indirectly to changes in cellular growth and energy metabolism.

2. Metabolic defects in nucleotide excision repair deficiency syndromes

Although the mutations causing the segmental progerias Cockayne syndrome (CS) and trichothiodystrophy (TTD) are known, how alterations in the associated nucleotide excision DNA repair proteins cause pleiotrophic disease symptoms including dwarfism and cachexia are not yet clear. In mouse models of these disorders, unrepaired endogenous DNA damage is linked to perturbations in energy metabolism and alterations in insulin/insulin-like growth factor-1 (IGF-1) signaling. Paradoxically, these changes resemble beneficial adaptive responses to DR associated with improved metabolic fitness and extended longevity. In this section, we will discuss perturbations in growth and energy metabolism associated with defects in NER proteins in human disease and mouse models, and the potential role of DNA damage in eliciting these changes.

2.1 Cockayne syndrome and trichothiodystrophy

NER is an evolutionarily conserved pathway required for the removal of UV-induced DNA damage. It is divided into two branches based on how the lesion is initially recognized. Global genome (GG)-NER can occur anywhere in the genome upon recognition of DNA helical distortions by the XPC/HR23B/CEN2 complex. Transcription-coupled (TC)-NER occurs only on the transcribed DNA strand and is initiated by the stalling of an elongating RNA polymerase, for example by steric hindrance at the site of a bulky adduct. TC-NER specific proteins CSA and CSB participate in the upstream events surrounding the stalling of an RNA polymerase at the site of DNA damage. Although both CSA and CSB are involved in ubiquitination and protein turnover – CSA is a component of a ubiquitin ligase complex (Groisman et al. 2003), and CSB contains a ubiquitin-binding domain required for UV damage repair (Anindya et al. 2010) - their exact roles in TC-NER remain unclear. Once the TC-NER or GG-NER machinery recognizes the lesion, the helicases XPB and XPD unwind the damaged DNA, allowing validation of the lesion by XPA, endonuclealytic cleavage of the phosphodiester backbone by XPG and XPF-ERCC1 and removal of the damaged oligonucleotide in preparation for repair DNA synthesis.

Mutations in CSA, CSB, XPG, XPD and XPB are associated with CS, a rare progressive disease characterized by photosensitivity, dwarfism, loss of subcutaneous fat and neurodegeneration. CS was first described by Edward Cockayne in 1936 (Cockayne 1936). To date, approximately 200 cases have been reported in the literature (Nance and Berry 1992; Ozdirim et al. 1996; Pasquier et al. 2006; Rapin et al. 2006). Despite UV sensitivity, CS is not associated with an elevated risk of skin cancer as observed in the related NER deficiency syndrome xeroderma pigmentosum (XP). Although there is a range in the onset and severity of CS, typical presentation involves normal in utero growth and birth weight followed by a profound postnatal growth failure within the first two years. This growth failure is also observed in the postnatal brain, resulting in developmental microcephaly and cognitive impairment. Neuropathological defects include demyelination and atrophy of white matter, calcification of the basal ganglia, cerebellar atrophy, demyelination of peripheral nerves, retinopathy, and neuronal loss in the inner ear (Weidenheim, Dickson, and Rapin 2009). Based on the involvement of white matter, CS is considered a form of leukodystrophy. Interestingly, such white matter diseases can be caused by various genetic defects in lysosome or peroxisome metabolism and typically present postnatally after normal birth and early development (Kohlschutter et al. 2010). Diabetes mellitus, early hypertension and atherosclerosis are also prevalent in CS (Rapin et al. 2006). Besides the nervous system and adipose tissue, other organ systems appear proportionately smaller in size yet unimpaired (Weidenheim, Dickson, and Rapin 2009). Death occurs around 12 years of age often from cachexia or an intercurrent illness such as respiratory infection.

The fact that weight is more affected than height in CS led to the use of the term cachexia, or wasting, in association with this disease (Nance and Berry 1992). Although it is not clear that lean mass is preferentially affected as is typical with cachexia, adipose tissue is clearly affected. CS is classified as a lipodystrophy, indicating the abnormal redistribution of fat. Subcutaneous fat loss leads to sunken eyes and a wizened appearance that are further defining characteristics of the disease. Adipocytes are a major site of energy storage in the form of triglycerides, as well as a source of lipokines involved in a variety of processes including appetite control, immune function and temperature regulation. CS patients presumably still have functioning adipocytes that can produce adipokines but do not store triglycerides for reasons that remain unclear. This is distinct from generalized lipoatrophy, in which adipocytes and associated adiopkines are lost, resulting in hyperlipidemia and insulin resistance despite the paucity of fat. Interestingly, lipids are also a major component of myelin sheaths that are lost in CS, although no connection between altered lipid metabolism and demyelination has been reported.

The cause of dwarfism in CS is not known; however there are no consistent data to suggest alteration of endocrine function (Rapin et al. 2006; Nance and Berry 1992). For example, growth hormone (GH) levels are normal to elevated. Whether or not transient perturbation of GH/IGF-1 signaling, which has been reported in mouse models (see below), is relevant in the human disease remains unknown.

Mutations in XPD and XPB, as well as another TFIIH component, p8, can cause another photosensitivity disorder with characteristic growth failure and neurological involvement known as TTD (Morice-Picard et al. 2009). Unlike CS, TTD patients present with characteristic brittle hair and nails caused by a transcriptional defect in terminally differentiating keratinocytes. Despite this difference, there are many similarities between the diseases as would be expected if they share a common basis in defective transcription-coupled DNA repair. As with CS, TTD shows no increase skin cancer risk despite photosensitivity. TTD patients also demonstrate dysmyelination and lipodystrophy. Despite the hypothesis that CS and TTD share a common basis in defect transcription-coupled DNA repair (Andressoo, Hoeijmakers, and Mitchell 2006), this is by no means the only hypothesis regarding the etiology of these diseases. For example, the requirement for the CAK complex of TFIIH in the phosphorylation and regulation of nuclear hormone receptors, which play a major role in cellular and organismal metabolism, has led to the competing hypothesis that disease symptoms are caused by defects in gene expression regulated by these transcriptional activators (Compe et al. 2007; Keriel et al. 2002; Brooks, Cheng, and Cooper 2008).

2.2 Mouse models of NER progeria

Mouse models of CS engineered by disabling the CSA or CSB genes share some characteristics of human CS but in a milder form. Knockout mice are born normally, but are photosensitive and display an age-dependent loss of photoreceptor cells (van der Horst et al. 2002; van der Horst et al. 1997). Although they develop normally, CSB mice remain lean in adulthood and have normal lifespans (Dolle et al. 2006). Interestingly, CSA and CSB mice are resistant to renal ischemia reperfusion injury, a form of acute oxidative and inflammatory stress, and display improved glucose tolerance and insulin sensitivity (Susa et al. 2009). Both of these phenotypes are typical of DR mice (Mitchell et al. 2009). TTD mice created by mutating residue 722 from an R to a W in the XPD C terminus faithfully recapitulate the brittle hair phenotype of the human TTD, but like the CS mice have an overall milder phenotype than the corresponding human disease (de Boer et al. 1998). TTD mice display end of life pathologies consistent with both accelerated aging (osteoporosis, aortic sarcopenia, lymphoid depletion) as well as DR (reduced inflammatory dermatitis, reduced pituitary adenoma, reduced subcutaneous fat) (Wijnhoven et al. 2005). Duodenal epithelial hyperplasia has been proposed to play a role in reduced food absorbance leading to the overall DR-like phenotype (Wijnhoven et al. 2005). XP-CS mice, engineered with a different point mutation in the XPD gene (G602D) associated in patients with the symptoms of both CS and XP also recapitulate the mild features of mouse CS as well as the severe skin cancer susceptibility of XP (Andressoo et al. 2006).

Another group of mouse models of NER deficiency share a more severe core phenotype of dwarfism, ataxia, failure to thrive and death before weaning at 3-4 weeks of age. This so-called "NER progeria" was first described in mice lacking the endonuclease Ercc1 (Melton et al. 1998; Weeda et al. 1997) and subsequently in a number of genetic models of NER deficiency, including CSB/XPA (Murai et al. 2001), XPA/TTD (de Boer et al. 1998), XPA/XPCS (Andressoo et al. 2006), CSB/XPC (Laposa, Huang, and Cleaver 2007) double homozygous mutants as well as XPG (Sun et al. 2003) and XPF (Tian et al. 2004) single homozygous mutants.

Common metabolic features of NER progeria in mice include reduced blood glucose and reduced insulin, disproportionate reduction of white adipose tissue weight, and accumulation of triglycerides in the liver (van de Ven et al. 2007). Although the cause of death is not clear, animals may inevitably succumb to hypoglycemia. Reduced food intake does not seem to be the cause of metabolic perturbations. Liver transcriptome analysis of *Ercc1-/-* and CSB/XPA mice revealed altered expression of genes involved in carbohydrate and oxidative metabolism and peroxisome biogenesis suggestive of increased glycogen synthesis, decreased glycolysis, and decreased oxidative metabolism (Niedernhofer et al. 2006). Global metabolic profiling by NMR revealed that *Ercc1-/-* mice have altered lipid and energy metabolism and a shift toward ketosis when compared to age-matched controls (Nevedomskaya et al. 2010). *Ercc1-/-* mice show several metabolic adaptations that resemble those seen in DR, including decreased LDL and VLDL, increased HDL, and decreased serum glucose (Nevedomskaya et al. 2010).

Another common feature of NER progeria that may underlie the growth retardation is reduced mRNA and serum protein expression of IGF-1 (Niedernhofer et al. 2006; van der Pluijm et al. 2007; van de Ven et al. 2006). Unlike long-lived endocrine deficient dwarfs (Ames, Snell) with reduced GH secretion due to defective anterior pituitary development (Bartke and Brown-Borg 2004), NER-deficient mice have an intact pituitary and normal to elevated GH levels, consistent with normal hypothalamic and pituitary function. Instead, GH receptor mRNA levels are reduced in multiple tissues, resulting in reduced GH-dependent IGF-1 production. Liver transcriptome analysis confirmed a general downregulation of multiple components of the postnatal GH/IGF-1 axis. Nonetheless, in select mouse models of severe NER progeria, effects on serum IGF-1 and glycemic index can be transient, occurring prior to weaning but normalizing in animals that survive this apparent developmental bottleneck (van de Ven et al. 2006).

Global profiling of gene expression in liver confirmed a significant overlap between NER progeria and long-lived dwarfism (Schumacher et al. 2008) consistent with the physiologic data. Paradoxically, the core feature of IGF-1 signaling attenuation increases lifespan in several species (Rincon et al. 2004; Longo and Finch 2003) but is associated with decreased longevity in NER progeria. Altered growth and energy metabolism has thus been interpreted as an adaptive response to endogenous genotoxic stress. Whether or not this response is maladaptive in this model is not known, but does appear to be so in mouse models of models of Hutchinson-Gilford progeria syndrome (HGPS) (Marino et al. 2010) as discussed below.

2.3 Evidence for a role of DNA repair in CD and TTD phenotypes

What is the evidence that defects in DNA repair, and in particular TC-NER, are causative of the pleiotropic disease symptoms including disturbances in growth and energy metabolism? Most NER proteins associated with disorders in man and mouse are multifunctional with distinct roles in several different cellular processes. For example, CSB was originally cloned as a TC-NER factor, but can also function in chromatin remodeling, transcriptional initiation (Le May, Mota-Fernandes et al. 2010), transcriptional elongation (Le May, Egly, and Coin 2010), BER via interactions with the BER glycosylase Ogg1 and stimulation of APE1 incision (Wong et al. 2007) and rRNA synthesis (Bradsher et al. 2002). Similarly, the TFIIH complex containing the XPB and XPD helicases plays a role in transcriptional initiation and activated transcription by a subset of nuclear hormone receptors (Keriel et al. 2002; Compe et al. 2007). Roles for many of these functions have been proposed to be causative of one or more symptoms of CS, TTD or XP. However, due in large part to the high degree of overlap between symptoms in multiple different mouse models, where the effects of homozygous mutations can be interrogated against a standardized genetic and environmental background, it has been hypothesized that these conditions have a common underlying cause (Andressoo, Hoeijmakers, and Mitchell 2006; van de Ven et al. 2007). Currently, the only known common function of each of the proteins, including CSA, CSB, XPD, XPB and XPG, is the transcription-coupled arm of NER. Based on current data, this makes a defect in

TC-NER a plausible cause of overlapping disease symptoms, but does not rule out common pathways that are currently unknown or untested for all relevant disease loci.

If indeed defects in the TC-NER pathway are causative of disease symptoms, what are the relevant endogenous DNA lesions? Most of what is known about the function of TC-NER proteins is derived from cell-based experiments with UV as the source of DNA damage. UV irradiation produces two types of bulky lesions which are substrates for NER; cyclobutane pyrimidine dimers, mainly removed by TC-NER and pyrimidine 6-4 pyrimidone photoproducts, typically processed by GG-NER. Indeed, cells deficient in CSB fail to repair cyclobutane dimers but repair 6-4 photoproducts efficiently (Barrett et al. 1991). UV light may possibly damage keratinocytes of CS patients, but has little capacity to induce lesions in other relevant tissues. Most bulky lesions are induced by exogenous sources, but some bulky lesions are created by endogenous sources (De Bont and van Larebeke 2004).

8,5′-cyclopurine-2′-deoxynucleaosides (cyPudNs) are endogenous lesions formed in DNA by the hydroxyl radical (Jaruga, Theruvathu, et al. 2004; Dizdaroglu et al. 1987). cyPudNs are chemically stable lesions which are expected to accumulate slowly and are candidates for lesions which could cause neurodegeneration (Kuraoka et al. 2000; Brooks 2008). cyPudNs block transcription and, unlike most oxidative DNA lesions, cyPudNs are repaired by NER rather than BER (Brooks et al. 2000; Kuraoka et al. 2000). *In vitro* assays using CHO and NER-deficient CHO cells show that ERCC1 and XPG are required for excision of the 8,5′-(S)-cyclo-2′deoxyadenosine (cyclo-dA) lesion, while BER glycosylases are not active on the cyclo-dA lesion (Brooks et al. 2000). Using a host cell reactivation assay, Brooks et. al. found that cyclo-dA is a substrate for NER *in vivo* (Brooks et al. 2000). Oxidative lesions are elevated in and may contribute to neurodegeneration (Kruman 2004). TC-NER may protect neurons from oxidative lesions, the accumulation of which may lead to the neuronal death observed in CS. Nonetheless, it remains controversial whether or not cells from CS patients or mice are hypersensitive to oxidative stress (van de Ven et al. 2006). Thus despite the growing literature on molecular functions of CSA, CSB and other TC-NER proteins, proof that unrepaired endogenous oxidative lesions cause CS and/or TTD is lacking. Identification of such a lesion and its target tissue awaits.

3. Metabolic defects in other DNA repair and maintenance disorders

A number of human syndromes and mouse models with defects in DNA damage repair and signaling also display perturbations in growth and energy metabolism. Some of these show characteristics of adaptive changes reminiscent of DR as described above in TC-NER syndromes, while others display insulin resistance and atherosclerosis resembling metabolic syndrome on the opposite end of the energy spectrum. In this section, we will describe a number of syndromes and/or mouse models with known defects in DNA repair, genome maintenance or DNA damage-related signal transduction with an emphasis on changes in growth, energy metabolism, adiposity and glucose homeostasis.

3.1 Hutchinson-Gilford Progeria Syndrome

Hutchinson-Gilford Progeria Syndrome (HGPS) is a rare autosomal dominant progeria characterized by failure to thrive, growth retardation unrelated to GH deficiency, baldness and decreased body fat without insulin resistance (Merideth et al. 2008). Atherosclerosis is thought to result from the general accelerated aging observed in all tissues and organs rather than from elevated serum lipoproteins (Al-Shali and Hegele 2004). Vascular disease and stroke are the main causes of death in HGPS, with a life expectancy of about 13 years of age (Merideth et al. 2008). HGPS is caused by a mutation in Lamin A, a component of the nuclear envelope, which leads to a truncated protein missing the Zpmste24 cleavage site (Merideth et al. 2008).

Mouse models deficient in Zmpste24 exhibit nuclear architecture abnormalities, severe growth retardation, loss of subcutaneous adipose tissue, accumulation of lipid in ectopic sites such as liver, and premature death (Pendas et al. 2002; Varela et al. 2005). Aberrations in cardiac muscle of Zmpste24 mice include thinning of the ventricular wall, muscle degeneration, increased inflammation and interstitial fibrosis, suggesting that cardiomyopathy and heart failure contribute to death in this model (Pendas et al. 2002). Zmpste24 mice exhibit increased autophagy in skeletal muscle, possibly due to decreased circulating glucose and insulin and increased adiponectin, resulting in AMPK activation and suppression of the mTOR pathway (Marino et al. 2008). Gene expression data of livers of Zmpste24 mice indicate a shift from glucose to lipid metabolism, a response also seen in starvation (Marino et al. 2008). Zmpste24 mice show decreased IGF-1 and GHR expression in the liver, along with suppressed levels of IGF-1 and increased levels of GH in the serum (Marino et al. 2010). Treatment of Zmpste24 mice with recombinant IGF-1 using a subcutaneous minipump rescues some of the progeroid phenotypes, resulting in improved body weight, increased subcutaneous fat, reduced kyphosis and reduced alopecia (Marino et al. 2010). Serum GH levels were restored (reduced to normal) and lifespan of Zmpste24 mice was expended by 18% by IGF-1 treatment (Marino et al. 2010). Thus, chronic perturbation of the somatotroph axis in response to defects in nuclear architecture has been interpreted as a maladaptive response that actually accelerates disease symptoms.

Does nuclear architecture have any impact on DNA damage repair or signaling? Evidence for a connection between nuclear architecture and DNA damage comes from cells of Zmpste24 deficient mice. These cells display increased chromosomal abnormalities and γ-H2AX phosphorylation indicative of greater DNA damage and reduced genomic stability (Liu et al. 2005). Fibroblasts from HGPS patients senesce prematurely, indicating a cell-autonomous alteration in proliferative capacity (Bridger and Kill 2004; Allsopp et al. 1992). Thus, alterations in nuclear architecture leading to chromosome instability can indirectly activate the DNA damage response (Liu et al. 2005; Verstraeten et al. 2007).

3.2 Werner syndrome

Werner syndrome is a segmental progeria characterized by short stature, early graying and loss of hair. There is no evidence for endocrine deficiency as an explanation for growth deficiency (Monnat 2010). Type 2 diabetes mellitus and dyslipidemia leading to atherosclerosis are also common features of Werner syndrome. Patients with Werner syndrome typically live into their mid-50s and die from premature cardiovascular disease or cancer (Huang et al. 2006; Martin 1985). Werner syndrome patients show accelerated brain accumulation of amyloid β peptide and hyperphosphorylated tau, both common in age-associated disorders (Leverenz, Yu, and Schellenberg 1998). Werner syndrome is also associated with loss of myelin fibers in both the central and peripheral nervous system (Umehara et al. 1993) although without the significant delays in neuronal development observed in CS. Werner syndrome is caused by a defect in Werner (WRN), a Rec-Q helicase which hydrolyzes ATP to separate double-stranded DNA for replication, recombination, transcription and repair (Monnat 2010). The WRN protein is also essential for maintaining chromosomal integrity through intact recombination or DNA replication (Monnat 2010).

Many features of Werner syndrome are faithfully recapitulated in a mouse model in which the WRN gene is lacking the helicase domain (WRN$^{\Delta hel/\Delta hel}$) (Huang et al. 2006; Lachapelle, Oesterreich, and Lebel 2011). WRN$^{\Delta hel/\Delta hel}$ mice have elevated levels of ROS and oxidative DNA damage in liver and heart, and elevated serum triglycerides, glucose and insulin; all of which return to wildtype level upon long-term vitamin C treatment (Lebel et al. 2010). WRN appears to play a role in protecting cells from oxidative damage, and the loss of WRN leads to changes resembling the metabolic syndrome.

3.3 Ataxia Telangiectasia
Deficiency in the DNA damage sensor ATM (Ataxia Telangiectasia Mutated) leads to ataxia telangiectasia (A-T). A-T is a rare autosomal disorder characterized by cerebellar ataxia, elevated cancer incidence, immune dysfunction and elevated sensitivity to ionizing radiation (Shackelford 2005). The life expectancy for patients with A-T is roughly 20 years (Chun and Gatti 2004). A-T patients display signs of premature aging as well as insulin resistance and lowered insulin receptor affinity (Lavin 2000). Mouse models of ATM deficiency show an age-dependent increase in blood glucose and decrease in insulin sensitivity, consistent with a conserved role of this protein in metabolic function (Miles et al. 2007). In an *ApoE$^{-/-}$* mouse model, haploinsufficiency of ATM leads to accelerated atherosclerosis and multiple features of metabolic syndrome relative to the *ApoE$^{-/-}$* mouse (Mercer et al. 2010).

3.4 Seckel syndrome
Stalled replication forks activate A-T and Rad-related protein (ATR), which leads to cell cycle checkpoint activation. Defective ATR signaling in humans causes Seckel syndrome, characterized by growth retardation and severe microcephaly (O'Driscoll and Jeggo 2008). While growth hormone secretion is normal, Seckel syndrome features high circulating IGF-1 levels and slightly decreased binding affinity for the IGF-1 receptor (Ducos et al. 2001; Schmidt et al. 2002). Whether this represents a constitutive defect in IGF-1 signalling or an adaptive response to a defective DNA damage response remains unknown.

3.5 TP53
Activation of the tumor suppressor p53 by genotoxic or other forms of stress can trigger various outcomes that reduce the chance of a damaged cell progressing into a tumor, ranging from cellular senescence to apoptosis. Besides its role in the response to genotoxic stress, p53 plays a central role in cellular energy metabolism through regulation of oxidative phosphorylation, glucose transporter expression and fatty acid synthase (Zhang, Qin, and Wang 2010). Mice engineered with defects in p53 are highly cancer prone, but also display a number of metabolic phenotypes. For example, phosphorylation of p53 at Ser18 by ATM is an important regulator of glucose homeostasis, as a S18A mutation renders mice insulin resistant (Armata et al. 2010). p53 is activated in adipose tissue upon high fat diet-induced obesity and insulin resistance in mice; inhibition of p53 in adipose tissue rescues senescence and insulin resistance in diabetic mice (Minamino et al. 2009). Taken together, these data suggest that p53 activation, for example by oxidative stress derived from over-nutrition and potentially by isolated DNA damage, can promote the onset of metabolic syndrome.

3.6 DNA-PK, KU

DNA-PK, Ku70 and Ku80 form a complex at double strand breaks to facilitate non-homologous end joining (NHEJ). Mice deficient in the catalytic subunit of DNA-PK (DNA-PKcs) exhibit accelerated aging, growth defects and decreased lifespan (Espejel et al. 2004). Mice deficient in Ku80 display premature aging symptoms including osteopenia, atrophic skin, hepatocellular degeneration and age-specific mortality; *Ku70-/-* mice display growth retardation (Gu et al. 1997; Vogel et al. 1999). Increased lymphoma and defects in B and T cells of DNA-PK, Ku70 and Ku80 mice are attributed to their lack of NHEJ resulting in deficient V(D)J recombination required for adaptive immunity; however, premature aging phenotypes are not seen in Rag-1 (V(D)J deficient) mice and thus not related to the lack of adaptive immunity and associated inflammation (Holcomb, Vogel, and Hasty 2007). Reduced size in Ku80 mice is not due to reduced IGF-1, but may instead be related to defects in cell-autonomous proliferation (van de Ven et al. 2006).

3.7 NEIL1 DNA glycosylase deficiency

NEIL1 glycoslyase is the homologue of the bacterial formamidopyrimidine DNA glycolyslase and initiates repair of oxidative lesions in BER, acting specifically on 2,6-diamino-4-hydroxy-5-formamidopyrimidine   and   4,6-diamino-5-formamidopyrimidine lesions (Jaruga, Birincioglu, et al. 2004). A mouse model deficient in NEIL-1 glycosylase develops severe obesity, dyslipidemia, fatty liver disease and hyperinsulinemia in the absence of exogenous oxidative stress (Vartanian et al. 2006). The development of metabolic syndrome in *NEIL1-/-* mice is accelerated on a high-fat diet, indicating NEIL1 absence renders mice more susceptible to oxidative stress-induced metabolic syndrome (Sampath et al. 2011). Although no human diseases are associated with deficiency of NEIL1, several polymorphisms of NEIL1 with different activities on oxidized bases are found in humans (Roy et al. 2007). Whether or not these polymorphisms may lead to susceptibility to metabolic disease is not understood.

3.8 SIRT6

SIRT6 is the mammalian homologue of yeast Sir2 and is an NAD-dependent histone deacetylase. SIRT6 was originally described as a component of the BER system, as SIRT6 deficient MEFs are hypersensitive to BER-lesion inducting agents such as methyl methanesulfonate and hydrogen peroxide; sensitivity was restored to that of wildtype by introducing the dRP lyase domain of Polβ (Mostoslavsky et al. 2006). Although no direct interaction between SIRT6 and BER factors has been reported to date, SIRT6 appears to impact DNA repair by stabilizing chromatin and facilitating DNA-PK dependent damage signaling (Lombard 2009; McCord et al. 2009). SIRT6 also influences metabolism both by deacetylating histone H3 lysine 9 and by repressing HIF1α to control the expression of glycolytic genes, which explains the glucose imbalance seen in SIRT6 knockout mice (Zhong et al. 2010). The SIRT6 phenotype is predominantly a metabolic one, with mice developing normally, although smaller than wildtypes, until 2 weeks of age, when they suffer from a degenerative wasting and severe hypoglycemia resulting in death (Mostoslavsky et al. 2006). Like NER progeria, SIRT6 knockout mice also have reduced serum IGF-1, likely contributing to their small size. Neural-specific deletion of SIRT6 does not rescue the postnatal growth failure, but does rescue the severe hypoglycemia that leads to death in full-body knockouts of SIRT 6 (Schwer et al. 2010; Mostoslavsky et al. 2006). Neural-specific

SIRT6 mice survive much longer than the whole-body knockouts, and by one year of age become obese (Schwer et al. 2010).

Syndrome	Affected gene	Metabolic feature
Cockayne Syndrome	CSA/CSB	Loss of subcutaneous fat
Trichothiodystrophy	XPB/XPD/TTDA	Loss of subcutaneous fat
Hutchinson-Gilford Progeria Syndrome	Lamin A	Loss of subcutaneous fat, atheroslcerosis
Werner Syndrome	WRN	Lipid accumulation in blood, insulin resistance
Ataxia telangiectasia	ATM	Insulin resistance
Seckel syndrome	ATR	Increased IGF-1

Table 1. Human DNA repair diseases resulting in aberrant metabolism.

4. Cell culture models

In cultured cells, a number of recent studies on gene expression, signal transduction and protein interaction networks upon genotoxic stress point to both direct and indirect links between various forms of DNA damage and pathways regulating growth and energy metabolism.

In mammals, organismal growth and metabolism are controlled by availability of nutrients and energy, which in turn influence secretion of circulating regulatory hormones including insulin from the pancreas, growth hormone from the pituitary, and growth-hormone dependent IGF-1 from the liver. Cellular responses to nutrients, energy and growth factor availability are controlled at the cell surface by receptor tyrosine kinases including the insulin receptor (IR) and IGF-1 receptor (IGF-1R). Binding of peptide hormones to their cognate receptors activates a signal transduction cascade resulting in the phosphorylation and activation of downstream kinases including AKT and mTOR. AKT exerts control over energy metabolism by phosphorylating and inactivating FOXO transcription factors as well as TSC1, a major negative regulator of mTOR. mTOR activation, which requires growth factors as well as nutrients (amino acids) and energy, results in phosphorylation and activation of ribosomal protein S6 kinase, promoting protein translation and increased cell size and growth. mTOR also phosphorylates and inactivates the translational repressor eIF-4E-binding protein 1 (4EBP1), further promoting protein synthesis.

The role of protein kinases in DNA repair and the DDR is firmly established. In response to ionizing radiation, DNA damage response proteins ATM and ATR phosphorylate checkpoint kinases Chk1 and Chk2, as well as p53 to block cell cycle progression (Stokes et al. 2007). The kinase DNA-PK, a PI3-type protein kinase in the same family as ATM and ATR, is directly involved in the repair of DNA double strand breaks through the process of NHEJ. However, each of these kinases can target additional substrates involved in growth and energy metabolism outside of canonical DNA repair and damage signaling pathways in response to growth factor stimulation. For example, DNA-PK is recruited by the upstream-stimulatory factor to the promoter of fatty acid synthase (FAS), the master regulator of fatty acid synthesis, upon insulin stimulation (Wong et al. 2009). DNA-PK is required for transient DNA breaks at the FAS promoter and transcription of FAS (Wong et al. 2009). ATM is required for phosphorylation of 4EBP1 on Ser 111 to promote protein anabolism upon insulin stimulation (Yang and Kastan 2000). This may be due indirectly to phosphorylation and inactivation of the mTOR repressor TSC2 by ATM (Alexander et al. 2010; Yang and Kastan 2000). ATM is also required for IGF-1 stimulated phosphorylation (activation) of AMPK, a cellular sensor of energy activated by low ATP/AMP ratios, to suppress energy-demanding processes such as cell growth in PANC and HeLa cells (Suzuki et al. 2004). ATM is also capable of inhibiting the stress signaling kinase JNK, whose activity is linked to several features of the metabolic syndrome (Schneider et al. 2006). Recently, ATM has been shown to be involved in the activation of autophagy through inhibition of mTOR (Alexander et al. 2010). DNA damage response proteins thus appear to be important regulators of cell growth and energy metabolism in response to environmental cues such as nutrient availability.

Importantly, there is mounting evidence that DDR proteins can also control these same metabolic pathways in response to DNA damage. One of the first clues was that ATM regulates expression of the IGF-1R in response to ionizing radiation (Peretz et al. 2001). Subsequent analysis of the ATM and ATR substrate pathway following ionizing radiation revealed several connections to the insulin-IGF-1-AKT pathway, including previously unidentified substrates insulin receptor substrate 2 (IRS2), AKT3 and its regulators HSP90 (heat shock protein 90) and PP2A (protein phosphatase 2A) (Matsuoka et al. 2007). Downstream targets of AKT including the transcription factor FOXO1, TSC1, S6K and 4E-BP1 were also identified as ATM and/or ATR substrates (Matsuoka et al. 2007). Cells lacking ATM demonstrate elevated mTOR and glycerophospholipid pathways when exposed to ionizing radiation (Varghese et al. 2010). Upon UV irradiation, DNA-PK is also required for translational reprogramming by directly or indirectly targeting the amino acid deprivation sensor GCN2 (Powley et al. 2009). The net outcome of this signal transduction cascade is to reduce general translation while at the same time to increase translation of proteins involved in adaptation to DNA damage, including NER proteins.

In addition to direct effects on cellular metabolism, activation of the DDR can trigger senescence-associated inflammatory cytokine secretion including IL-6 that can have an indirect effect on metabolism (Rodier et al. 2009). In 3T3-L1 adipocytes, for example, IL-6 inhibits phosphoenolpyruvate carboxykinase, which is required for triglyceride biosynthesis, thus increasing fatty acid mobilization (Feingold et al. 2011).

Another target of DNA damage-induced signal transduction is the tumor suppressor p53. p53 is normally a short-lived protein, but stabilization by phosphorylation promotes its activity as a transcriptional activator of cell-cycle inhibitors such as p21. p53 is stabilized as a result of multiple forms of stress, including genotoxic stress from ionizing radiation, ultraviolet radiation and ROS. In addition to cell cycle targets, p53 targets include genes involved directly in glycolysis (repression of phosphoglycerate mutase, (Kondoh et al. 2007)), and indirectly in respiration (activation of synthesis of cytochrome oxidase 2, a factor involved in COX assembly (Matoba et al. 2006)). In both cases, loss of p53 results in an increased glycolytic rate and decreased oxidative metabolism as is typically seen in cancer cells. TIGAR, another p53 target, is activated by low levels of stress and functions to repress glycolysis and to increase flux through the pentose phosphate pathway, resulting in increased generation of reduced glutathione, reduced ROS levels and protection from apoptosis (Bensaad et al. 2006). In some cells, glucose utilization by glycolysis competes with the pentose phosphate pathway responsible for generating NADPH reducing equivalents. Because NADPH is required for production of one of the major cellular antioxidants, reduced glutathione, increased glycolysis can come at the expense of increased, rather than decreased, ROS. However, it is worth pointing out that this may be cell-type specific, as in other cells reduced glycolysis results in increased apoptosis.

ATR may be the kinase responsible for phosphorylating and stabilizing p53 in response to genotoxic stress (Colman, Afshari, and Barrett 2000). ATR is recruited to stalled replication forks by the single strand DNA binding protein RPA and the ATR-interacting protein ATRIP. Single-stranded DNA regions serve as a platform for RPA-ATRIP-ATR recruitment in the context of stalled elongating replication machinery (Ljungman 2007). p53 can be also be stabilized even in the absence of DNA damage by inhibiting transcriptional elongation by RNA PolII (Bode and Dong 2004; Ljungman 2007). Thus, lesions that block an elongating RNA PolII and activate TC-NER can also signal through p53. Interestingly, the production of UV-induced DNA damage foci in quiescent fibroblasts requires ATR and is defective in primary cells from patients with Seckel syndrome (O'Driscoll et al. 2003).

In cells deficient in TC-NER, unrepaired UV-induced lesions cause downregulation of both the GHR and IGF-1R (Garinis et al. 2009). This is consistent with the finding in NER progeroid mice of reduced insulin/IGF-1 signaling (Niedernhofer et al. 2006; van der Pluijm et al. 2007; van de Ven et al. 2006), and suggests that this effect can be cell autonomous *in vivo* rather than driven primarily by neuronal or neuroendocrine control. Interestingly, downregulation of growth receptors upon UV treatment was not inhibited *in vitro* by inhibitors of AKT, MAPK or JAK, but whether it requires DDR signaling through ATM, ATR or DNA-PK is not reported (Garinis et al. 2009). The identity of the signaling pathway from the lesion to receptor downregulation is currently not known.

In addition to impacting cellular metabolism by activating signal transduction pathways, DNA damage repair pathways can also directly affect cellular energy status. PARP is activated upon oxidative base damage and consumes both ATP and NAD+ in the polyadenylation of various local substrates (Gagne et al. 2006), thus reducing available cellular energy currencies. Depending on the amount of damage and level of PARP activation, cellular energy stores can be depleted to pathological levels resulting in cell death. In the absence of exogenous DNA damage, PARP ablation results in increased NAD+ levels and increased activation of the NAD+-dependent deacetylase SIRT1, phenocopying aspects of SIRT1 deacetylase activation on mitochondrial metabolism (Bai et al. 2011). Thus, PARP provides a link between DNA damage and energy metabolism through direct effects on energy currencies as well as indirect effects of NAD+ and ATP dependent enzymes.

5. Conclusions

Cellular energy metabolism is a major source of ROS that can damage cellular components, including DNA. Oxidative DNA damage can in turn activate the DDR, a network of repair and signaling activities required for damage removal and stress adaptation. Inborn errors in DNA damage repair and signaling in human syndromes and mouse models typically display pathologies consistent with perturbation of growth and energy metabolism, including dwarfism and changes in insulin signaling and lipid accumulation. Interestingly, some disorders present with phenotypes reminiscent of the maladaptive response to nutrient/energy excess seen in metabolic syndrome. For example, in in A-T and Werner syndrome, these symptoms include dyslipidemia and insulin resistance. In other disorders, including mouse models of CS and TTD, symptoms appear on the opposite end of the nutrient/energy spectrum, with hypoglycemia, increased insulin sensitivity and reduced adiposity reminiscent of the beneficial adaptations to DR. Over time, however, chronic activation of adaptations such as reduced IGF-1 that may be beneficial in the context of a wildtype mammal on a restricted diet may in fact become maladaptive in the context of genome instability. For example, mouse models of severe NER progeria have reduced IGF-1, but nonetheless have shortened lifespans, while restoration of IGF-1 levels in a mouse model of HGPS ameliorates disease symptoms. On the cellular level, recent data suggest that proteins involved in the DNA damage response can exert both direct and indirect control over pathways involved in energy metabolism and substrate utilization, including insulin and IGF-1 signaling. Which of these genetic defects leads to constitutive alterations in metabolic processes and which to adaptive responses to genotoxic stress remains to be fully elucidated. Furthermore, to what degree unrepaired DNA damage itself serves as the trigger for metabolic changes, and the identity of the causative lesion, is in most cases unknown. In conclusion, despite recent emerging data on a connection between the DNA damage response and energy metabolism, there is a relative dearth of studies on cellular or organismal energy metabolism in the context of genome instability disorders, with much remaining to be done in this burgeoning field.

6. References

Al-Shali, K. Z., and R. A. Hegele. 2004. Laminopathies and atherosclerosis. *Arteriosclerosis, thrombosis, and vascular biology* 24 (9):1591-5.

Alexander, A., S. L. Cai, J. Kim, A. Nanez, M. Sahin, K. H. MacLean, K. Inoki, K. L. Guan, J. Shen, M. D. Person, D. Kusewitt, G. B. Mills, M. B. Kastan, and C. L. Walker. 2010. ATM signals to TSC2 in the cytoplasm to regulate mTORC1 in response to ROS. *Proceedings of the National Academy of Sciences of the United States of America* 107 (9):4153-8.

Allsopp, R. C., H. Vaziri, C. Patterson, S. Goldstein, E. V. Younglai, A. B. Futcher, C. W. Greider, and C. B. Harley. 1992. Telomere length predicts replicative capacity of human fibroblasts. *Proceedings of the National Academy of Sciences of the United States of America* 89 (21):10114-8.

Andressoo, J. O., J. H. Hoeijmakers, and J. R. Mitchell. 2006. Nucleotide excision repair disorders and the balance between cancer and aging. *Cell cycle* 5 (24):2886-8.

Andressoo, J. O., J. R. Mitchell, J. de Wit, D. Hoogstraten, M. Volker, W. Toussaint, E. Speksnijder, R. B. Beems, H. van Steeg, J. Jans, C. I. de Zeeuw, N. G. Jaspers, A. Raams, A. R. Lehmann, W. Vermeulen, J. H. Hoeijmakers, and G. T. van der Horst. 2006. An Xpd mouse model for the combined xeroderma pigmentosum/Cockayne syndrome exhibiting both cancer predisposition and segmental progeria. *Cancer cell* 10 (2):121-32.

Anindya, R., P. O. Mari, U. Kristensen, H. Kool, G. Giglia-Mari, L. H. Mullenders, M. Fousteri, W. Vermeulen, J. M. Egly, and J. Q. Svejstrup. 2010. A ubiquitin-binding domain in Cockayne syndrome B required for transcription-coupled nucleotide excision repair. *Molecular cell* 38 (5):637-48.

Armata, H. L., D. Golebiowski, D. Y. Jung, H. J. Ko, J. K. Kim, and H. K. Sluss. 2010. Requirement of the ATM/p53 tumor suppressor pathway for glucose homeostasis. *Mol Cell Biol* 30 (24):5787-94.

Bai, P., C. Canto, H. Oudart, A. Brunyanszki, Y. Cen, C. Thomas, H. Yamamoto, A. Huber, B. Kiss, R. H. Houtkooper, K. Schoonjans, V. Schreiber, A. A. Sauve, J. Menissier-de

Murcia, and J. Auwerx. 2011. PARP-1 Inhibition Increases Mitochondrial Metabolism through SIRT1 Activation. *Cell metabolism* 13 (4):461-8.

Barrett, S. F., J. H. Robbins, R. E. Tarone, and K. H. Kraemer. 1991. Evidence for defective repair of cyclobutane pyrimidine dimers with normal repair of other DNA photoproducts in a transcriptionally active gene transfected into Cockayne syndrome cells. *Mutation research* 255 (3):281-91.

Bartke, A., and H. Brown-Borg. 2004. Life extension in the dwarf mouse. *Curr Top Dev Biol* 63:189-225.

Beckman, K. B., and B. N. Ames. 1998. The free radical theory of aging matures. *Physiol Rev* 78 (2):547-81.

Bensaad, K., A. Tsuruta, M. A. Selak, M. N. Vidal, K. Nakano, R. Bartrons, E. Gottlieb, and K. H. Vousden. 2006. TIGAR, a p53-inducible regulator of glycolysis and apoptosis. *Cell* 126 (1):107-20.

Bode, A. M., and Z. Dong. 2004. Post-translational modification of p53 in tumorigenesis. *Nature reviews. Cancer* 4 (10):793-805.

Bradsher, J., J. Auriol, L. Proietti de Santis, S. Iben, J. L. Vonesch, I. Grummt, and J. M. Egly. 2002. CSB is a component of RNA pol I transcription. *Molecular cell* 10 (4):819-29.

Bridger, J. M., and I. R. Kill. 2004. Aging of Hutchinson-Gilford progeria syndrome fibroblasts is characterised by hyperproliferation and increased apoptosis. *Exp Gerontol* 39 (5):717-24.

Brooks, P. J. 2008. The 8,5'-cyclopurine-2'-deoxynucleosides: candidate neurodegenerative DNA lesions in xeroderma pigmentosum, and unique probes of transcription and nucleotide excision repair. *DNA repair* 7 (7):1168-79.

Brooks, P. J., T. F. Cheng, and L. Cooper. 2008. Do all of the neurologic diseases in patients with DNA repair gene mutations result from the accumulation of DNA damage? *DNA repair* 7 (6):834-48.

Brooks, P. J., D. S. Wise, D. A. Berry, J. V. Kosmoski, M. J. Smerdon, R. L. Somers, H. Mackie, A. Y. Spoonde, E. J. Ackerman, K. Coleman, R. E. Tarone, and J. H. Robbins. 2000. The oxidative DNA lesion 8,5'-(S)-cyclo-2'-deoxyadenosine is repaired by the nucleotide excision repair pathway and blocks gene expression in mammalian cells. *The Journal of biological chemistry* 275 (29):22355-62.

Chun, H. H., and R. A. Gatti. 2004. Ataxia-telangiectasia, an evolving phenotype. *DNA repair* 3 (8-9):1187-96.

Cockayne, E. A. 1936. Dwarfism with retinal atrophy and deafness. *Arch Dis Child* 11 (61):1-8.

Colman, M. S., C. A. Afshari, and J. C. Barrett. 2000. Regulation of p53 stability and activity in response to genotoxic stress. *Mutation research* 462 (2-3):179-88.

Compe, E., M. Malerba, L. Soler, J. Marescaux, E. Borrelli, and J. M. Egly. 2007. Neurological defects in trichothiodystrophy reveal a coactivator function of TFIIH. *Nature neuroscience* 10 (11):1414-22.

de Boer, J., J. de Wit, H. van Steeg, R. J. Berg, H. Morreau, P. Visser, A. R. Lehmann, M. Duran, J. H. Hoeijmakers, and G. Weeda. 1998. A mouse model for the basal transcription/DNA repair syndrome trichothiodystrophy. *Molecular cell* 1 (7):981-90.

De Bont, R., and N. van Larebeke. 2004. Endogenous DNA damage in humans: a review of quantitative data. *Mutagenesis* 19 (3):169-85.

Dizdaroglu, M., M. L. Dirksen, H. X. Jiang, and J. H. Robbins. 1987. Ionizing-radiation-induced damage in the DNA of cultured human cells. Identification of 8,5-cyclo-2-deoxyguanosine. *The Biochemical journal* 241 (3):929-32.

Dolle, M. E., R. A. Busuttil, A. M. Garcia, S. Wijnhoven, E. van Drunen, L. J. Niedernhofer, G. van der Horst, J. H. Hoeijmakers, H. van Steeg, and J. Vijg. 2006. Increased genomic instability is not a prerequisite for shortened lifespan in DNA repair deficient mice. *Mutat Res* 596 (1-2):22-35.

Ducos, B., S. Cabrol, M. Houang, L. Perin, M. Holzenberger, and Y. Le Bouc. 2001. IGF type 1 receptor ligand binding characteristics are altered in a subgroup of children with intrauterine growth retardation. *J Clin Endocrinol Metab* 86 (11):5516-24.

Espejel, S., M. Martin, P. Klatt, J. Martin-Caballero, J. M. Flores, and M. A. Blasco. 2004. Shorter telomeres, accelerated ageing and increased lymphoma in DNA-PKcs-deficient mice. *EMBO Rep* 5 (5):503-9.

Feingold, K. R., A. Moser, J. K. Shigenaga, and C. Grunfeld. 2011. Inflammation inhibits the expression of phosphoenolpyruvate carboxykinase in liver and adipose tissue. *Innate Immun*.

Fontana, L., and S. Klein. 2007. Aging, adiposity, and calorie restriction. *Jama* 297 (9):986-94.

Gagne, J. P., M. J. Hendzel, A. Droit, and G. G. Poirier. 2006. The expanding role of poly(ADP-ribose) metabolism: current challenges and new perspectives. *Curr Opin Cell Biol* 18 (2):145-51.

Garinis, G. A., L. M. Uittenboogaard, H. Stachelscheid, M. Fousteri, W. van Ijcken, T. M. Breit, H. van Steeg, L. H. Mullenders, G. T. van der Horst, J. C. Bruning, C. M. Niessen, J. H. Hoeijmakers, and B. Schumacher. 2009. Persistent transcription-blocking DNA lesions trigger somatic growth attenuation associated with longevity. *Nature cell biology* 11 (5):604-15.

Groisman, R., J. Polanowska, I. Kuraoka, J. Sawada, M. Saijo, R. Drapkin, A. F. Kisselev, K. Tanaka, and Y. Nakatani. 2003. The ubiquitin ligase activity in the DDB2 and CSA complexes is differentially regulated by the COP9 signalosome in response to DNA damage. *Cell* 113 (3):357-67.

Gu, Y., K. J. Seidl, G. A. Rathbun, C. Zhu, J. P. Manis, N. van der Stoep, L. Davidson, H. L. Cheng, J. M. Sekiguchi, K. Frank, P. Stanhope-Baker, M. S. Schlissel, D. B. Roth, and F. W. Alt. 1997. Growth retardation and leaky SCID phenotype of Ku70-deficient mice. *Immunity* 7 (5):653-65.

Holcomb, V. B., H. Vogel, and P. Hasty. 2007. Deletion of Ku80 causes early aging independent of chronic inflammation and Rag-1-induced DSBs. *Mechanisms of ageing and development* 128 (11-12):601-8.

Hotamisligil, G. S. 2006. Inflammation and metabolic disorders. *Nature* 444 (7121):860-7.

Huang, S., L. Lee, N. B. Hanson, C. Lenaerts, H. Hoehn, M. Poot, C. D. Rubin, D. F. Chen, C. C. Yang, H. Juch, T. Dorn, R. Spiegel, E. A. Oral, M. Abid, C. Battisti, E. Lucci-Cordisco, G. Neri, E. H. Steed, A. Kidd, W. Isley, D. Showalter, J. L. Vittone, A. Konstantinow, J. Ring, P. Meyer, S. L. Wenger, A. von Herbay, U. Wollina, M. Schuelke, C. R. Huizenga, D. F. Leistritz, G. M. Martin, I. S. Mian, and J. Oshima. 2006. The spectrum of WRN mutations in Werner syndrome patients. *Hum Mutat* 27 (6):558-67.

Jaruga, P., M. Birincioglu, T. A. Rosenquist, and M. Dizdaroglu. 2004. Mouse NEIL1 protein is specific for excision of 2,6-diamino-4-hydroxy-5-formamidopyrimidine and 4,6-diamino-5-formamidopyrimidine from oxidatively damaged DNA. *Biochemistry* 43 (50):15909-14.

Jaruga, P., J. Theruvathu, M. Dizdaroglu, and P. J. Brooks. 2004. Complete release of (5'S)-8,5'-cyclo-2'-deoxyadenosine from dinucleotides, oligodeoxynucleotides and DNA, and direct comparison of its levels in cellular DNA with other oxidatively induced DNA lesions. *Nucleic acids research* 32 (11):e87.

Keriel, A., A. Stary, A. Sarasin, C. Rochette-Egly, and J. M. Egly. 2002. XPD mutations prevent TFIIH-dependent transactivation by nuclear receptors and phosphorylation of RARalpha. *Cell* 109 (1):125-35.

Kohlschutter, A., A. Bley, K. Brockmann, J. Gartner, I. Krageloh-Mann, A. Rolfs, and L. Schols. 2010. Leukodystrophies and other genetic metabolic leukoencephalopathies in children and adults. *Brain Dev* 32 (2):82-9.

Kondoh, H., M. E. Lleonart, D. Bernard, and J. Gil. 2007. Protection from oxidative stress by enhanced glycolysis; a possible mechanism of cellular immortalization. *Histol Histopathol* 22 (1):85-90.

Kruman, II. 2004. Why do neurons enter the cell cycle? *Cell Cycle* 3 (6):769-73.

Kuraoka, I., C. Bender, A. Romieu, J. Cadet, R. D. Wood, and T. Lindahl. 2000. Removal of oxygen free-radical-induced 5',8-purine cyclodeoxynucleosides from DNA by the nucleotide excision-repair pathway in human cells. *Proceedings of the National Academy of Sciences of the United States of America* 97 (8):3832-7.

Lachapelle, S., S. Oesterreich, and M. Lebel. 2011. The Werner syndrome helicase protein is required for cell proliferation, immortalization, and tumorigenesis in Scaffold Attachment Factor B1 deficient mice. *Aging (Albany NY)* 3 (3):277-90.

Laposa, R. R., E. J. Huang, and J. E. Cleaver. 2007. Increased apoptosis, p53 up-regulation, and cerebellar neuronal degeneration in repair-deficient Cockayne syndrome mice. *Proceedings of the National Academy of Sciences of the United States of America* 104 (4):1389-94.

Lavin, M. F. 2000. An unlikely player joins the ATM signalling network. *Nature cell biology* 2 (12):E215-7.

Le May, N., J. M. Egly, and F. Coin. 2010. True lies: the double life of the nucleotide excision repair factors in transcription and DNA repair. *Journal of nucleic acids* 2010.

Lebel, M., L. Massip, C. Garand, and E. Thorin. 2010. Ascorbate improves metabolic abnormalities in Wrn mutant mice but not the free radical scavenger catechin. *Ann N Y Acad Sci* 1197:40-4.

Leverenz, J. B., C. E. Yu, and G. D. Schellenberg. 1998. Aging-associated neuropathology in Werner syndrome. *Acta Neuropathol* 96 (4):421-4.

Liu, B., J. Wang, K. M. Chan, W. M. Tjia, W. Deng, X. Guan, J. D. Huang, K. M. Li, P. Y. Chau, D. J. Chen, D. Pei, A. M. Pendas, J. Cadinanos, C. Lopez-Otin, H. F. Tse, C. Hutchison, J. Chen, Y. Cao, K. S. Cheah, K. Tryggvason, and Z. Zhou. 2005. Genomic instability in laminopathy-based premature aging. *Nature medicine* 11 (7):780-5.

Ljungman, M. 2007. The transcription stress response. *Cell Cycle* 6 (18):2252-7.

Lodish, H., ed. 2000. *Molecular Cell Biology*. 4 ed. New York: W.H. Freeman and Company.

Lombard, D. B. 2009. Sirtuins at the breaking point: SIRT6 in DNA repair. *Aging (Albany NY)* 1 (1):12-6.

Longo, V. D., and C. E. Finch. 2003. Evolutionary medicine: from dwarf model systems to healthy centenarians? *Science* 299 (5611):1342-6.

Marino, G., A. P. Ugalde, A. F. Fernandez, F. G. Osorio, A. Fueyo, J. M. Freije, and C. Lopez-Otin. 2010. Insulin-like growth factor 1 treatment extends longevity in a mouse model of human premature aging by restoring somatotroph axis function.

Proceedings of the National Academy of Sciences of the United States of America 107 (37):16268-73.

Marino, G., A. P. Ugalde, N. Salvador-Montoliu, I. Varela, P. M. Quiros, J. Cadinanos, I. van der Pluijm, J. M. Freije, and C. Lopez-Otin. 2008. Premature aging in mice activates a systemic metabolic response involving autophagy induction. *Human molecular genetics* 17 (14):2196-211.

Martin, G. M. 1985. Genetics and aging; the Werner syndrome as a segmental progeroid syndrome. *Adv Exp Med Biol* 190:161-70.

Matoba, S., J. G. Kang, W. D. Patino, A. Wragg, M. Boehm, O. Gavrilova, P. J. Hurley, F. Bunz, and P. M. Hwang. 2006. p53 regulates mitochondrial respiration. *Science* 312 (5780):1650-3.

Matsuoka, S., B. A. Ballif, A. Smogorzewska, E. R. McDonald, 3rd, K. E. Hurov, J. Luo, C. E. Bakalarski, Z. Zhao, N. Solimini, Y. Lerenthal, Y. Shiloh, S. P. Gygi, and S. J. Elledge. 2007. ATM and ATR substrate analysis reveals extensive protein networks responsive to DNA damage. *Science* 316 (5828):1160-6.

McCay, C.M., M.F. Crowel, and L.A. Maynard. 1935. The effect of retarded growth upon the length of the life span and upon the ultimate body size. *J Nutr* 10:63-79.

McCord, R. A., E. Michishita, T. Hong, E. Berber, L. D. Boxer, R. Kusumoto, S. Guan, X. Shi, O. Gozani, A. L. Burlingame, V. A. Bohr, and K. F. Chua. 2009. SIRT6 stabilizes DNA-dependent protein kinase at chromatin for DNA double-strand break repair. *Aging (Albany NY)* 1 (1):109-21.

Melton, D. W., A. M. Ketchen, F. Nunez, S. Bonatti-Abbondandolo, A. Abbondandolo, S. Squires, and R. T. Johnson. 1998. Cells from ERCC1-deficient mice show increased genome instability and a reduced frequency of S-phase-dependent illegitimate chromosome exchange but a normal frequency of homologous recombination. *J Cell Sci* 111 (Pt 3):395-404.

Mercer, J. R., K. K. Cheng, N. Figg, I. Gorenne, M. Mahmoudi, J. Griffin, A. Vidal-Puig, A. Logan, M. P. Murphy, and M. Bennett. 2010. DNA damage links mitochondrial dysfunction to atherosclerosis and the metabolic syndrome. *Circulation research* 107 (8):1021-31.

Merideth, M. A., L. B. Gordon, S. Clauss, V. Sachdev, A. C. Smith, M. B. Perry, C. C. Brewer, C. Zalewski, H. J. Kim, B. Solomon, B. P. Brooks, L. H. Gerber, M. L. Turner, D. L. Domingo, T. C. Hart, J. Graf, J. C. Reynolds, A. Gropman, J. A. Yanovski, M. Gerhard-Herman, F. S. Collins, E. G. Nabel, R. O. Cannon, 3rd, W. A. Gahl, and W. J. Introne. 2008. Phenotype and course of Hutchinson-Gilford progeria syndrome. *N Engl J Med* 358 (6):592-604.

Miles, P. D., K. Treuner, M. Latronica, J. M. Olefsky, and C. Barlow. 2007. Impaired insulin secretion in a mouse model of ataxia telangiectasia. *Am J Physiol Endocrinol Metab* 293 (1):E70-4.

Minamino, T., M. Orimo, I. Shimizu, T. Kunieda, M. Yokoyama, T. Ito, A. Nojima, A. Nabetani, Y. Oike, H. Matsubara, F. Ishikawa, and I. Komuro. 2009. A crucial role for adipose tissue p53 in the regulation of insulin resistance. *Nature medicine* 15 (9):1082-7.

Mitchell, J. R., M. Verweij, K. Brand, M. van de Ven, N. Goemaere, S. van den Engel, T. Chu, F. Forrer, C. Muller, M. de Jong, W. van Ijcken, J. N. Ijzermans, J. H. Hoeijmakers, and R. W. de Bruin. 2009. Short-term dietary restriction and fasting precondition against ischemia reperfusion injury in mice. *Aging Cell.*

Monnat, R. J., Jr. 2010. Human RECQ helicases: roles in DNA metabolism, mutagenesis and cancer biology. *Semin Cancer Biol* 20 (5):329-39.

Morice-Picard, F., M. Cario-Andre, H. Rezvani, D. Lacombe, A. Sarasin, and A. Taieb. 2009. New clinico-genetic classification of trichothiodystrophy. *Am J Med Genet A* 149A (9):2020-30.

Mostoslavsky, R., K. F. Chua, D. B. Lombard, W. W. Pang, M. R. Fischer, L. Gellon, P. Liu, G. Mostoslavsky, S. Franco, M. M. Murphy, K. D. Mills, P. Patel, J. T. Hsu, A. L. Hong, E. Ford, H. L. Cheng, C. Kennedy, N. Nunez, R. Bronson, D. Frendewey, W. Auerbach, D. Valenzuela, M. Karow, M. O. Hottiger, S. Hursting, J. C. Barrett, L. Guarente, R. Mulligan, B. Demple, G. D. Yancopoulos, and F. W. Alt. 2006. Genomic instability and aging-like phenotype in the absence of mammalian SIRT6. *Cell* 124 (2):315-29.

Murai, M., Y. Enokido, N. Inamura, M. Yoshino, Y. Nakatsu, G. T. van der Horst, J. H. Hoeijmakers, K. Tanaka, and H. Hatanaka. 2001. Early postnatal ataxia and abnormal cerebellar development in mice lacking Xeroderma pigmentosum Group A and Cockayne syndrome Group B DNA repair genes. *Proceedings of the National Academy of Sciences of the United States of America* 98 (23):13379-84.

Nance, M. A., and S. A. Berry. 1992. Cockayne syndrome: review of 140 cases. *Am J Med Genet* 42 (1):68-84.

Nevedomskaya, E., A. Meissner, S. Goraler, M. de Waard, Y. Ridwan, G. Zondag, I. van der Pluijm, A. M. Deelder, and O. A. Mayboroda. 2010. Metabolic profiling of accelerated aging ERCC1 d/- mice. *J Proteome Res* 9 (7):3680-7.

Niedernhofer, L. J., G. A. Garinis, A. Raams, A. S. Lalai, A. R. Robinson, E. Appeldoorn, H. Odijk, R. Oostendorp, A. Ahmad, W. van Leeuwen, A. F. Theil, W. Vermeulen, G. T. van der Horst, P. Meinecke, W. J. Kleijer, J. Vijg, N. G. Jaspers, and J. H. Hoeijmakers. 2006. A new progeroid syndrome reveals that genotoxic stress suppresses the somatotroph axis. *Nature* 444 (7122):1038-43.

O'Driscoll, M., and P. A. Jeggo. 2008. The role of the DNA damage response pathways in brain development and microcephaly: insight from human disorders. *DNA repair* 7 (7):1039-50.

O'Driscoll, M., V. L. Ruiz-Perez, C. G. Woods, P. A. Jeggo, and J. A. Goodship. 2003. A splicing mutation affecting expression of ataxia-telangiectasia and Rad3-related protein (ATR) results in Seckel syndrome. *Nat Genet* 33 (4):497-501.

Ozdirim, E., M. Topcu, A. Ozon, and A. Cila. 1996. Cockayne syndrome: review of 25 cases. *Pediatr Neurol* 15 (4):312-6.

Pasquier, L., V. Laugel, L. Lazaro, H. Dollfus, H. Journel, P. Edery, A. Goldenberg, D. Martin, D. Heron, M. Le Merrer, P. Rustin, S. Odent, A. Munnich, A. Sarasin, and V. Cormier-Daire. 2006. Wide clinical variability among 13 new Cockayne syndrome cases confirmed by biochemical assays. *Arch Dis Child* 91 (2):178-82.

Pendas, A. M., Z. Zhou, J. Cadinanos, J. M. Freije, J. Wang, K. Hultenby, A. Astudillo, A. Wernerson, F. Rodriguez, K. Tryggvason, and C. Lopez-Otin. 2002. Defective prelamin A processing and muscular and adipocyte alterations in Zmpste24 metalloproteinase-deficient mice. *Nat Genet* 31 (1):94-9.

Peretz, S., R. Jensen, R. Baserga, and P. M. Glazer. 2001. ATM-dependent expression of the insulin-like growth factor-I receptor in a pathway regulating radiation response. *Proceedings of the National Academy of Sciences of the United States of America* 98 (4):1676-81.

Powley, I. R., A. Kondrashov, L. A. Young, H. C. Dobbyn, K. Hill, I. G. Cannell, M. Stoneley, Y. W. Kong, J. A. Cotes, G. C. Smith, R. Wek, C. Hayes, T. W. Gant, K. A. Spriggs, M. Bushell, and A. E. Willis. 2009. Translational reprogramming following UVB irradiation is mediated by DNA-PKcs and allows selective recruitment to the polysomes of mRNAs encoding DNA repair enzymes. *Genes & development* 23 (10):1207-20.

Randle, P. J., P. B. Garland, C. N. Hales, and E. A. Newsholme. 1963. The glucose fatty-acid cycle. Its role in insulin sensitivity and the metabolic disturbances of diabetes mellitus. *Lancet* 1 (7285):785-9.

Rapin, I., K. Weidenheim, Y. Lindenbaum, P. Rosenbaum, S. N. Merchant, S. Krishna, and D. W. Dickson. 2006. Cockayne syndrome in adults: review with clinical and pathologic study of a new case. *J Child Neurol* 21 (11):991-1006.

Rincon, M., R. Muzumdar, G. Atzmon, and N. Barzilai. 2004. The paradox of the insulin/IGF-1 signaling pathway in longevity. *Mechanisms of ageing and development* 125 (6):397-403.

Rodier, F., J. P. Coppe, C. K. Patil, W. A. Hoeijmakers, D. P. Munoz, S. R. Raza, A. Freund, E. Campeau, A. R. Davalos, and J. Campisi. 2009. Persistent DNA damage signalling triggers senescence-associated inflammatory cytokine secretion. *Nature cell biology* 11 (8):973-9.

Roy, L. M., P. Jaruga, T. G. Wood, A. K. McCullough, M. Dizdaroglu, and R. S. Lloyd. 2007. Human polymorphic variants of the NEIL1 DNA glycosylase. *The Journal of biological chemistry* 282 (21):15790-8.

Sampath, H., A. K. Batra, V. Vartanian, J. R. Carmical, D. Prusak, I. B. King, B. Lowell, L. F. Earley, T. G. Wood, D. L. Marks, A. K. McCullough, and R. Stephen L. 2011. Variable penetrance of metabolic phenotypes and development of high-fat diet-induced adiposity in NEIL1-deficient mice. *Am J Physiol Endocrinol Metab* 300 (4):E724-34.

Schmidt, A., A. Chakravarty, E. Brommer, B. D. Fenne, T. Siebler, P. De Meyts, and W. Kiess. 2002. Growth failure in a child showing characteristics of Seckel syndrome: possible effects of IGF-I and endogenous IGFBP-3. *Clin Endocrinol (Oxf)* 57 (2):293-9.

Schneider, J. G., B. N. Finck, J. Ren, K. N. Standley, M. Takagi, K. H. Maclean, C. Bernal-Mizrachi, A. J. Muslin, M. B. Kastan, and C. F. Semenkovich. 2006. ATM-dependent suppression of stress signaling reduces vascular disease in metabolic syndrome. *Cell metabolism* 4 (5):377-89.

Schumacher, B., I. van der Pluijm, M. J. Moorhouse, T. Kosteas, A. R. Robinson, Y. Suh, T. M. Breit, H. van Steeg, L. J. Niedernhofer, W. van Ijcken, A. Bartke, S. R. Spindler, J. H. Hoeijmakers, G. T. van der Horst, and G. A. Garinis. 2008. Delayed and accelerated aging share common longevity assurance mechanisms. *PLoS Genet* 4 (8):e1000161.

Schwer, B., B. Schumacher, D. B. Lombard, C. Xiao, M. V. Kurtev, J. Gao, J. I. Schneider, H. Chai, R. T. Bronson, L. H. Tsai, C. X. Deng, and F. W. Alt. 2010. Neural sirtuin 6 (Sirt6) ablation attenuates somatic growth and causes obesity. *Proceedings of the National Academy of Sciences of the United States of America* 107 (50):21790-4.

Shackelford, R. E. 2005. Pharmacologic manipulation of the ataxia-telangiectasia mutated gene product as an intervention in age-related disease. *Med Hypotheses* 65 (2):363-9.

Stokes, M. P., J. Rush, J. Macneill, J. M. Ren, K. Sprott, J. Nardone, V. Yang, S. A. Beausoleil, S. P. Gygi, H. Livingstone, H. Zhang, R. D. Polakiewicz, and M. J. Comb. 2007. Profiling of UV-induced ATM/ATR signaling pathways. *Proceedings of the National Academy of Sciences of the United States of America* 104 (50):19855-60.

Sun, X. Z., Y. N. Harada, R. Zhang, C. Cui, S. Takahashi, and Y. Fukui. 2003. A genetic mouse model carrying the nonfunctional xeroderma pigmentosum group G gene. *Congenit Anom (Kyoto)* 43 (2):133-9.

Susa, D., J. R. Mitchell, M. Verweij, M. van de Ven, H. Roest, S. van den Engel, I. Bajema, K. Mangundap, J. N. Ijzermans, J. H. Hoeijmakers, and R. W. de Bruin. 2009. Congenital DNA repair deficiency results in protection against renal ischemia reperfusion injury in mice. *Aging Cell* 8 (2):192-200.

Suzuki, A., G. Kusakai, A. Kishimoto, Y. Shimojo, T. Ogura, M. F. Lavin, and H. Esumi. 2004. IGF-1 phosphorylates AMPK-alpha subunit in ATM-dependent and LKB1-independent manner. *Biochemical and biophysical research communications* 324 (3):986-92.

Tian, M., R. Shinkura, N. Shinkura, and F. W. Alt. 2004. Growth retardation, early death, and DNA repair defects in mice deficient for the nucleotide excision repair enzyme XPF. *Mol Cell Biol* 24 (3):1200-5.

Tieu, K., C. Perier, C. Caspersen, P. Teismann, D. C. Wu, S. D. Yan, A. Naini, M. Vila, V. Jackson-Lewis, R. Ramasamy, and S. Przedborski. 2003. D-beta-hydroxybutyrate rescues mitochondrial respiration and mitigates features of Parkinson disease. *The Journal of clinical investigation* 112 (6):892-901.

Tyner, S. D., S. Venkatachalam, J. Choi, S. Jones, N. Ghebranious, H. Igelmann, X. Lu, G. Soron, B. Cooper, C. Brayton, S. Hee Park, T. Thompson, G. Karsenty, A. Bradley, and L. A. Donehower. 2002. p53 mutant mice that display early ageing-associated phenotypes. *Nature* 415 (6867):45-53.

Umehara, F., M. Abe, M. Nakagawa, S. Izumo, K. Arimura, K. Matsumuro, and M. Osame. 1993. Werner's syndrome associated with spastic paraparesis and peripheral neuropathy. *Neurology* 43 (6):1252-4.

van de Ven, M., J. O. Andressoo, V. B. Holcomb, P. Hasty, Y. Suh, H. van Steeg, G. A. Garinis, J. H. Hoeijmakers, and J. R. Mitchell. 2007. Extended longevity mechanisms in short-lived progeroid mice: identification of a preservative stress response associated with successful aging. *Mechanisms of ageing and development* 128 (1):58-63.

van de Ven, M., J. O. Andressoo, V. B. Holcomb, M. von Lindern, W. M. Jong, C. I. De Zeeuw, Y. Suh, P. Hasty, J. H. Hoeijmakers, G. T. van der Horst, and J. R. Mitchell. 2006. Adaptive stress response in segmental progeria resembles long-lived dwarfism and calorie restriction in mice. *PLoS Genet* 2 (12):e192.

van de Ven, Marieke, Jaan-Olle Andressoo, Valerie B. Holcomb, Marieke von Lindern, Willeke Jong, Chris I. De Zeeuw, Yousin Suh, Paul Hasty, Jan H. J. Hoeijmakers, Gijsbertus T. J. van der Horst, and James R. Mitchell. 2006. Adaptive stress response in segmental progeria resembles long-lived dwarfism and calorie restriction in mice. *PLoS Genetics* preprint (2006):e192.

van der Horst, G. T., L. Meira, T. G. Gorgels, J. de Wit, S. Velasco-Miguel, J. A. Richardson, Y. Kamp, M. P. Vreeswijk, B. Smit, D. Bootsma, J. H. Hoeijmakers, and E. C. Friedberg. 2002. UVB radiation-induced cancer predisposition in Cockayne syndrome group A (Csa) mutant mice. *DNA repair* 1 (2):143-57.

van der Horst, G. T., H. van Steeg, R. J. Berg, A. J. van Gool, J. de Wit, G. Weeda, H. Morreau, R. B. Beems, C. F. van Kreijl, F. R. de Gruijl, D. Bootsma, and J. H. Hoeijmakers. 1997. Defective transcription-coupled repair in Cockayne syndrome B mice is associated with skin cancer predisposition. *Cell* 89 (3):425-35.

van der Pluijm, I., G. A. Garinis, R. M. Brandt, T. G. Gorgels, S. W. Wijnhoven, K. E. Diderich, J. de Wit, J. R. Mitchell, C. van Oostrom, R. Beems, L. J. Niedernhofer, S.

Velasco, E. C. Friedberg, K. Tanaka, H. van Steeg, J. H. Hoeijmakers, and G. T. van der Horst. 2007. Impaired genome maintenance suppresses the growth hormone--insulin-like growth factor 1 axis in mice with Cockayne syndrome. *PLoS biology* 5 (1):e2.

Varela, I., J. Cadinanos, A. M. Pendas, A. Gutierrez-Fernandez, A. R. Folgueras, L. M. Sanchez, Z. Zhou, F. J. Rodriguez, C. L. Stewart, J. A. Vega, K. Tryggvason, J. M. Freije, and C. Lopez-Otin. 2005. Accelerated ageing in mice deficient in Zmpste24 protease is linked to p53 signalling activation. *Nature* 437 (7058):564-8.

Varghese, R. S., A. Cheema, P. Cheema, M. Bourbeau, L. Tuli, B. Zhou, M. Jung, A. Dritschilo, and H. W. Ressom. 2010. Analysis of LC-MS data for characterizing the metabolic changes in response to radiation. *J Proteome Res* 9 (5):2786-93.

Vartanian, V., B. Lowell, I. G. Minko, T. G. Wood, J. D. Ceci, S. George, S. W. Ballinger, C. L. Corless, A. K. McCullough, and R. S. Lloyd. 2006. The metabolic syndrome resulting from a knockout of the NEIL1 DNA glycosylase. *Proceedings of the National Academy of Sciences of the United States of America* 103 (6):1864-9.

Verstraeten, V. L., J. L. Broers, F. C. Ramaekers, and M. A. van Steensel. 2007. The nuclear envelope, a key structure in cellular integrity and gene expression. *Curr Med Chem* 14 (11):1231-48.

Vogel, H., D. S. Lim, G. Karsenty, M. Finegold, and P. Hasty. 1999. Deletion of Ku86 causes early onset of senescence in mice. *Proc Natl Acad Sci U S A* 96 (19):10770-5.

Weeda, G., I. Donker, J. de Wit, H. Morreau, R. Janssens, C. J. Vissers, A. Nigg, H. van Steeg, D. Bootsma, and J. H. J. Hoeijmakers. 1997. Disruption of mouse ERCC1 results in a novel repair syndrome with growth failure, nuclear abnormalities and senescence. *Curr Biol* 7 (6):427-39.

Weidenheim, K. M., D. W. Dickson, and I. Rapin. 2009. Neuropathology of Cockayne syndrome: Evidence for impaired development, premature aging, and neurodegeneration. *Mechanisms of ageing and development* 130 (9):619-36.

Wijnhoven, S. W., R. B. Beems, M. Roodbergen, J. van den Berg, P. H. Lohman, K. Diderich, G. T. van der Horst, J. Vijg, J. H. Hoeijmakers, and H. van Steeg. 2005. Accelerated aging pathology in ad libitum fed Xpd(TTD) mice is accompanied by features suggestive of caloric restriction. *DNA repair* 4 (11):1314-24.

Wong, H. K., M. Muftuoglu, G. Beck, S. Z. Imam, V. A. Bohr, and D. M. Wilson, 3rd. 2007. Cockayne syndrome B protein stimulates apurinic endonuclease 1 activity and protects against agents that introduce base excision repair intermediates. *Nucleic acids research* 35 (12):4103-13.

Wong, R. H., I. Chang, C. S. Hudak, S. Hyun, H. Y. Kwan, and H. S. Sul. 2009. A role of DNA-PK for the metabolic gene regulation in response to insulin. *Cell* 136 (6):1056-72.

Yang, D. Q., and M. B. Kastan. 2000. Participation of ATM in insulin signalling through phosphorylation of eIF-4E-binding protein 1. *Nature cell biology* 2 (12):893-8.

Zhang, X. D., Z. H. Qin, and J. Wang. 2010. The role of p53 in cell metabolism. *Acta Pharmacol Sin* 31 (9):1208-12.

Zhong, L., A. D'Urso, D. Toiber, C. Sebastian, R. E. Henry, D. D. Vadysirisack, A. Guimaraes, B. Marinelli, J. D. Wikstrom, T. Nir, C. B. Clish, B. Vaitheesvaran, O. Iliopoulos, I. Kurland, Y. Dor, R. Weissleder, O. S. Shirihai, L. W. Ellisen, J. M. Espinosa, and R. Mostoslavsky. 2010. The histone deacetylase Sirt6 regulates glucose homeostasis via Hif1alpha. *Cell* 140 (2):280-93.

4

DNA Damage and mRNA Levels of DNA Base Excision Repair Enzymes Following H$_2$O$_2$ Challenge at Different Temperatures

Kyungmi Min and Susan E. Ebeler

Department of Viticulture & Enology, University of California, Davis
USA

1. Introduction

Our cells are continuously exposed to endogenous and exogenous oxidizing agents that can damage DNA leading to disruption of transcription, translation, and DNA replication (Davies, 2000). Accordingly, protective mechanisms, including the presence of cellular antioxidants and induction of enzymatic repair of damaged lesions, are necessary in order to survive in this oxidizing environment. When damaged DNA lesions are not prevented or properly repaired, they can cause mutations that increase the risk of degenerative diseases.

The baseline level of oxidative damage associated with normal cellular processes has been estimated as high as 1 base modification per 130,000 bases in nuclear DNA (Davies, 2000). However, high levels of reactive oxygen species (ROS) result in an increase in modified DNA levels. Overall more than 20 modified DNA base lesions have been identified, including 8-oxoguanine which is the most abundant DNA adduct (Cooke et al., 2003). In addition, ROS can attack DNA, generating strand breaks, sugar damage and DNA-protein cross-links. A single strand break (SSB) is a discontinuity in the sugar-phosphate backbone of one strand of a DNA duplex leaving modified ends which inhibit or block DNA polymerases and DNA ligases (Caldecott, 2001). SSBs can be produced directly from ROS attack, indirectly from DNA repair processes, by direct disintegration of deoxyribose, or by abortive DNA topoisomerase 1 activity (Dianov & Parsons, 2007; Leppard & Campoux, 2005).

DNA repair mechanisms to maintain the genomic integrity have been described. DNA base lesions and single strand breaks resulting from ROS-induced oxidative attack are mainly repaired through the base excision repair (BER) pathway (reviewed in (Caldecott, 2003; de Murcia & Menissier de Murcia, 1994; Dianov & Parsons, 2007; Wilson, 2007)). In order to repair DNA base lesions, BER is initiated by specific DNA glycosylases. For example, human 8-oxoguanine DNA-glycosylase 1 (hOGG1), a bifunctional glycosylase, recognizes and cleaves 8-oxoguanine and also catalyzes 3' of the abasic site (AP site). Following this initiation step, AP-endonuclease I (APE1) cleaves the AP site making a gap between the DNA 3'-OH and the 5'-phosphate. The SSBs, produced either directly from ROS attack or indirectly from DNA repair processes, can then be recognized by the enzyme poly (ADP-ribose) polymerase-1 (PARP1). Binding of PARP-1 to the AP sites stimulates the formation of poly (ADP-ribose) polymers and dissociation of PARP-1 from the DNA-recruiting BER proteins at the damage site. DNA polymerase β fills the gap by DNA synthesis. Finally the resulting nick is sealed by DNA ligase, completing the short-patch repair pathway. In this pathway X-ray cross-complementing 1 (XRCC1) plays a major role in facilitating the interaction among the proteins involved in the BER pathway such as APE1, DNA polymerase β and DNA ligase III (Caldecott, 2003). Depending on the nature of AP sites, some AP sites are repaired by the long-patch repair pathway requiring different enzymes including flap endonuclease and DNA ligase I. Even though the basic DNA repair mechanisms are well described, recent evidence suggests that DNA repair mechanisms are quite complicated with more than 100 proteins involved in the repair of various lesions (Wood et al., 2001).

Deficiencies in DNA repair systems have been shown in several types of cancer (Langland et al., 2002; Lynch & Smyrk, 1996; Marchetto et al., 2004). However, whether such deficiencies in DNA repair enzymes are associated with single nucleotide polymorphisms (SNPs) is still arguable.

Several studies have examined the DNA repair capacity of different cells upon exposure to environmental agents such as oxidants or antioxidants (Astley et al., 2002; Collins et al., 1995, 2003; Torbergsen & Collins, 2000). Most studies have either only monitored DNA damage or determined the mRNA expression levels of DNA repair enzymes, mostly hOGG1, in order to elucidate the role of oxidants or antioxidants on DNA repair activity. However, monitoring only DNA damage for DNA repair kinetics reflects more global effects instead of specific aspects of repair (Berwick & Vineis, 2000). In addition, the exact relationships between oxidative stress, DNA damage and induction of the mRNA expression levels of repair enzymes including hOGG1 is unclear (Hodges & Chipman, 2002; Kim et al., 2001) although hOGG1 has been shown to be inducible responding to various oxidative conditions (Kim et al., 2001; Lan et al., 2003).

As these previous studies indicate, multiple methods and markers of DNA damage and repair may be needed in order to explain molecular responses to DNA damaging agents. Furthermore, information is still lacking about the rate of DNA repair immediately following treatment with oxidants or antioxidants; this information may be important in determining steady-state damage levels following induction of oxidative stress (Collins & Harrington, 2002). Therefore the current study was undertaken to better understand the relationship between cellular DNA damage and induction of mRNA expression of repair enzymes following acute oxidant treatment using Caco-2 cells (human colon cancer cells). Oxidant (H_2O_2) treated cells were monitored over an extended recovery period, and both DNA damage levels and mRNA levels of several DNA BER enzymes (hOGG1, APE1, PARP1, XRCC1) were quantified over time in order to better understand DNA repair kinetics and the molecular responses to an oxidative DNA damaging agent.

2. Materials and methods

2.1 Chemicals and reagents

Caco-2 cells were generously donated by Dr. Bo Lonnerdal (University of California, Davis). Hydrogen peroxide, penicillin and streptomycin were purchased from Sigma-Aldrich (St. Louis, MO). Minimum essential medium (MEM) with Earl's salts, including 1-glutamine and 0.25% trypsin-EDTA solution, were from Gibco (Invitrogen, Carlsbad, CA). Fetal bovine serum was obtained from Gemini (West Sacramento, CA). For the single cell gel electrophoresis assay, a commercial kit was purchased from Trevigen Co. (Gaithersburg, MD). For real time PCR, reverse transcription kits and SYBR Green PCR master mix were purchased from Applied Biosystems (Foster City, CA) and Roche (Mannheim, Germany), respectively.

2.2 Cell culture and treatments

Caco-2 cells were grown in MEM, supplemented with 10% (v/v) fetal bovine serum, L-glutamine, 1% penicillin and streptomycin (10 units/mL and 1 mg/mL respectively) at 37°C in a humidified environment composed of 5% CO$_2$ and 95% air; the growing medium was changed every two days. Cells were subcultured at 80-90% confluency. After seeding onto a 100 mm cell culture plate with a density of 5×10^6 cells/plate, cells were grown for one day and treated with fresh hydrogen peroxide (100 µM) for 30 min at 37°C, a physiologically relevant temperature, or for 10 min at 4°C, a condition where DNA repair should be minimized. After washing with phosphate buffered saline (PBS), cells were incubated in growing medium (including serum) at 37°C for up to 5 h. For the cells treated with oxidant at 37°C, they were further incubated for 8 hours in order to confirm the mRNA expression pattern of some DNA repair genes. Some cells were collected for comet assay and the others were collected for RNA extraction. Each experimental treatment was performed in duplicate on 3 different days.

2.3 Measurement of DNA damage

After incubation in growing medium for 0-5 h, cells were harvested with trypsin-EDTA solution, washed twice with ice-cold PBS, and cell viability was determined with the trypan blue exclusion test. The single cell gel electrophoresis (comet assay) procedure was based on methods of Singh et al. with slight modifications (Singh et al., 1988). A commercial comet assay kit was used to measure strand breaks following the manufacturer's protocols. Briefly, cells were diluted with PBS in order to have a cell density of 1× 10^5 cells/mL and embedded into low melting point agarose on comet slides. Embedded cells were lysed in lysis solution (including 1% sodium lauryl sarcosinate) for 1 hour and unwound in alkaline solution (300 mM NaOH, 1 mM EDTA, pH > 13). Subsequently, electrophoresis was performed for 30 min at 300 mA. Cells were neutralized by washing with water, dried following immersion in ethanol, and kept at room temperature in the dark until silver staining. Silver stained cells were imaged using a Nikon E600 with a Leica LEI-750 camera.

Images were analyzed by measuring % tail DNA of each cell using CometScore software (version 1.5, www.autocomet.com). Cells (75 total) were collected from 2 slides per treatment and the whole procedure for DNA damage measurement was repeated three times independently. Slides were coded and counted blindly; after imaging and counting, slides were decoded in order to quantify differences among samples.

2.4 Measurement of expression of DNA repair enzymes
2.4.1 Total RNA extraction

Total RNA was extracted from Caco-2 cells using Trizol (Invitrogen, Grand Island, NY) according to the manufacturer's instructions. The concentrations of extracted RNA were determined using a NanoDrop spectrophotometer (NanoDrop Technologies, Wilmington,

DE) with the quality of RNA determined from the absorbance ratio of $A_{260}/A_{280} > 1.8$ and confirmed by gel electrophoresis. Extracted RNA was preserved at -80°C until used. cDNA was synthesized using 5 μg total RNA, oligo $d(T)_{16}$ primers, and MultiScribe Reverse Transcriptase (Applied Biosystems, Foster City, CA). Reverse transcription was performed by following the manufacturer's protocol.

2.4.2 Real-time quantitative RT-PCR (qRT-PCR)

In order to detect DNA repair enzyme genes (hOGG1, APE1, PARP1 and XRCC1) and β-actin (used as a reference gene), qRT-PCR was performed using SYBR Green PCR Master Mix reagents (Roche, Mannheim, Germany) on a PRISM 7700 Sequence Detection System (Applied Biosystems, Foster City, CA). Specific primers for each gene are shown in Table1. Real time quantitative RT-PCR (real time qRT-PCR) was performed through the amplification for 40 cycles of 95°C (30 sec), 58°C (30 sec) and 60°C (1 min) after activation of enzyme at 95°C (10 min). The data were normalized using β-actin as an internal standard. Relative fold changes were calculated using the formula of $2^{-\Delta\Delta Ct}$ by comparing mRNA levels to the control. Triplicate qRT-PCR analyses were run for each sample.

Primers		Sequences (5′→ 3′)	Size (bp)	References
β-actin	Forward	TCACCCAACACTGTGCCCATCTACGA	180	Mambo et al., 2005
	Reverse	TCGGTGAGGATCTTCATGAGGTA		
hOGG1	Forward	GCGACTGCTGCGACAAGAC	250	Chevillard et al., 1998
	Reverse	TCGGGCACTGGCACTCAC		
APE1	Forward	GAG TAA GAC GGC CGC AAA GAA AAA	296	Collins et al., 2003
	Reverse	CCG AAG GAG CTG ACC AGT ATT GAT		
PARP1	Forward	CAA CTT TGC TGG GAT CCT GT	185	Mayer et al., 2002
	Reverse	TGT TTC CAA GGG CAA CTT CT		
XRCC1	Forward	CGC TGG GGA GCA AGA CTA TG	517	Noe et al., 2004
	Reverse	CAA ATC CAA CTT CCT CTT CC′		

Table 1. Primers of DNA repair enzyme genes and reference gene for RT-PCR analysis.

2.5 Statistical analysis

Each experiment was performed three times independently. Statistical evaluations were performed with GraphPad Prism (GraphPad software, San Diego, CA). One-way analysis of variance (ANOVA) was used to determine the significance of the experimental variables.

Mean values for each treatment were compared with the Dunnett's multiple comparison post-test at a 95% confidence interval. Student's t-test was used to compare effects of the temperature.

3. Results

Caco-2 cells were treated with sublethal concentrations (100 μM) of hydrogen peroxide at two different temperatures. This concentration of hydrogen peroxide showed no significant effects on the viability of Caco-2 cells under these experimental conditions and was confirmed to generate significant DNA damage including DNA SSBs and oxidative DNA adducts (Min & Ebeler, 2009). Oxidant treatment at 4°C for 10 min has been adopted in several previous studies to reduce DNA repair and so was adopted in this study as a comparison treatment where DNA repair should be minimized (Astley et al., 2002; Collins et al., 1995). The higher temperature (37°C) was used to represent physiological temperature conditions. Neither condition affected cell viability in the present study (data not shown). Levels of DNA damage (SSBs) was monitored over time by comet assay and mRNA levels of several BER enzymes were correspondingly determined by real time qRT-PCR.

Fig. 1 shows DNA damage levels during the recovery time following oxidant treatment at 4°C. Immediately after hydrogen peroxide treatment (time 0), DNA damage increased significantly. Levels of damage then decreased consistently throughout the recovery period. Fig. 2 shows corresponding levels of mRNA for several DNA BER enzymes following oxidant challenge at 4°C. Except for XRCC1, mRNA levels for all DNA repair enzymes varied significantly during the recovery time following oxidant treatment ($p < 0.05$). mRNA levels of PARP1 increased immediately after oxidant treatment at time 0. In contrast, expression levels of hOGG1, which cleaves the 8-oxoguanine lesion, decreased initially (0 h) and remained lower than control throughout the recovery period. APE1 expression also decreased initially (0 h) but then increased again over the recovery period following treatment at 4°C.

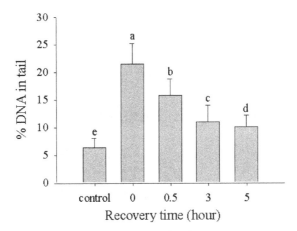

Fig. 1. DNA damage under oxidant challenge at 4°C. Bars represent mean ± SD. Bars not sharing a letter are significantly different ($P < 0.05$) (for each time, n=6 independent replications x 2 slides per replication).

Fig. 3 and 4 show DNA damage change and corresponding mRNA levels of DNA repair enzymes following oxidant challenge at 37°C. Levels of DNA damage increased significantly immediately following hydrogen peroxide treatment although the amount of damage was less than that of cells treated with oxidant at 4°C (t-test; p < 0.001) (Fig.3). The level of DNA damage decreased by 39% during the first 0.5 h, a rate of decrease that was faster than that observed following oxidant treatment at 4°C. However, the level of DNA damage did not maintain this rapid decrease over an extended period and DNA damage actually increased slightly after 3 h. Nonetheless, the level of damage was still lower than that at 0 h and levels of damaged DNA again decreased at 5 h.

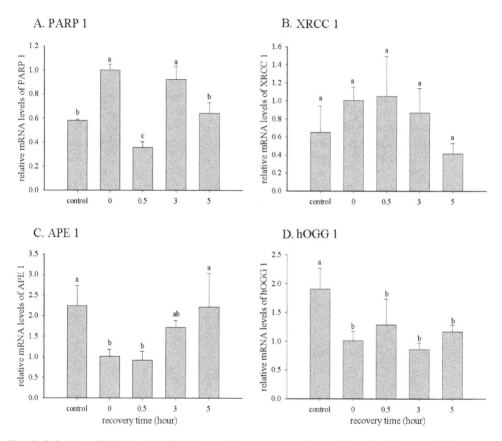

Fig. 2. Relative mRNA levels of DNA repair enzymes under oxidant challenge at 4°C. Levels are reported relative to 0 time. Bars represent mean ± SD. Bars not sharing a letter are significantly different (P < 0.05) (for each time, n=3 independent replications and qRT-PCR was analyzed in triplicate for each sample).

Unlike at 4°C mRNA levels did not change significantly for any of the repair enzymes immediately (0 h) after hydrogen peroxide treatment at 37°C (Fig. 4). However, hOGG1 levels did increase at 0.5 h and then gradually decreased during the recovery. XRCC1 levels also decreased late in the recovery period. On the other hand, APE1 expression increased late in the recovery time (3-5 h) and showed an approximately inverse relationship with hOGG1 levels. mRNA expression levels of PARP1, a SSB recognizing enzyme, changed dynamically at 4°C however, at 37°C PARP1 levels generally were maintained at the basal levels except for decreases which occurred at 3 and 5 h (Fig. 4).

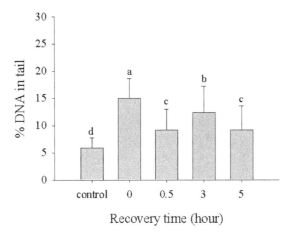

Fig. 3. DNA damage under oxidant challenge at 37°C. Bars represent mean ± SD. Bars not sharing a letter are significantly different (P < 0.05) (for each time, n=6 independent replications x 2 slides per replication).

4. Discussion

SSBs are a common type of DNA damage produced not only by ROS directly, but also indirectly during DNA repair processes. Moreover, no matter what the origins of SSBs are, SSBs are mostly repaired by the BER pathway. In this study, acute oxidative stress was induced in the Caco-2 cells by H₂O₂ treatment. Hydrogen peroxide has been shown previously to generate significant DNA damage including DNA base lesions and SSBs (Cantoni et al., 1987; Dizdaroglu, 1994; Min & Ebeler, 2009). In order to obtain a more complete picture of the cellular response to DNA damaging agents, DNA damage as a function of SSBs and corresponding mRNA expression levels of DNA repair enzymes were monitored. The measured DNA damage is the result of a balance between production of breaks by specific DNA base lesion glycosylases and the sealing of gaps by polymerases and ligases (Cantoni et al., 1987). Among DNA BER enzymes, PARP1, which recognizes and binds to AP sites, and XRCC1, a coordinating protein of the DNA BER pathway, were evaluated here. In addition, hOGG1, a glycosylase which cleaves 8-oxoguanine, and APE1, an endonuclease which cleaves AP sites, were also monitored. We examined DNA damage and repair at two different temperatures. Several studies have induced DNA damage at low temperature in order to minimize the possibilities of DNA repair (Astley et al., 2002; Collins et al., 1995). Accordingly our study adopted low temperature as a reference condition and also monitored responses at 37°C in order to elucidate the biochemical responses to DNA damaging agents at physiological temperature.

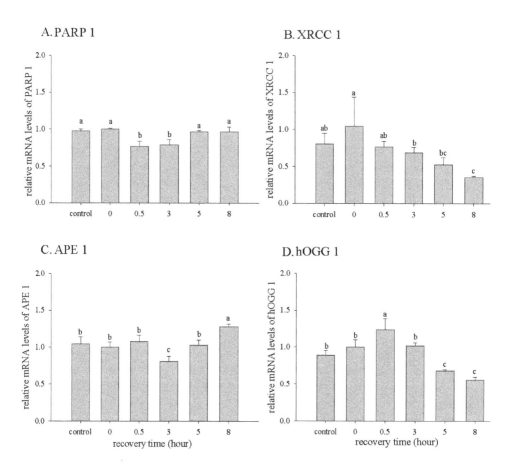

Fig. 4. Relative mRNA levels of DNA repair enzymes under oxidant challenge at 37°C. Levels are reported relative to the 0 time. Bars represent mean ± SD. Bars not sharing a letter are significantly different (P < 0.05) (for each time, n=3 independent treatments and qRT-PCR was analyzed in triplicate for each sample).

Higher levels of DNA damage followed by steady repair over time were observed following oxidant treatment at 4°C compared to treatment at 37°C. Foray et al. (1995) have shown more DNA double strand breaks at 4°C compared to 37°C following ionizing radiation, consistent with our study using a chemical oxidant. In our study, mRNA levels of PARP1 responded quickly to increased DNA damage at 4°C while the expression levels of hOGG1 and APE1 decreased immediately following oxidant treatment. Early decreases of APE 1 have been shown by Morita-Fujimura et al. after cold-injury induced brain trauma in mice (Morita-Fujimura et al., 1999). The increase of PARP1 immediately after oxidant treatment and the late gradual increase of APE1 may be factors contributing to the decrease in DNA damage (i.e., increase in repair) over time following the low temperature oxidant challenge. Therefore, although low temperature is typically associated with reduced metabolic and enzymatic activity, the effects of cold temperature on DNA damage appear to be complex and more investigations are needed to understand the effects of cold temperature on DNA damage and subsequent repair activity.

Levels of SSBs initially and over time, were different following oxidant challenge at 37°C compared to oxidant challenge at 4°C. It is possible that DNA repair was actually initiated during the hydrogen peroxide treatment at the higher temperature resulting in lower DNA damage levels immediately after oxidant treatment. This could at least partially account for the lower level of damage observed at 0 h compared to the treatment at 4°C. In addition, mRNA expression patterns of the repair genes were different from those at 4°C. For example, increased levels of hOGG1 within the first 0.5 h following oxidant challenge were consistent with greater DNA repair (i.e., decreased levels of DNA damage) that was observed following oxidant treatment at 37°C. The inverse relationship between APE1 and hOGG1 mRNA levels from 3 to 8 h at 37°C is consistent with hOGG1 producing AP sites which then induce mRNA production of APE1 (Hill et al., 2001).

Measuring the mRNA expression levels of DNA BER genes has been indicated to be a sensitive end point for determining the effects of chronic oxidative stress to DNA (Rusyn et al., 2004). In addition, consistent with our results following oxidant challenge at 37°C expression of hOGG1 mRNA, has been shown to be inducible responding to various conditions and reflecting DNA repair, at least initially. However, our results indicate that no single gene reflects the overall DNA repair response at any one point in time following oxidant treatment and it is difficult to fully relate changes in mRNA expression levels to the observed DNA damage repair kinetics.

5. Conclusions

Our study indicates that DNA damage induced by oxidant at physiological temperature (37°C) is lower as compared to damage at low temperatures. In addition, the pattern of mRNA expression of DNA repair processing enzymes is different over time following treatment. Some of the changes in DNA damage levels over the extended recovery period could be associated with the overall pattern of mRNA expression of several DNA repair enzymes, however, our results indicate that an individual gene alone may not accurately reflect the overall DNA repair capacity. Our study also indicates that protocols using low temperatures to minimize DNA repair may actually result in conditions that enhance DNA damage and result in very different repair kinetics than those that occur at a physiologic temperature. Experimental protocols should be carefully evaluated and interpreted if nonphysiologic conditions are used. Further studies comparing oxidative damage, mRNA expression and protein/enzyme levels and their activity are needed in order to fully understand the molecular responses to DNA damaging agents in the DNA damage/repair processes under variety of conditions.

6. Acknowledgments

We thank Dr. Bo Lonnerdal for use of cell culture facilities and Dr. David Mills for providing access to the RT-PCR instrument. We also thank Dr. Jong-Min Baek (Genomics Facility, UC Davis) for discussing qRT-PCR results. This study was funded by a Wine Spectator Scholarship for Kyungmi Min.

7. References

Astley, S. B, Elliott, R. M., Archer, D. B, & Southon, S. (2002). Increased cellular carotenoid levels reduce the persistence of DNA single-strand breaks after oxidative challenge. *Nutr. Cancer*, 43, 2, pp. 202-213.

Berwick, M., & Vineis, P. (2000). Markers of DNA repair and susceptibility to cancer in humans: an epidemiologic review. *J. Natl. Cancer Inst.*, 92, 11, pp. 874-897.

Caldecott, K. W. (2001). Mammalian DNA single-strand break repair: an X-ra(y)ted affair. *Bioessays*, 23, 5, pp. 447-455.

Caldecott, K. W. (2003). XRCC1 and DNA strand break repair. *DNA Repair* (Amst), 2, 9, pp. 955-969.

Cantoni, O., Murray, D., & Meyn, R. E. (1987). Induction and repair of DNA single-strand breaks in EM9 mutant CHO cells treated with hydrogen peroxide. *Chem. Biol. Interact.*, 63, 1, pp. 29-38.

Chevillard, S., Radicella, J. P., Levalois, C., Lebeau, J., Poupon, M. F., Oudard, S., Dutrillaux, B., & Boiteux, S. (1998). Mutations in OGG1, a gene involved in the repair of oxidative DNA damage, are found in human lung and kidney tumours. *Oncogene*, 16, 23, pp. 3083-3086.

Collins, A. R., Harrington, V., Drew, J., & Melvin, R. (2003). Nutritional modulation of DNA repair in a human intervention study. *Carcinogenesis*, 24, 3, pp. 511-515.

Collins, A. R., Ma, A. G., & Duthie, S. J. (1995). The kinetics of repair of oxidative DNA damage (strand breaks and oxidised pyrimidines) in human cells. *Mutat. Res.*, 336, 1, pp. 69-77.

Collins, A., & Harrington, V. (2002). Repair of oxidative DNA damage: assessing its contribution to cancer prevention. *Mutagenesis*, 17, 6, pp. 489-493.

Cooke, M. S., Evans, M. D., Dizdaroglu, M., & Lunec, J. (2003). Oxidative DNA damage: mechanisms, mutation, and disease. *FASEB J.*, 17, 10, pp. 1195-1214.

Davies, K. J. (2000). Oxidative stress, antioxidant defenses, and damage removal, repair, and replacement systems. *IUBMB Life*, 50, 4-5, pp. 279-289.

de Murcia, G., & Menissier de Murcia, J. (1994). Poly(ADP-ribose) polymerase: a molecular nick-sensor. *Trends Biochem. Sci.*, 19, 4, pp. 172-176.

Dianov, G. L. & Parsons, J. L. (2007). Co-ordination of DNA single strand break repair. *DNA Repair* (Amst), 6, 4, pp. 454-460.

Dizdaroglu, M. (1994). Chemical determination of oxidative DNA damage by gas chromatography-mass spectrometry. *Methods Enzymol.*, 234, pp. 3-16.

Foray, N., Arlett, C. F., & Malaise, E. P. (1995). Dose-rate effect on induction and repair rate of radiation-induced DNA double-strand breaks in a normal and an ataxia telangiectasia human fibroblast cell line. *Biochimie*, 77, 11, pp. 900-905.

Hill, J. W., Hazra, T. K., Izumi, T., & Mitra, S. (2001). Stimulation of human 8-oxoguanine-DNA glycosylase by AP-endonuclease: potential coordination of the initial steps in base excision repair. *Nucleic Acids Res.* 29, 2, pp. 430-438.

Hodges, N. J., & Chipman, J. K. (2002). Down-regulation of the DNA-repair endonuclease 8-oxo-guanine DNA glycosylase 1 (hOGG1) by sodium dichromate in cultured human A549 lung carcinoma cells. *Carcinogenesis*, 23, 1, pp. 55-60.

Kim, H. N., Morimoto, Y., Tsuda, T., Ootsuyama, Y., Hirohashi, M., Hirano, T., Tanaka, I., Lim, Y., Yun, I. G., & Kasai, H. (2001). Changes in DNA 8-hydroxyguanine levels, 8-

hydroxyguanine repair activity, and hOGG1 and hMTH1 mRNA expression in human lung alveolar epithelial cells induced by crocidolite asbestos. *Carcinogenesis*, 22, 2, pp. 265-269.

Lan, J., Li, W., Zhang, F., Sun, F. Y., Nagayama, T., O'Horo, C., & Chen, J. (2003). Inducible repair of oxidative DNA lesions in the rat brain after transient focal ischemia and reperfusion. *J. Cereb. Blood Flow Metab.*, 23, 11, pp. 1324-1339.

Langland, G., Elliott, J., Li, Y., Creaney, J., Dixon, K., & Groden, J. (2002). The BLM helicase is necessary for normal DNA double-strand break repair. *Cancer Res.*, 62, 10, pp. 2766-2770.

Leppard, J. B., & Champoux, J. J. (2005). Human DNA topoisomerase I: relaxation, roles, and damage control. *Chromosoma*, 114, 2, pp. 75-85.

Lynch, H. T., & Smyrk, T. (1996). Hereditary nonpolyposis colorectal cancer (Lynch syndrome). An updated review. *Cancer*, 78, 6, pp. 1149-1167.

Mambo, E., Chatterjee, A., de Souza-Pinto, N. C., Mayard, S., Hogue, B. A. Hoque, M. O., Dizdaroglu, M., Bohr, V. A., & Sidransky, D. (2005). Oxidized guanine lesions and hOgg1 activity in lung cancer. *Oncogene*, 24, 28, pp. 4496-4508.

Marchetto, M. C., Muotri, A. R., Burns, D. K., Friedberg, E. C., & Menck, C. F. (2004). Gene transduction in skin cells: preventing cancer in xeroderma pigmentosum mice. *Proc. Natl. Acad. Sci. U S A*, 101, 51, pp. 17759-17764.

Mayer, C., Popanda, O., Zelezny, O., von Brevern, M. C., Bach, A., Bartsch, H., & Schmezer, P. (2002). DNA repair capacity after gamma-irradiation and expression profiles of DNA repair genes in resting and proliferating human peripheral blood lymphocytes. *DNA Repair* (Amst), 1, 3, pp. 237-250.

Min, K. & Ebeler, S. E. (2009). Quercetin inhibits hydrogen peroxide-induced DNA damage and enhances DNA repair in Caco-2 cells. *Food Chem. Tox.*, 47, pp. 2716-2722.

Morita-Fujimura, Y., Fujimura, M., Kawase, M., & Chan, P. H. (1999). Early decrease in apurinic/apyrimidinic endonuclease is followed by DNA fragmentation after cold injury-induced brain trauma in mice. *Neuroscience*, 93, 4, pp. 1465-1473.

Noe, V., Penuelas, S., Lamuela-Raventos, R. M., Permanyer, J., Ciudad, C. J., Izquierdo-Pulido, M. (2004). Epicatechin and a cocoa polyphenolic extract modulate gene expression in human Caco-2 cells. *J. Nutr.*, 134, 10, pp. 2509-2516.

Rusyn, I., Asakura, S., Pachkowski, B., Bradford, B. U., Denissenko, M. F., Peters, J. M., Holland, S. M., Reddy, J. K., Cunningham, M. L., & Swenberg, J. A. (2004). Expression of base excision DNA repair genes is a sensitive biomarker for in vivo detection of chemical-induced chronic oxidative stress: identification of the molecular source of radicals responsible for DNA damage by peroxisome proliferators. *Cancer Res.* 64, 3, pp. 1050-1057.

Singh, N. P., McCoy, M. T., Tice, R. R., & Schneider, E. L. (1988). A simple technique for quantitation of low levels of DNA damage in individual cells. *Exp. Cell Res.*, 175, 1, pp. 184-191.

Torbergsen, A. C., & Collins, A. R. (2000). Recovery of human lymphocytes from oxidative DNA damage; the apparent enhancement of DNA repair by carotenoids is probably simply an antioxidant effect. *Eur. J. Nutr.*, 39, 2, pp. 80-85.

Wilson, D. M & Bohr, V. A. (2007). The mechanics of base excision repair, and its relationship to aging and disease. *DNA Repair* (Amst), 6, 4, pp. 544-559.

Wood, R. D., Mitchell, M., Sgouros, J., & Lindahl, T. (2001). Human DNA repair genes, *Science*, 291, 5507, pp. 1284-1289.

Part 3

Infection, Inflammation and DNA Repair

5

The Role of DNA Repair Pathways in Adeno-Associated Virus Infection and Viral Genome Replication / Recombination / Integration[1]

Kei Adachi[1,2] and Hiroyuki Nakai[1,2]
[1]Department of Microbiology and Molecular Genetics
University of Pittsburgh School of Medicine
USA

1. Introduction

Cellular DNA is constantly being damaged not only by extrinsic factors such as ionizing radiation and environmental carcinogens but also by intrinsic agents such as reactive oxygen species arising during normal cellular metabolism. Of the myriad of DNA lesions, inflicted by extrinsic and intrinsic genome damaging agents, DNA double strand break (DSB) is the most threatening. Replication fork arrest at DNA lesions could also be a threat since stalled replication forks, if fail to restart appropriately, induce DNA strand breaks. When cells encounter such strand breaks and other types of DNA damage, they mount a DNA damage response (DDR) (Harper & Elledge, 2007) that senses DNA damage and initiates a cascade of signal transduction pathways consequently culminating in cell cycle arrest, DNA repair and/or apoptosis when the DNA lesions become irreparable. Although cells are equipped with such DNA damage sensing and repair machinery primarily to handle damaged cellular DNA, triggers and receivers of DDR are not necessarily the cells' own genetic materials. DDR can also be provoked by essentially non-damaged DNA exogenously introduced into cells, most commonly viral genetic materials in nature and recombinant DNA (*e.g.*, viral vectors for gene delivery) in laboratory.

During virus-host interaction, viruses manipulate DDR upon infection of cells in a way that benefits their life cycles, while host cells fight against them to eliminate the invaders. DDR is detrimental to viral life cycles in many instances; therefore, DDR is often viewed as an innate antiviral host defense mechanism. For example, adenoviruses express viral proteins that block

---

[1] Abbreviations: AAV, adeno-associated virus; ATM, Ataxia telangiectasia mutated; ATR, Ataxia telangiectasia and Rad3 related; ATR-IP, ATR-interacting protein; BLM, Bloom syndrome protein; CARE, the cis-acting replication element within the p5 promoter; DDR, DNA damage response; DNA-PKcs, DNA-dependent protein kinase catalytic subunit; ds, double-stranded; DSB, double strand break; HR, homologous recombination; MRN, Mre11/Rad50/NBS1; NHEJ, non-homologous end joining; rAAV, recombinant AAV; RBS, Rep-binding site; RPA, replication protein A; SCID, severe combined immune deficiency; ss, single-stranded; TopBP1, DNA topoisomerase II-binding protein 1; WRN, Warner protein; wtAAV, wild type AAV. The demarcation between wtAAV and rAAV is often not important. If this is the case, AAV without wt or r prefix is used.
[2] Current affiliation: *Department of Molecular & Medical Genetics, Oregon Health & Science University School of Medicine, USA*

the cellular non-homologous end joining (NHEJ) pathway, which, unless inactivated, concatemerizes viral genomes and prohibits viral genome packaging into virions (Evans & Hearing, 2005; Stracker et al., 2002). Viruses may also take advantage of DDR in their life cycle as seen in retroviruses, which exploit the NHEJ pathway to complete insertion of their genomic materials into host cellular DNA (Daniel et al., 1999; Li et al., 2001). Similar but distinct types of "intervention" by viruses on DDR have been found in many other viruses (Lilley et al., 2007; Weitzman et al., 2004, 2010). Thus, understanding DDR and DNA repair machinery is imperative for elucidating the biology of viruses and viral vectors, and conversely, studying virus biology provides new insights into fundamental biological processes elicited by DNA damage. In this context, interactions between viruses and host DDR and DNA repair machinery have recently gained attention and established a new area of basic research. Importantly, this field of study is relevant to gene therapy research in overcoming its limitations and drawbacks and improving the current molecular therapy approaches.

Adeno-associated virus (AAV) represents a good example for exploring this new research field, which studies the interactions between viruses and DNA repair machinery. AAV has become increasingly popular as a promising gene delivery vehicle. Wild type AAV (wtAAV) is replication defective and recombinant AAV (rAAV) is devoid of virally encoded genes. Despite their replication-defective nature and/or lack of expression of viral proteins, there are significant interactions between virus and host DNA repair machinery, which determine the fates of the virus and the host cells following infection. In this chapter, we provide an overview of how wtAAV and rAAV alter the fate of the host cells through DDR, and how DDR processes the viral genomic DNA by exerting DNA repair machinery to establish the lytic and latent life cycles of wtAAV and transduction of rAAV.

2. Adeno-associated virus (AAV)

Adeno-associated virus (AAV) is a non-enveloped replication-defective animal virus of approximately 20 nm in diameter (Figure 1a). It belongs to Dependovirus, a genus of the family Parvoviridae, which has a viral capsid in the simplest icosahedral shape composed of 60 units of viral structural proteins. Productive AAV replication requires co-infection of a helper virus such as adenoviruses and herpesviruses. A virion has an approximately 5-kb single-stranded DNA genome of either plus or minus polarity at an equal probability. AAV serotype 2 and many other serotypes are prevalent in human populations worldwide and up to 80% of adult humans have been infected with AAV in their childhood (Boutin et al., 2010; Calcedo et al., 2009; Erles et al., 1999). AAV is generally considered as a non-pathogenic virus, and clinical relevance of AAV infection in humans appears to be limited to male infertility (Erles et al., 2001), early miscarriage in pregnant women (Burguete et al., 1999; Pereira et al., 2010) and protection against cervical cancer (Su & Wu, 1996; Walz & Schlehofer, 1992) although some studies have shown negative results (Strickler et al., 1999). The current relevance of AAV in biological and medical research primarily stems from its benefits as a tool for gene delivery and genetic engineering of the cellular genome and as a refined agent for inducing DDR without damaging the cellular genome (Table 1).

2.1 Wild type adeno-associated virus serotype 2 (wtAAV2)
2.1.1 Structural organization of wtAAV2
AAV was first identified as a contaminant in adenovirus stocks in early 1960s (Atchison et al., 1965). Since infectious wild type AAV2 (wtAAV2) clones were generated from

The Role of DNA Repair Pathways in Adeno-Associated Virus Infection and Viral Genome
Replication / Recombination / Integration

75

AAV-derived agents and tools	Applications
rAAV of any serotypes	• Delivery of exogenous genetic materials to cells with no toxicity • Targeted genetic manipulation of cells (*i.e.*, precise introduction of insertion, deletion or a small mutation at a defined location in the cellular genome in a predicted manner) • Introduction of DDR without damaging the cellular genome • Identification of DNA breakage sites in the cellular genome
wtAAV2	• Introduction of DDR without damaging the cellular genome • Tumor cell-specific killing
Rep68/78	• Site-specific insertion of exogenous genetic materials at the AAVS1 site in the human chromosome 19q13.42

Table 1. AAV as biological agents and tools

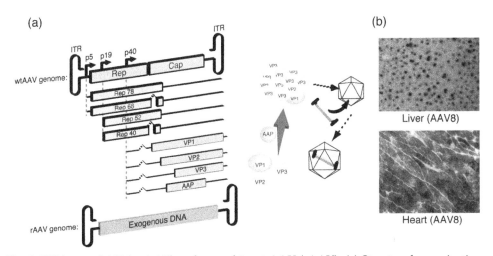

Fig. 1. Wild-type AAV (wtAAV) and recombinant AAV (rAAV). (a) Structural organization of wtAAV and rAAV. wtAAV genome is a single-stranded DNA with ITRs at the both ends. The two viral genes (the *rep* and *cap* genes) encode five non-structural (Rep and AAP) and three structural (VP) proteins, and they are controlled by the three viral promoters (p5, p19, and p40). AAV virion particle consists of VP1, VP2, and VP3. AAP supports assembly of VP proteins. rAAV genome is devoid of the viral components except for the ITRs, and contains an exogenous DNA of interest. (b) Representative photomicrographs of XGal-stained sections of the murine liver and heart transduced AAV8-EF1α-nlslacZ and AAV8-CMV-lacZ vectors at a high dose (7.2.x 10^{12} viral particles per mouse), respectively. All the hepatocytes and cardiomyocytes express the lacZ marker gene product, which turns transduced cells blue by the XGal staining.

recombinant plasmids (Samulski et al., 1982), AAV2 has been most extensively studied for viral capsid structure, genome organization, virally encoded protein functions, AAV life cycle and infection pathways (reviewed in Berns & Parrish, 2007; Carter et al., 2009; Smith & Kotin, 2002). WtAAV2 has a single-stranded DNA genome of 4679 nucleotides (nt) in length (GenBank accession no. AF043303) that comprises the region encoding 2 viral genes (e.g., the rep and the cap genes), their promoters (p5, p19 and p40 promoters), a polyadenylation signal, and two 145-nt inverted terminal repeats (ITR) forming T-shaped DNA hairpins at each viral genome terminus (Figure 1a). WtAAV2 expresses a total of 3 structural proteins (VP1, VP2 and VP3 from the cap gene) and 5 non-structural proteins (Rep40, Rep52, Rep68, and Rep78 from the rep gene and AAP from an alternative open reading frame from the cap gene). VP proteins form the AAV viral capsids while Rep proteins play roles in viral genome replication, packaging and site-specific viral genome integration at the AAVS1 site in the human chromosome 19 (Kotin et al., 1990, 1992). AAP protein (AAP stands for assembly-activating protein), which was identified in 2010, plays a role in directing VP proteins to nucleolus, the organelle where new AAV virions assemble (Sonntag et al., 2010).

2.1.2 The viral life cycle of wtAAV2

The life cycle of wtAAV2 consists of the lytic and the latent phases. Following infection through its surface receptors including heparan sulfate proteoglycan (Summerford & Samulski, 1998), wtAAV2 viral particles are carried to the nucleus where single-stranded viral genomes are released from virions into nucleoplasm. When an adenovirus co- or super-infects cells that are infected with wtAAV2, adenovirus helper functions are supplied and wtAAV2 enters the lytic phase where productive viral genome replication takes place. Adenoviral E1a, E1b55k, E4orf6, DNA-binding protein (DPB), and virus-associated RNA I (VAI-RNA) have been identified as the helper functions required for the growth of wtAAV2 and rAAV (Berns & Parrish, 2007; Geoffroy & Salvetti, 2005). In the lytic cycle, there are significant interactions between viral components and host DDR mediated by adenoviral E1 and E4 gene products and AAV large Rep proteins (i.e., Rep68/78). The interactions are primarily aimed at blocking the cell cycle and suppressing the NHEJ DNA repair pathway (more details are described in 3.2.).

In the absence of helper virus co-infection, most of the viral genomes are lost during cell division in dividing cells because they do not replicate or segregate together with the cellular genome into daughter cells. However, a certain proportion of AAV genomes establishes a latent phase by integration into the cellular genome, particularly at the AAVS1 site located within the human chromosome 19q13.42 (Kotin et al., 1992; Samulski et al., 1991). The AAVS1 site has a 33-nt DNA sequence within the myosin binding subunit (MBS) 85 gene and this short DNA sequence serves as the target for the site-specific integration (Linden et al., 1996b; Tan et al., 2001). The site-specific integration process requires expression of Rep68/78, which binds to a GCTC repeat element termed Rep binding site (RBS) and creates a nick at a nearby 3'-CCGGT/TG-5', designated terminal resolution site (trs). A set of these two recognition sequences is located within the AAV-ITR and the AAVS1 site (Brister & Muzyczka, 1999; McCarty et al., 1994). Several cellular factors have been shown to modulate Rep68/78-mediated site-specific integration (Figure 2b), although the experimental observations appear to be in conflict in some aspects. High mobility group protein 1 (HMG1) binds to Rep78,

The Role of DNA Repair Pathways in Adeno-Associated Virus Infection and Viral Genome
Replication / Recombination / Integration

77

enhances its RBS binding and nicking activities, and promotes site-specific integration at the AAVS1 site (Costello et al., 1997). In addition, the human immunodeficiency virus type 1 (HIV-1) TAR RNA binding protein 185 (TRP-185) binds to the RBS within the AAVS1 site, interact with Rep68, enhances Rep68's helicase activity, and controls selection of AAV genome integration sites within the AAVS1 locus (Figure 2b) (Yamamoto et al., 2007). This mode of latency is unique to wtAAV2 among the animal viruses, and is the case at least in cultured cells. In latently-infected human tissues, a majority of wtAAV2 genomes persist as circular genomes and no site-specific integration has been demonstrated even by sensitive PCR-based assays (Schnepp et al., 2005); therefore, the significance of the site-specific integration of wtAAV2 in natural infection in humans remains elusive.

2.1.3 wtAAV2 viral components that evoke DDR

Among the viral components, large Rep proteins, the cis-acting replication element (CARE) within the p5 promoter (Fragkos et al., 2008; Francois et al., 2005; Nony et al., 2001; Tullis & Shenk, 2000), AAV-ITR, and the unusual single-stranded nature of the viral genome are particularly important in AAV-evoked DDR and interaction with DNA repair machinery. These elements could potentially activate DDR without AAV viral genome replication.

2.2 Recombinant AAV (rAAV) vectors

Recombinant AAV (rAAV) vectors are genetically-engineered viral agents that carry heterologous DNA to be delivered to target cells and are devoid of all the viral genome sequence except for the 145-nt (ITR) at each genome terminus. Until early 2000s, rAAV vectors were primarily derived from AAV2 due to the limited availability of alternative serotypes at that time. rAAV2 vectors have a broad host range and outstanding ability to deliver genes of interest to both dividing and non-dividing cells of various types *in vitro*. However, rAAV2 exhibits limited transduction efficiency in tissues and organs *in vivo* when administered in experimental animals. This drawback of rAAV2 has recently been overcome by the discovery of new serotypes exemplified by AAV serotypes 8 and 9 (AAV8 and AAV9) (Gao et al., 2002, 2004). rAAV vectors derived from serotypes alternative to AAV2 have become widely available at present and been shown to exhibit unprecedented robust transduction in various tissues and organs by intravascular injection of the vector (Figure 1b) (Foust et al., 2009; Ghosh et al., 2007; Inagaki et al., 2006; Nakai et al., 2005a; Sarkar et al., 2006; Vandendriessche et al., 2007; Wang et al., 2005). It should be noted that alternative serotype rAAV vectors are in general those containing a rAAV2 viral genome encapsidated with an alternative serotype viral coat (*i.e.*, pseudoserotyped rAAV2 vectors) (Rabinowitz et al., 2002). Therefore, they are often referred to as AAV2/8 and AAV2/9 (genotype/serotype) when rAAV2 genome is contained in AAV8 and AAV9 viral coats, respectively. In addition to the exploitation of AAV capsids derived from various serotypes and variants present in nature, recent advances in genetic engineering of viral capsids aiming for the creation of specific cell type/tissue-targeting vectors have significantly broadened the utility of this vector system (Asokan et al., 2010; Excoffon et al., 2009; Koerber et al., 2009; Yang et al., 2009). Double-stranded (ds) rAAV vectors and gene targeting rAAV vectors are also worthy of note. Ds rAAV contains a ds viral genome in place of a single-stranded (ss) DNA

(McCarty, 2008). Because ds rAAV vectors overcome the rate-limiting step in transduction, *i.e.*, conversion from ss to ds DNA in infected cells, they exhibit a 1-2 log higher transduction efficiency than that achievable with the conventional ss vectors (McCarty et al., 2003; Wang et al., 2003). Gene-targeting rAAV vectors have the ability to introduce genomic alterations precisely and site-specifically at high frequencies of up to 1% (Russell & Hirata, 1998; Vasileva & Jessberger, 2005), which is several logs higher than that achievable by the conventional homologous recombination (HR) approaches (Thomas & Capecchi, 1987) (please refer to 3.5 for more details). Nonetheless, even if rAAV vectors are devoid of several key components that trigger DDR (*i.e.*, large Rep expression and the CARE), establishment of rAAV transduction heavily relies on the interactions between rAAV viral genomes and DNA repair machinery irrespective of serotypes or nature of viral genomes (*i.e.*, ss rAAV or ds rAAV).

3. AAV and DNA repair pathways

An overview of AAV and DNA repair pathways is summarized in Figure 2.

3.1 AAV-evoked DDR
3.1.1 Earlier evidence for the role of DDR in the AAV genome processing

Although the interplay between virus and DDR is a relatively new area of research, earlier studies indicated potential roles of DDR in the AAV life cycle or viral genome processing. The first indicative evidence came from the observation that cells treated with a wide variety of genotoxic agents including UV irradiation and carcinogens such as hydroxyurea could support wtAAV2 genome replication in the absence of helper virus co-infection (Yakinoglu et al., 1988; Yakobson et al., 1987, 1989). Subsequently, such treatment was found to augment rAAV2 transduction efficiency in both dividing and non-dividing cells with the latter showing a more dramatic enhancing effect (Alexander et al., 1994; Russell et al., 1995). These earlier observations suggested that activated DNA repair pathways following DNA damage induced by genotoxic treatment somehow facilitated the conversion of rAAV genomes from ss to ds DNA by second-strand synthesis (Figure 2f, g and h) (Ferrari et al., 1996; Fisher et al., 1996). As mentioned earlier, the formation of ds AAV genomes is a critical step for wtAAV to initiate productive infection and for rAAV to undergo abortive infection and express transgene products. A better response to the treatment in non-dividing cells conforms to the idea that DNA repair pathways are constitutively activated to a greater extent in dividing cells. Such activation is required to repair DNA replication errors that occur naturally and unavoidably. Although the underlying mechanism of this effect still remains elusive, one can speculate that up-regulation of DNA repair pathways increases the pool of cellular factors required for AAV genome processing. Alternatively, factors inhibitory for wtAAV genome replication or rAAV transduction may become sequestered from AAV genomes to multiple DNA repair foci formed on the damaged cellular genome (Figure 2f and g). A recent observation that the MRN complex and ATM, the major DDR proteins, have an inhibitory effect on rAAV transduction supports the latter model (Cataldi & McCarty 2010; Cervelli et al., 2008; Choi et al., 2006; Sanlioglu et al., 2000; Schwartz et al., 2007).

The Role of DNA Repair Pathways in Adeno-Associated Virus Infection and Viral Genome
Replication / Recombination / Integration

79

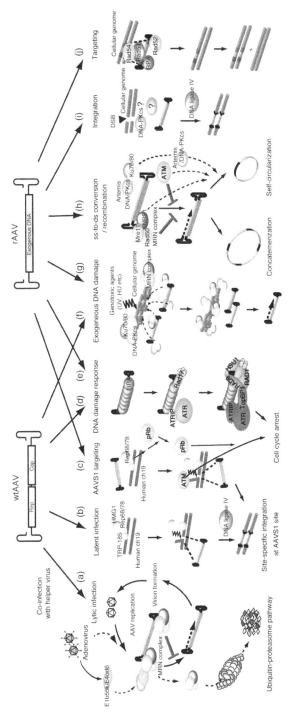

Fig. 2. A hypothetical model of the interactions between DNA damage responses (DDRs), DNA repair proteins and AAV genomes. (a) In the presence of adenovirus co-infection, adenoviral E1B55k/E4orf6 degrades and E4orf3 mislocates the MRN complex bound to AAV-ITR, allowing efficient second-strand synthesis and subsequent genome replication. (b) In the absence of helper virus co-infection, AAV Rep68/78 introduces a nick at the AAVS1 site in the human chromosome 19q13.42, where wtAAV2 genome integrates. It has been shown that TRP-185 and HMG1 proteins modulate this process. (c) Expression of Rep68/78 supplied in trans, mediates site-specific integration of rAAV (AAVS1 targeting) and/or activates the ATM pathway. Over-expression of Rep68/78 activates both pRb and ATM pathways, resulting in a complete block of the cell cycle in the S phase. (d, e) Activation of the ATR pathway by wtAAV2 or rAAV genome results in the G2/M arrest. (f, g) Genotoxic treatment damages the cellular genome at multiple locations, to which the inhibitory MRN complex and DNA-PK (Ku proteins and DNA-PKcs) are presumed to be sequestered from AAV genomes, allowing processing of viral genomes toward wtAAV2 replication and rAAV transduction. (h) The MRN complex and Ku bind to rAAV genome and suppress rAAV transduction. ATM may also have an inhibitory effect. The MRN complex, ATM and Artemis/DNA-PKcs promote generation of circular monomers via intramolecular recombination of rAAV genomes. (i) rAAV genomes integrate at pre-existing breaks in the cellular genome via NHEJ pathway(s). DNA-PKcs is dispensable but it could influence the efficiency of viral genome integration. (j) The Rad51/Rad54-mediated HR pathway mediates efficient rAAV gene targeting. In the pathways a, f, g, and h, dashed arrows extending from AAV-ITR indicate leading strands generated by a second-strand synthesis mechanism. In the pathway h, either or both of the second-strand synthesis mechanism and annealing of complementary ss DNA genomes convert ss genomes to ds DNA.

3.1.2 DNA repair proteins associated with AAV genomes in cells

AAV is composed of only two elements, VP proteins that form viral capsids and a single-stranded viral genomic DNA. VP proteins primarily determine biological properties of various AAV serotypes; *i.e.*, how AAV particles reach cells, enter cells, traffic in cytoplasm and nucleoplasm, and uncoat virion shells to release viral genomes. At present there is no evidence indicating that the above-mentioned AAV infection pathways driven by the capsid trigger DDR. AAV-evoked DDR is all about the cellular responses against AAV viral genomes except for wtAAV2, which expresses Rep68/78 proteins that also trigger DDR. It is plausible that the structure of single-stranded DNA with T-shaped hairpin termini, which is unusual and is not present in the cellular genome, is recognized as damaged DNA and triggers DDR. Direct evidence for the association of AAV genomes with DNA repair machinery has obtained in chromatin immunoprecipitation (ChIP) studies where AAV genomes and their associated cellular factors were crosslinked by formalin and precipitated together using antibodies specific to DNA repair proteins. To date, the MRN complex, Ku86, Rad52, RPA and DNA polymerase delta have been identified as factors bound to ss AAV genomes (Cervelli et al., 2008; Jurvansuu et al., 2005; Zentilin et al., 2001). In addition, immunofluorescence microscopy has revealed that the MRN complex, ATR, TopBP1, BLM, Brca1, Rad17, RPA, and Rad51 are recruited to the discrete nuclear foci where AAV genomes accumulate (Cervelli et al., 2008; Jurvansuu et al., 2005). Table 2 summarizes the roles of DNA repair proteins in AAV infection/transduction, AAV genome self-circularization, and AAV genome integration into the host genome.

3.1.3 AAV genome activates ATR-mediated DDR

Although not exclusive, the DNA repair proteins found to be associated with AAV genomes described in 3.1.2 are those involved in the ATR-mediated DDR that is triggered by stalled replication forks (Figure 2d and e) (reviewed in Branzei & Foiani, 2010 and Shiotani & Zou, 2009). At stalled replication forks, ss DNA regions become coated with RPA. RPA then recruits ATR-ATRIP and the Rad17 complex to the damaged site. The Rad17 complex subsequently recruits the ring-shaped trimeric Rad9/Rad1/Hus1 (9-1-1) complex, and finally ATR-ATRIP kinase becomes activated by TopBP1 recruited to the site and sends a DNA damage checkpoint signal (Figure 2d and e). In addition, Mre11 has also been reported to relocalize to stalled replication forks to a limited extent (Mirzoeva & Petrini, 2003). AAV-ITR exhibits a close structural similarity to stalled replication forks in that it contains both ss DNA regions and ss DNA-ds DNA junctions. This strongly supports a model in which AAV-ITR is recognized as a stalled replication fork and triggers the checkpoint response via ATR kinase. The actual activation of the ATR pathway by AAV genomes has been confirmed by the demonstration that the ATR-downstream effector proteins; *i.e.*, Chk1 and RPA, become phosphorylated in cells infected with wtAAV2 or UV-irradiated wtAAV2, both of which are devoid of the ability to replicate or express viral genes in the system used for the experiment (Fragkos et al., 2008; Ingemarsdotter et al., 2010; Jurvansu et al., 2005, 2007). Interestingly, rAAV2 genome devoid of the 55-nt CARE within the p5 promoter does not evoke the ATR-mediated checkpoint signal, and it has been shown that co-existence of both ITR and CARE in an AAV genome is essential for the activation (Fragkos et al., 2008). The consequence of the AAV genome-evoked ATR-mediated DDR is G2/M cell cycle arrest in wild type cells, while it leads to cell death in p53-deficient cells (Ingemarsdotter et al., 2010; Jurvansuu et al., 2007) (please see 3.1.4. for more details). Cell cycle arrest in the late S and/or G2 phases following infection of wtAAV2 or UV-irradiated wtAAV2 was observed

The Role of DNA Repair Pathways in Adeno-Associated Virus Infection and Viral Genome
Replication / Recombination / Integration

81

Protein	Effects of deficiency[2]						Note	References[3]
	In vitro			In vivo				
	T	C	I	T	C	I		
Artemis			↓	↓				1
ATM	↑	↓/↑→	↑	↓				2, 3, 4, 5
ATR	↑/→	→	→				wtAAV2-evoked signal ↑	5
BLM		↓						4
Chk1							wtAAV2-evoked signal ↑	14, 15
DNA-PKcs	↓	↓	↓/↑	↓	↓	↑/→	rAAV2 genome replication ↓ when deficient wtAAV2 genome replication ↑ when deficient	1, 4, 5, 6, 7, 8, 15
Ku70/80(86)	↑	→					wtAAV2 genome replication ↓ when deficient Targeting efficiency ↑ when deficient	3, 4
ligase IV		→	↓					4, 8
MDC1	↑							9
MRN	↑	↓			→			9, 4, 10
Rad52	↓			→	→			3, 16
Rad54B							Targeting efficiency ↓ when deficient	11
Rad54L							Targeting efficiency ↓ when deficient	11
WRN		↓						4
XRCC3		→					Targeting efficiency ↓ when deficient	4, 11
pRb							Induction of cell death when deficient	12, 13
p21							Induction of cell death when deficient	12, 13
p53							Induction of cell death when deficient	12, 13

Table 2. DNA repair and AAV

in an earlier study although how and what DDR is involved was not known at that time (Winocour et al., 1988).

3.1.4 AAV genome-evoked DDR leading to cell death

A unique aspect of AAV-evoked DDR is the ability to induce cell death without productive viral genome amplification, viral gene expression or cellular DNA damage, when cells are devoid of p53 expression. In 2001, Raj et al. reported an unexpected experimental observation that wtAAV2 infection of an osteosarcoma cell line that lacks expression of functional p53 leads to cell death through apoptosis or mitotic catastrophe, whereas the wild type control cells merely undergo a transient cell cycle arrest in the G2 phase (Raj et al., 2001). Mitotic catastrophe is an ill-defined term describing an apoptosis-like cell death during mitosis that takes place even in the presence of unrepaired DNA damage (Castedo et al., 2004; Vakifahmetoglu et al., 2008). This p53 deficiency-dependent cell killing effect was

---

[2] Observed effects caused by deficiency or knockdown are summarized. T, transduction efficiency; C, AAV genome self- circularization efficiency; I, AAV genome integration efficiency. In the table, arrows indicate an increase (↑), a decrease (↓) or no change (→).

[3] References cited are as follows: 1, Inagaki et al., 2007b; 2, Sanlioglu et al., 2000; 3, Zentilin et al., 2001; 4, Choi et al., 2006; 5, Cataldi et al., 2010; 6, Song et al., 2006; 7, Choi et al., 2010; 8, Daya et al., 2009; 9, Cervelli et al., 2008; 10, Schwartz et al., 2007; 11, Vasileva et al., 2006; 12, Garner et al., 2007; 13, Raj et al., 2001; 14, Schwartz et al., 2009; 15, Collaco et al., 2009; 16, Nakai, unpublished.

also observed when cells were infected with UV-irradiated wtAAV2 or microinjected with a 145-nt AAV2-ITR oligonucleotide, demonstrating that the unusual structure of the AAV2-ITR sequence itself is the culprit (Raj et al., 2001). Initially it was presumed that infection of wtAAV2 activates the ATM-p53-mediated DDR, which in turn increases and decreases the levels of p21 and CDC25C, respectively, resulting in the G2 arrest (Raj et al., 2001). Although the mechanism of p53 deficiency-dependent cell killing by AAV genomes still remains elusive, a series of subsequent studies on this phenomenon has revealed at least three potentially independent AAV-evoked pathways leading to cell death: the pathways involving (1) p53-p21-pRb, (2) p84N5 via caspase 6, and (3) ATR-Chk1. In the first mechanism, AAV-evoked DDR signal is transduced to a potent antiapoptotic proteins, pRb, via p53 and p21. Therefore, cells defective in this pathway fail to transduce the DDR signal to pRb, leading to apoptosis (Garner et al., 2007). In the second mechanism, functional defect of the p53-p21-pRb pathway allows activation of the nuclear death domain protein p84N5, which otherwise is inhibited by association with pRb (Doostzadeh-Cizeron et al., 1999). The activated p84N5 then induces apoptosis via caspase-6 (Garner et al., 2007). In the third mechanism, AAV genomes activate ATR, which in turn phosphorylates Chk1, causing a transient cell cycle arrest in the G2 phase. In the absence of p53, cells fail to sustain the G2 arrest following degradation of the unstable Chk1, progress suicidally into mitosis, and die via mitotic catastrophe associated with centriole overduplication and the subsequent formation of multipolar mitotic spindles (Ingemarsdotter et al., 2010; Jurvansuu et al., 2007). Whether all of the pathways or only some of them are triggered by AAV genomes remains unknown at present.

3.1.5 AAV2 Rep68/78-evoked DDR
In addition to AAV genome as a trigger of DDR, AAV2 large Rep proteins (*i.e.*, Rep68/78) themselves also evoke DDR independent of AAV genome. In the lytic phase of the AAV life cycle where cells are co-infected with a helper virus, Rep proteins are strongly expressed and exert many functions in the network of cellular proteins and viral factors derived from adenovirus or other helpers. Rep proteins can also be expressed without helper virus infection but only to a limited extent due in part to the large Reps' ability to negatively regulate their own promoter (p5) and the promoter for the small Rep proteins (p19) (Beaton et al., 1989; Kyostio et al., 1994). The significance of Rep68/78 expression in the absence of helper viruses reside in a series of the AAVS1-targeting approaches that exploit wtAAV2's ability to introduce exogenously derived DNA into the AAVS1 site in a site-specific manner (Figure 2c) (Henckaerts & Linden, 2010; Linden et al., 1996a). In these approaches, a donor vector in any context (*e.g.*, plasmid DNA, adenoviral vectors or rAAV) containing a gene of interest and RBS is delivered to human cells where AAV2 large Rep expression is supplied by the same vector or a separate one. The AAV2-ITR sequence is commonly used as an RBS-containing cis element; however, the p5 promoter also serves as an alternative (Philpott et al., 2002).

It has been known that Rep68/78 shows significant cellular toxicity due to the strong antiproliferative action of the protein (Yang et al., 1994). Rep78 completely blocks the cell cycle in the S phase (Saudan et al., 2000). Studies have shown that Rep78 exerts two independent but complementing DDR-associated cellular signal transduction pathways to arrest the cell cycle. The two pathways are the pRb pathway and the ATM-Chk2 pathway (Berthet et al., 2005). In the first pRb pathway, Rep78 expression leads to an increased level of the cyclin-dependent kinase inhibitor p21 and accumulation of hypophosphorylated pRb,

The Role of DNA Repair Pathways in Adeno-Associated Virus Infection and Viral Genome
Replication / Recombination / Integration

83

the active form of pRb protein (Berthet et al., 2005; Saudan et al., 2000) (Figure 2c). Consequently, cellular proteins that control cell cycle progression such as cyclin A, cyclin B1, and Cdc2, are down-regulated, resulting in slowing down the cell cycle (Saudan et al., 2000). Supporting this model, this effect is substantially attenuated in pRb-deficient mouse embryonic fibroblasts (Saudan et al., 2000). An increased amount of p21 might explain the inability to phosphorylate pRb upon large Rep expression, but the transcriptional activation of p21 has been shown to occur via a p53-independent pathway (Hermanns et al., 1997). In the second ATM-Chk2 pathway, the DNA-nicking activity of Rep68/78 creates multiple damaged sites in the cellular genome, which activates the ATM-Chk2 pathway and arrests the cell cycle (Figure 2c) (Berthet et al., 2005). Large Rep proteins create a break in only one strand of two-stranded DNA, which is not a type of damage that usually activates ATM. It is currently unknown how Rep68/78-induced DNA damage triggers this pathway. Worthy to note, activation of either one of the above-mentioned two pathways by itself is not sufficient for the complete block of the cell cycle, which is attainable by Rep68/78 expression (Berthet et al., 2005). It appears that there would be many other Rep68/78-associated DNA repair pathways that have yet to be identified. This is because a recent study using a tandem affinity purification (TAP) approach has demonstrated physical interaction of Rep78 with many DNA repair-associated proteins including DNA-dependent protein kinase catalytic subunit (DNA-PKcs), minichromosome maintenance (MCM) proteins, Ku70/80, proliferating cell nuclear antigen (PCNA), RPA, and structural maintenance of chromosome 2 (SMC2) (Nash et al., 2009).

3.2 wtAAV2 genome replication and DNA repair pathways

In the lytic phase of the wtAAV2 life cycle, viral genome replication requires co-infection of a helper virus. Since human adenoviruses have been most extensively studied in the context of AAV virology, this section specifically focuses on the interplay between wtAAV2, human adenoviruses, and DNA repair machinery. The adenoviral components required in the lytic infection are E1a, E1b55k, E4orf6, DBP, and VAI. A series of adenovirus/AAV co-infection studies has provided significant insights into how DDR and DNA repair machinery play roles in AAV genome replication in the presence of adenovirus helper functions (Collaco et al., 2009; Schwartz et al., 2009). It has been shown that adenoviral E1b55k/E4orf6 degrades the MRN complex via the ubiquitin-proteasome pathway and E4orf3 mislocalizes the MRN complex to aggresome, abrogating the MRN function in triggering the ATM and ATR pathways (Figure 2a) (Collaco et al., 2009). In addition, E4orf6 dissociates ligase IV from ligase IV/XRCC complex and degrades it (Jayaram et al., 2008). The main consequence of this adenoviral manipulation of DDR is inhibition on NHEJ, which prevents concatemeric adenoviral genome formation and promotes adenoviral genome replication and packaging. Although it remains elusive how beneficial the inhibition of NHEJ is in the AAV lytic life cycle, the significance of E1b/E4-mediated degradation of MRN complex in the wtAAV2 lytic cycle has been revealed by the observation that the MRN complex binds to AAV-ITR and inhibits wtAAV2 genome replication and rAAV vector transduction (Cervelli et al., 2008; Schwartz et al., 2007). Along the same line, the observation that cells deficient in ATM exhibit a higher rAAV transduction efficiency (Sanlioglu et al., 2000) might be explainable on the assumption that lack of ATM would be an equivalent to inactivation of the MRN complex because the MRN complex serves as a damage sensor that activates the ATM pathway (Carson et al., 2003). It is tempting to propose that dislocation of the MRN complex and other inhibitory factors from AAV genomes to the sites in the cellular genome where genome integrity is more severely threatened, is the mechanism for the augmentation of wtAAV2 genome replication and rAAV vector transduction by genotoxic treatment (Figure 2g). Suppression of the NHEJ pathway that involves DNA-PKcs and Ku proteins, however, may or may not be beneficial, because one study has shown that deficiency of these proteins both resulted in impaired rAAV2 genome replication (Choi et al., 2010) whereas another study has reported that siRNA-mediated knockdown of DNA-PKcs enhanced wtAAV2 genome replication (Collaco et al., 2009).

In addition to the adenovirus-evoked DDR, productive wtAAV2 viral genome replication triggers DDR distinct from that observed in adenovirus only infection (Collaco et al., 2009; Schwartz et al., 2009). Adenovirus-wtAAV2 co-infection results in much more pronounced activation of ATM and the checkpoint kinases, Chk1 and Chk2. This activation occurs independently of the MRN complex; therefore, the activation sustains even if MRN complex starts being degraded by adenoviral E1b/E4 proteins (Collaco et al., 2009). Other DDR substrate proteins RPA, NBS1 and H2AX become phosphorylated as the lytic phase progresses (Collaco et al., 2009; Schwartz et al., 2009). It has been shown that AAV genome replication is essential and sufficient to induce the DDR signal transduction cascade observed in the adenovirus co-infection, and Rep proteins does not play a role in the activation of DDR (Collaco et al., 2009; Schwartz et al., 2009). Among the three phosphatidylinositol 3-kinase-like kinases (PIKKs) that initiate signal transduction (*i.e.*, ATM, ATR and DNA-PKcs), ATM and DNA-PKcs are the primary kinases that phosphorylate downstream DDR substrates, and ATR appears to play only a minor role in the lytic phase of the AAV life cycle (Collaco et al., 2009; Schwartz et al., 2009). Although the significance of the DDR in the AAV lytic cycle remains unclear, the activation of the ATM pathway appears to be beneficial for AAV genome replication (Collaco et al., 2009).

3.3 rAAV genome recombination and DNA repair pathways
3.3.1 rAAV genome processing is mediated solely by DNA repair machinery

After entering nuclei, rAAV virion shells break down, releasing single-stranded (ss) vector genomes into nucleoplasm, which subsequently convert to various forms of double-stranded (ds) genomes (Deyle & Russell, 2009; Schultz & Chamberlain, 2008). It should be noted that rAAV does not express any viral gene products that can process viral genomes such as recombinases and integrases; therefore the processing of viral genomes must heavily depend on DNA repair machinery. In addition, unlike the battle between adenovirus and the host DNA repair systems as described in 3.2, rAAV has no means to manipulate DNA repair pathways once viral genomes evoke DDR. Unless rAAV genomes have been processed to completion into stable ds DNA with no free ends, DDR would remain activated due to the continued presence of viral DNA in an unusual structure presenting a single strand with free ends. In mammalian cells, extrachromosomal free DNA ends at ds rAAV genome termini as well as those in ds linear plasmid DNA, when exogenously delivered, appear to be removed primarily by ligating two free ends and making a single continuous ds DNA strand via NHEJ and/or occasionally HR rather than by DNA degradation (Nakai et al., 2003b; Nakai, unpublished observation). In this sense, the rAAV genomes processed into various forms in their latency could be viewed as byproducts that have been created and disposed of by a cellular defense mechanism against potentially toxic exogenous agents.

The Role of DNA Repair Pathways in Adeno-Associated Virus Infection and Viral Genome
Replication / Recombination / Integration

85

3.3.2 Single-to-double-stranded rAAV genome conversion and DNA repair machinery

How ss rAAV genomes become ds DNA is not completely understood but the process involves the following two mechanisms; second-strand synthesis (Ferrari et al., 1996; Fisher et al., 1996; Zhong et al., 2008; Zhou et al., 2008) and annealing of plus and minus strands (Hauck et al., 2004; Nakai et al., 2000). It has been shown that, upon rAAV infection, the MRN complex becomes activated, physically associates with AAV2-ITR and inhibits wtAAV2 replication and rAAV transduction (Figure 2a and h) (Cervelli et al., 2008; Schwartz et al., 2007); therefore, MRN appears to have some role in the conversion of ss to ds DNA. ATM has also been suggested to be a cellular factor that inhibits the single-to-double-stranded genome conversion because transduction efficiency with ss rAAV is significantly enhanced in ATM-deficient cells *in vitro* (Figure 2h) (Sanlioglu et al., 2000). However, a recent study has proposed an ATM-mediated gene silencing model rather than the mechanism involving the second-strand synthesis to explain the ATM's inhibitory effect. This model stems from the observation that, in the absence of ATM, ds rAAV transduction was enhanced as well, indicating that an alternative mechanism other than second-strand synthesis is involved (Cataldi & McCarty, 2010). Another factor that is known to inhibit this process is tyrosine-phosphorylated FKBP52, which binds to AAV-ITR and inhibits second-strand synthesis (Qing et al., 2001). Its dephosphorylation by T-cell protein tyrosine phosphatase (TC-PTP) dissociates FKBP52 from AAV-ITR, allowing the formation of ds genomes (Qing et al., 2003). *In vitro* AAV replication studies have identified the DNA polymerase that catalyzes second-strand synthesis as DNA polymerase δ (Nash et al., 2007), which is a polymerase that fills a single-stranded DNA gap created during the nuclear excision repair (Torres-Ramos et al., 1997). Physical association of DNA polymerase δ and AAV genome has also been demonstrated (Jurvansuu et al., 2005). At present it remains elusive whether and how the above-mentioned signal kinases (*i.e.*, MRN and ATM) and effectors (FKBP52 and DNA polymerase δ) are linked in the rAAV-evoked DDR.

3.3.3 Extrachromosomal rAAV genome recombination and DNA repair machinery

In addition to the above-mentioned single-to-double-stranded genome conversion, rAAV genomes are further processed into the following stable ds forms by intra- or inter-molecular DNA recombination mediated solely by DNA repair machinery, and establish the latent infection. The viral genome forms in the latent phase include ds circular monomers, large concatemers (circular and/or linear), and rAAV proviral genomes that are stably integrated into the host cellular genome at low frequencies (Deyle & Russell, 2009; Schultz & Chamberlain, 2008). It has not been determined when the rAAV genome recombination takes place, which may be either before, at, or after completion of the single-to-double-stranded genome conversion. In dividing cells, extrachromosomal genomes are lost because they do not replicate episomally, whereas they can be stabilized and maintained as chromatin in quiescent cells in animal tissues (Penaud-Budloo et al., 2008). Earlier studies indicated that the formation of large concatemeric rAAV genomes is important for transgene expression; however, accumulated observations might favor a model in which extrachromosomal circular monomer genomes, not large concatemers or integrated forms, are primarily responsible for persistent and stable transgene expression in rAAV-transduced animal tissues (Nakai et al., 2001; Nakai et al., 2002; Nathwani et al., 2011).

In extrachromosomal rAAV genome recombination, AAV-ITR plays a pivotal role in mediating recombination. Although it has yet to be elucidated how DDR is evoked by rAAV genomes in the context of rAAV genome recombination, it is not unreasonable to speculate that the T-shaped hairpin structure within the AAV-ITR and/or ss DNA-ds DNA junctions in the stem of the hairpin DNA trigger DDR. A set of DNA repair proteins, which includes DNA-PKcs, Artemis, ATM, MRN, BLM, and WRN (Figure 2h), has been found to be involved in rAAV genome recombination (Cataldi & McCarty, 2010; Choi et al., 2006; Duan et al., 2003; Inagaki et al., 2007b; Nakai et al., 2003b; Sanlioglu et al., 2000; Song et al., 2001). Deficiency of these proteins impairs intramolecular recombination of ss rAAV and/or ds rAAV genomes via the AAV-ITR sequence. DNA-PKcs and Artemis are the two major components in the classical NHEJ pathway of DSB repair. Artemis, when activated by DNA-PKcs, possesses an endonuclease activity and resolves DNA hairpin loops and flaps formed at broken DNA ends to facilitate ds DNA end joining (Ma et al., 2005). BLM and WRN are members of the RecQ family of DNA helicases. They unwind ds DNA to ensure the formation of proper recombination intermediates, and mediate a various types of DNA transactions, mainly HR (Bernstein et al., 2010). MRN is a multifaceted protein complex that functions as a primary sensor of DSB, binds DNA lesion, recruits ATM, and processes DNA ends by utilizing the Mre11 endo- and exo-nuclease activity that creates recombinogenic 3' single-stranded tails (Williams et al., 2010). The initial study of the structure of ITR-ITR junction sequences revealed that the majority of the recombination junctions in ds circular monomer genomes exhibited a 165-nt double-D ITR structure, the hallmark of HR (Duan et al., 1999; Xiao et al., 1997). This indicates that HR is the major pathway for intra- and inter-molecular genome recombination events. Supporting this view, Rad52, which is a key player in HR, was identified as a protein that binds to rAAV genomes in cultured cells (Zentilin et al., 2001). Interestingly, deficiency of Rad52 does not affect rAAV transduction efficiency or genome processing in murine liver (Nakai, unpublished observation). It remains possible that HR plays a major role in rAAV genome recombination at least under certain cellular environment; however, accumulated observations by us and others rather support a model in which NHEJ is the major pathway for extrachromosomal rAAV genome recombination. In the absence of DNA-PKcs or Artemis, intramolecular recombination is significantly impaired in cultured cells and animal tissues (Cataldi & McCarty, 2010; Duan et al., 2003; Inagaki et al., 2007b; Nakai et al., 2003b; Song et al., 2001), and the footprints on junction DNA are quite consistent with NHEJ-mediated recombination, showing nucleotide deletions of various degrees with occasional microhomology at junctions (Inagaki et al., 2007b). Interestingly, intra- and inter-molecular recombination events that form ds circular monomers and ds concatemers, respectively, are differentially regulated by different DNA repair pathways (Figure 2h). Intramolecular recombination heavily depends on the Artemis/DNA-PKcs-dependent NHEJ pathway, while the NHEJ pathways that mediate intermolecular recombination are redundant because intermolecular recombination occurs efficiently in the absence of DNA-PKcs or Artemis (Inagaki et al., 2007b). The DNA-PKcs or Artemis-independent NHEJ might be those involving ATM and/or MRN (Cataldi & McCarty, 2010; Choi et al., 2006; Duan et al., 2003; Inagaki et al., 2007b; Nakai et al., 2003b; Sanlioglu et al., 2000; Song et al., 2001). Alternatively, HR might be the major pathway for intermolecular rAAV recombination. This model stems from the observation that recombination between two homologous AAV-ITRs derived from the same serotype is preferred to that between two non-homologous AAV-ITRs derived from different serotypes (Yan et al., 2007). The ATR pathway does not appear to be involved in extrachromosomal rAAV genome recombination (Cataldi & McCarty, 2010).

How DNA-PKcs and Artemis process rAAV genome termini and mediate recombination has been extensively studied in the context of murine tissues. In DNA-PKcs or Artemis-deficient SCID mice, ds linear rAAV genomes with covalently closed hairpin caps at genome termini accumulate in rAAV-transduced tissues (Figure 3b). In SCID mouse thymi, V(D)J recombination is impaired resulting in accumulation of covalently-sealed hairpin intermediates at V(D)J coding ends in the T cell receptor gene (Rooney et al., 2002; Roth et al., 1992) (Figure 3a). These two phenomena are essentially the same in that if hairpin structures at DNA ends are not cleaved by the Artemis/DNA-PKcs endonuclease activity, covalently closed DNA ends accumulate without undergoing further recombination. Therefore, intramolecular recombination most likely uses the same Artemis/DNA-PKcs-dependent NHEJ pathway used for V(D)J recombination. It is not easy to determine GC-rich AAV-ITR hairpin DNA structures at sequencing levels; however this shortcoming has been overcome by exploiting the bisulfite PCR technique. Utilizing this method, the primary cleavage site by the Artemis/DNA-PKcs endonuclease activity has been mapped to the 5' end of the 3-base AAA loop at the AAV-ITR hairpin tips (Figure 3b) (Inagaki et al., 2007b). In DNA-PKcs-deficient SCID mouse tissues, the relative proportion of rAAV genome recombination junctions exhibiting the hallmark of HR increases, indicating compensatory activation of HR in the absence of DNA-PKcs in quiescent cells in animal tissues (Nakai, unpublished observation). In this regard, worthy of note are the following observations made by us and others that DNA repair pathways might somehow be linked to epigenetic modifications of rAAV genomes. We have found that the cytomegalovirus (CMV) immediately early gene promoter in rAAV genome can be significantly silenced in Artemis- or DNA-PKcs-deficient mouse muscle (Nakai, unpublished observation). Recently, Cataldi et al. reported that the CMV promoter is somewhat silenced in ATM-proficient murine fibroblasts compared to that in ATM-deficient cells (Cataldi & McCarty, 2010). These observations imply that rAAV genome recombination via NHEJ generates more functionally active genomes than HR presumably due to a difference in epigenetic modifications of rAAV genomes (Cataldi & McCarty, 2010).

3.4 rAAV genome integration and DNA repair pathways

rAAV is devoid of Rep68/78 expression; therefore, it lacks the ability to integrate into the cellular genome site specifically. In addition, rAAV does not harness machinery designed specifically for integration into the cellular genome. rAAV vectors are generally considered as episomal vectors, but they do integrate into the cellular genome of both dividing and non-dividing cells at low frequencies (Deyle & Russell, 2009; McCarty et al., 2004). This process is entirely dependent on the host cellular DNA repair machinery. Although it is not easy to determine the frequency of rAAV genome integration in each case and it may vary depending on the amount of rAAV genomes delivered to cells, integration has been reported to occur at approximately ~0.1% of total input rAAV genomes (Russell et al., 1994) or up to ~4% of cell population in rAAV-infected cultured cells (Cataldi & McCarty, 2010), or at approximately 0.1% of rAAV-transduced hepatocytes when rAAV is injected into newborn mice (Inagaki et al., 2008). rAAV genome integration occurs at nonrandom sites in both cultured cells and somatic cells in animals. The preferred genomic sites for integration include the 45s pre-ribosomal RNA gene, transcriptionally active genes, DNA palindromes, CpG islands, and the neighborhood of transcription start sites (Inagaki et al., 2007a; Miller et al., 2005; Nakai et al., 2003a). Although the mechanism of integration remains largely unknown, it has been presumed that input rAAV genomes are fortuitously captured at pre-

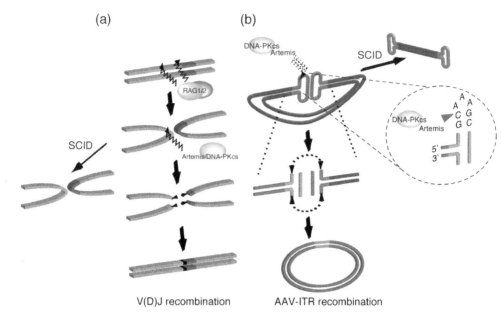

Fig. 3. A similarity of Artemis / DNA-PKcs-mediated hairpin cleavage in V(D)J recombination and AAV-ITR recombination. (a) During V(D)J recombination, the recombination activating gene products, Rag1 and Rag2 endonucleases, cleave the immunoglobulin and T cell receptor genes, forming covalently closed hairpin loops at cleaved DNA ends. Artemis/DNA-PKcs complex resolves the hairpin loops, which triggers the subsequent recombination between the two coding ends via the classical NHEJ DNA repair pathway. In cells deficient in either Artemis or DNA-PKcs (SCID phenotype), hairpin coding ends remain unrecombined and accumulate. (b) The same Artemis/DNA-PKcs-dependent NHEJ pathway mediates intramolecular AAV-ITR recombination, forming circular monomer genomes. Intermolecular AAV-ITR recombination occurs independently of Artemis/DNA-PKcs. A red arrowhead indicates the primary target for Artemis/DNA-PKcs-mediated cleavage. In SCID mouse tissues, ds linear rAAV genomes with covalently closed AAV-ITR hairpin caps accumulate.

existing breaks in the cellular genome when the DNA breaks are repaired by DNA repair machinery, which establishes rAAV integration. This model has been supported by the observations that rAAV genome integrations are frequently found at I-SceI-induced DSBs in the cellular genome (Miller et al., 2004) and genotoxic treatments can increase integration rates (Russell et al., 1995). Clinically, rAAV vectors are generally considered to be safe; however, one study has shown that vector genome integration could cause insertional mutagenesis leading to hepatocarcinogenesis in a mouse model (Donsante et al., 2007).

The detailed analyses of rAAV vector genome-cellular genome junction sequences in cultured cells and murine tissues have provided significant insights into which and how DNA repair pathways play roles in rAAV integration (Inagaki et al., 2007a; Miller et al., 2005; Nakai et al., 2005b). rAAV integration does not take place in a neat cut-and-paste fashion and always accompanies various degrees of deletions in rAAV genome terminal sequences and the cellular genomes around integration sites. Complex genomic

The Role of DNA Repair Pathways in Adeno-Associated Virus Infection and Viral Genome
Replication / Recombination / Integration

89

rearrangements are not rare and integration often causes a chromosomal translocation. All of these observations fit very well with a model in which NHEJ mediates rAAV integration. A series of studies has shown that DNA-PKcs has negative or positive effects on integration depending on the experimental systems used (Figure 2i). In a cell-free *in vitro* rAAV integration system, ss rAAV integration frequency increases and decreases by the addition of DNA-PKcs antibody and purified DNA-PKcs, respectively, leading to a conclusion that DNA-PKcs inhibits rAAV integration (Song et al., 2004). Whereas, in a cell culture system using DNA-PKcs-proficient M059K and deficient M059J cells, DNA-PKcs has been shown to enhance integration of both ss rAAV and ds rAAV (Cataldi & McCarty, 2010; Daya et al., 2009). In the context of animal experiment, Song et al. have exploited a two-thirds partial hepatectomy approach and shown that rAAV genomes integrate in DNA-PKcs-deficient SCID mouse livers at a significantly greater frequency than that of wild type control animals (*i.e.*, >50% in SCID versus <10% in wild type mice) (Song et al., 2004). Whereas, our most recent study has indicated that this effect could be observed at a limited range of liver transduction levels, and deficiency of DNA-PKcs may not have a generalized effect on rAAV integration frequency (Adachi & Nakai, unpublished observation). Nonetheless, a high-throughput ss rAAV integration site analysis in mouse liver, muscle and heart has successfully identified many rAAV integration sites in both wild type and SCID mouse tissues. This indicates that DNA-PKcs itself does not play a direct role in the process of rAAV genome integration (Figure 2i) (Inagaki et al., 2007a). Other DNA repair proteins that might participate in the rAAV genome integration process include ATM, which also shows varying effects on integration in cell culture experiments depending on the types of cells and rAAV (*i.e.*, ss versus ds rAAV) (Cataldi & McCarty, 2010; Sanlioglu et al., 2000). Interestingly, our study has implied that rAAV genomes more preferably integrate in the cellular genome than remain as extrachromosomal genomes when murine hepatocytes receive a minimum rAAV dose to establish latency (Adachi & Nakai, unpublished observation). This observation indicates that different DDRs are evoked and recruit different DNA repair machinery depending on the amount of DDR triggers in a cell. Collectively, at this point, there is no consensus model that explains which and how DNA repair pathways mediate rAAV integration. As for the integration of rAAV at the AAVS1 site in the presence of Rep68/78 expression, DNA-PKcs enhances site-specific integration of ss rAAV but not ds rAAV, indicating differential effects of DNA repair proteins in the Rep-mediated integration (Daya et al., 2009).

3.5 rAAV-mediated gene targeting and DNA repair pathways

HR mediated by the conventional vector systems occurs with efficiencies of a range of 10^{-6} to 10^{-7}. In this regard, rAAV has become increasingly popular as the most efficient tool to precisely introduce defined DNA modifications at the target site in the cellular genome with remarkably high efficiencies of up to 1% in the cell population (Hendrie & Russell, 2005; Khan et al., 2011; Russell & Hirata, 1998; Vasileva & Jessberger, 2005). Targeting efficiencies could be increased further by 60-100 fold or more by introducing a DSB at the target site with a site-specific endonuclease (Miller et al., 2003; Porteus et al., 2003). This system, named the gene targeting rAAV vector system, has been applied in various disciplines, not only for gene therapy (Chamberlain et al., 2004) but also for generating knockout animals (Sun et al., 2008) and other types of basic research (Khan et al., 2011). Gene targeting rAAV serves as a donor vector that carries a DNA segment homologous to the chromosomal target sequence with a desired modification being introduced. The length of the homology arms can be 1.7

kb or potentially shorter, which is an advantage over the conventional targeting vectors that require a longer homologous DNA sequence (Hirata & Russell, 2000). Despite significant advance in the applications of the system, the underlying mechanism for rAAV-mediated gene targeting is poorly understood. As described above, rAAV does not harness any machinery designed specifically for mediating highly efficient gene targeting. The unusual structure of viral genome DNA is the only element that makes the system much more efficient than the conventional approaches.

The mechanism of rAAV-mediated gene targeting has just begun to be partly elucidated. Studies have indicated that the single-stranded nature of gene-targeting rAAV is key to efficient gene targeting reactions. Experimental evidence has come from the observation that, when mixtures of gene-targeting ss rAAV and ds rAAV vectors were used, gene correction rates correlated with the amounts of ss rAAV but not ds rAAV within the mixtures (Hirata & Russell, 2000). Another study took advantage of recombinant minute virus of mice (rMVM), a rAAV-like parvovirus-based vector that predominantly packages viral genomes of minus polarity and does rarely undergo second-strand synthesis to form ds viral genomes. When reporter cells were infected with gene-targeting rMVM vectors containing either the coding or noncoding strand of a transgene cassette, a significant difference in targeting efficiencies was revealed between the two, indicating that ss viral genomes are the substrate (Hendrie et al., 2003). However, a recent study points out limitations in the previously used assay systems and argues against the above model because ds rAAV has also been found to mediate gene targeting at a higher level compared with the ss rAAV control (Hirsch et al., 2010). Although the nature of gene targeting substrates may be a subject of debate, it is clear that rAAV genome integration and rAAV-mediated gene targeting use different DNA repair pathways. Genotoxic treatment, which significantly augments rAAV genome integrations, does not affect gene targeting efficiency (Hirata & Russell, 2000). In addition, rAAV gene targeting occurs preferentially in S-phase cells and does not take place at an appreciable level in terminally differentiated murine skeletal muscle fibers (Liu et al., 2004; Trobridge et al., 2005). Moreover, the cell cycle dependence has not clearly been demonstrated in rAAV integration and a study has demonstrated a readily appreciable level of rAAV integration in terminally differentiated cardiomyocytes and skeletal myofibers (Inagaki et al., 2007a). Collectively, NHEJ appears to be the major DNA repair pathway involved in rAAV integration while rAAV-mediated gene targeting uses HR. It has been demonstrated that RAD51/RAD54 pathway of HR is required for efficient rAAV-mediated gene targeting (Figure 2j), and deficiency of either of the NHEJ proteins, DNA-PKcs and Ku70, enhances the targeting rates (Fattah et al., 2008; Vasileva et al., 2006). Although the DNA-PKcs effect appears to be a cell-type dependent phenomenon (Fattah et al., 2008), the observations underscore the significant contribution of the HR pathways in rAAV-mediated gene targeting. Manipulation of HR and NHEJ pathways with small molecules will offer a novel and effective means to further improve rAAV-mediated gene targeting approaches to genetically engineer cellular genomes.

4. AAV as a tool for studying damaged DNA sites, DDR, and DNA repair pathways

AAV has provided the most powerful means to deliver genetic materials to a broad range of cell and tissue/organ types without toxicity and to introduce sequence modifications at defined locations. What has made AAV more attractive is its utility as an unprecedented research tool to study molecular and cellular biology, where gene delivery is not a primary goal. As described in 3.1.3 and 3.1.4, AAV has been successfully exploited as a refined agent that can trigger DDR toward cell cycle arrest and apoptosis. AAV can deliver an element that triggers DDR (*e.g.*, stalled replication forks) extrachromosomally with minimal transcriptional responses (McCaffrey et al., 2008) and without damaging the cellular genome. Although the phenomena observed in the AAV-based system may not necessarily recapitulate what takes place when the cellular DNA is damaged, it is assumed that molecularly defined extrachromosomal DDR triggers would provide a simple and less complicated means to study cellular responses to DNA damage. In addition, AAV has been exploited to study potential differences in DNA repair pathways among various tissues in the context of living animals. This type of study has demonstrated that, in hepatocytes, there is significant redundancy of Artemis/DNA-PKcs-independent NHEJ pathways that process hairpin DNA ends, while such redundancy is not observed in skeletal myofibers or cardiomyocytes in mice (Inagaki et al., 2007b). Moreover, AAV has recently emerged as a powerful tool to identify DNA sites damaged either endogenously or exogenously by genotoxic treatment or agents. Using rAAV as a tool to label pre-existing damaged DNA sites, a study has shown that DNA palindromes with an arm length of $\geq$ 20 base pairs in the cellular genome represent the sites susceptible to breakage in mouse tissues (Inagaki et al., 2007a). Another study has taken a similar AAV-based labeling approach and demonstrated frequent off-target cleavage of the cellular genome by a rare cutting endonuclease, I-SceI, following expression of I-SceI in cells (Petek et al., 2010). Perhaps applications of AAV in biological and medical research will not be limited to the disciplines described above and will continue to expand with the advent of novel rAAV vector technologies.

5. Conclusions

The virus-host interaction from a viewpoint of viral components and DNA repair machinery is an emerging research area that would offer unprecedented means to study both virology and molecular and cellular biology. The interaction in this aspect is most studied with adenoviruses, herpesviruses, and retroviruses including human immunodeficiency virus. These viruses have evolved sophisticated machinery to benefit them by manipulating or controlling DDR, DNA repair machinery, and the cell cycle. In this regard, AAV (*i.e.*, wtAAV and rAAV) represents a unique viral agent in that Rep proteins are the sole viral components that interact with DNA repair machinery and rAAV expresses no such component. Despite the seemingly simple nature of AAV, there are significant virus-host interactions that involve DDR and DNA repair machinery in AAV infection, and we have just begun to appreciate them as summarized in this chapter. There has been an increasing interest in AAV primarily as a promising gene delivery vector and more recently as a new tool to study DNA damage, DDR, and DNA repair machinery. Studying AAV from various scientific aspects including virology, immunology, physiology, gene therapy, DNA damage, DDR, DNA repair, genomic instability, carcinogenesis, and so on, would significantly advance our knowledge about AAV and could solve unanswered fundamental biological questions that are difficult to address by the conventional approaches.

6. Acknowledgment

Preparation of this chapter is in part supported by the National Institutes of Health (R01 DK078388). The authors are most grateful to Christopher Naitza and Baskaran Rajasekaran for their invaluable assistance in preparation of the manuscript. The authors apologize to investigators whose papers relevant to the topic of this chapter were not cited due to space constraints or inadvertent oversight.

7. References

Alexander, I. E., Russell, D. W. & Miller, A. D. (1994). DNA-damaging agents greatly increase the transduction of nondividing cells by adeno-associated virus vectors. *Journal of Virology*, Vol.68, No.12, pp. 8282-8287, ISSN 0022-538X

Asokan, A., Conway, J. C., Phillips, J. L., Li, C., Hegge, J., Sinnott, R., Yadav, S., DiPrimio, N., Nam, H. J., Agbandje-McKenna, M., McPhee, S., Wolff, J. & Samulski, R. J. (2010). Reengineering a receptor footprint of adeno-associated virus enables selective and systemic gene transfer to muscle. *Nature Biotechnology*, Vol.28, No.1, pp. 79-82, ISSN 1546-1696

Atchison, R. W., Casto, B. C. & Hammon, W. M. (1965). Adenovirus-associated defective virus particles. *Science*, Vol.149, pp. 754-756, ISSN 0036-8075

Beaton, A., Palumbo, P. & Berns, K. I. (1989). Expression from the adeno-associated virus p5 and p19 promoters is negatively regulated in trans by the rep protein. *Journal of Virology*, Vol.63, No.10, pp. 4450-4454, ISSN 0022-538X

Berns, K. I. & Parrish C. R.. (2007). Parvoviridae, In *Fields VIROLOGY*, vol.2, 5th ed., D. M. Knipe, P. M. Howley, D. E. Griffin, R. A. Lamb, M. A. Martin, B. Roizman, and S. E. Straus (eds.), pp. 2437-2477, LIPPINCOTT WILLIAMS & WILKINS, ISBN 0-7817-1832-5, Philadelphia, PA.

Bernstein, K. A., Gangloff, S. & Rothstein, R. (2010). The recq DNA helicases in DNA repair. *Annual Review of Genetics*, Vol.44, pp. 393-417, ISSN 1545-2948

Berthet, C., Raj, K., Saudan, P. & Beard, P. (2005). How adeno-associated virus rep78 protein arrests cells completely in s phase. *Proceedings of the National Academy of Sciences of the United States of America*, Vol.102, No.38, pp. 13634-13639, ISSN 0027-8424

Boutin, S., Monteilhet, V., Veron, P., Leborgne, C., Benveniste, O., Montus, M. F. & Masurier, C. (2010). Prevalence of serum igg and neutralizing factors against adeno-associated virus (aav) types 1, 2, 5, 6, 8, and 9 in the healthy population: Implications for gene therapy using aav vectors. *Human Gene Therapy*, Vol.21, No.6, pp. 704-712, ISSN 1557-7422

Branzei, D. & Foiani, M. (2010). Maintaining genome stability at the replication fork. *Nature Reviews Molecular Cell Biology*, Vol.11, No.3, pp. 208-219, ISSN 1471-0080

Brister, J. R. & Muzyczka, N. (1999). Rep-mediated nicking of the adeno-associated virus origin requires two biochemical activities, DNA helicase activity and transesterification. *Journal of Virology*, Vol.73, No.11, pp. 9325-9336, ISSN 0022-538X

Burguete, T., Rabreau, M., Fontanges-Darriet, M., Roset, E., Hager, H. D., Koppel, A., Bischof, P. & Schlehofer, J. R. (1999). Evidence for infection of the human embryo with adeno-associated virus in pregnancy. *Human Reproduction*, Vol.14, No.9, pp. 2396-2401, ISSN 0268-1161

Calcedo, R., Vandenberghe, L. H., Gao, G., Lin, J. & Wilson, J. M. (2009). Worldwide epidemiology of neutralizing antibodies to adeno-associated viruses. *Journal of Infectious Diseases*, Vol.199, No.3, pp. 381-390, ISSN 0022-1899

The Role of DNA Repair Pathways in Adeno-Associated Virus Infection and Viral Genome
Replication / Recombination / Integration

93

Carson, C. T., Schwartz, R. A., Stracker, T. H., Lilley, C. E., Lee, D. V. & Weitzman, M. D. (2003). The mre11 complex is required for atm activation and the g2/m checkpoint. *EMBO Journal*, Vol.22, No.24, pp. 6610-6620, ISSN 0261-4189

Carter, B. J., Burstein, H. & Peluso, R. W. (2009). Adeno-associated virus and AAV vectors for gene delivery, In: Gene and cell therapy, N. S. Templeton, (ed.), pp. 115-157, CRC press, ISBN 978-0-8493-8768-5, Boca Raton, FL.

Castedo, M., Perfettini, J. L., Roumier, T., Andreau, K., Medema, R. & Kroemer, G. (2004). Cell death by mitotic catastrophe: A molecular definition. *Oncogene*, Vol.23, No.16, pp. 2825-2837, ISSN 0950-9232

Costello, E., Saudan, P., Winocour, E., Pizer, L. & Beard, P. (1997). High mobility group chromosomal protein 1 binds to the adeno-associated virus replication protein (rep) and promotes rep-mediated site-specific cleavage of DNA, atpase activity and transcriptional repression. EMBO Journal, Vol. 16, No. 19, pp. 5943-5954, ISSN 0261-4189

Cataldi, M. P. & McCarty, D. M. (2010). Differential effects of DNA double-strand break repair pathways on single-strand and self-complementary adeno-associated virus vector genomes. *Journal of Virology*, Vol.84, No.17, pp. 8673-8682, ISSN 1098-5514

Cervelli, T., Palacios, J. A., Zentilin, L., Mano, M., Schwartz, R. A., Weitzman, M. D. & Giacca, M. (2008). Processing of recombinant aav genomes occurs in specific nuclear structures that overlap with foci of DNA-damage-response proteins. *Journal of Cell Science*, Vol.121, No.Pt 3, pp. 349-357, ISSN 0021-9533

Chamberlain, J. R., Schwarze, U., Wang, P. R., Hirata, R. K., Hankenson, K. D., Pace, J. M., Underwood, R. A., Song, K. M., Sussman, M., Byers, P. H. & Russell, D. W. (2004). Gene targeting in stem cells from individuals with osteogenesis imperfecta. *Science*, Vol.303, No.5661, pp. 1198-1201, ISSN 1095-9203

Choi, V. W., McCarty, D. M. & Samulski, R. J. (2006). Host cell DNA repair pathways in adeno-associated viral genome processing. *Journal of Virology*, Vol.80, No.21, pp. 10346-10356, ISSN 0022-538X

Choi, Y. K., Nash, K., Byrne, B. J., Muzyczka, N. & Song, S. (2010). The effect of DNA-dependent protein kinase on adeno-associated virus replication. *PLoS ONE*, Vol.5, No.12, pp. e15073, ISSN 1932-6203

Collaco, R. F., Bevington, J. M., Bhrigu, V., Kalman-Maltese, V. & Trempe, J. P. (2009). Adeno-associated virus and adenovirus coinfection induces a cellular DNA damage and repair response via redundant phosphatidylinositol 3-like kinase pathways. *Virology*, Vol.392, No.1, pp. 24-33, ISSN 1096-0341

Daniel, R., Katz, R. A. & Skalka, A. M. (1999). A role for DNA-pk in retroviral DNA integration. *Science*, Vol.284, No.5414, pp. 644-647, ISSN 0036-8075

Daya, S., Cortez, N. & Berns, K. I. (2009). Adeno-associated virus site-specific integration is mediated by proteins of the nonhomologous end-joining pathway. *Journal of Virology*, Vol.83, No.22, pp. 11655-11664, ISSN 1098-5514

Deyle, D. R. & Russell, D. W. (2009). Adeno-associated virus vector integration. *Current Opinion Molecular Therapy*, Vol.11, No.4, pp. 442-447, ISSN 2040-3445

Donsante, A., Miller, D. G., Li, Y., Vogler, C., Brunt, E. M., Russell, D. W. & Sands, M. S. (2007). Aav vector integration sites in mouse hepatocellular carcinoma. *Science*, Vol.317, pp. 477, ISSN 1095-9203

Doostzadeh-Cizeron, J., Evans, R., Yin, S. & Goodrich, D. W. (1999). Apoptosis induced by the nuclear death domain protein p84n5 is inhibited by association with rb protein. *Molecular Biology of the Cell*, Vol.10, No.10, pp. 3251-3261, ISSN 1059-1524

Duan, D., Yan, Z., Yue, Y. & Engelhardt, J. F. (1999). Structural analysis of adeno-associated virus transduction circular intermediates. *Virology*, Vol.261, No.1, pp. 8-14, ISSN 0042-6822

Duan, D., Yue, Y. & Engelhardt, J. F. (2003). Consequences of DNA-dependent protein kinase catalytic subunit deficiency on recombinant adeno-associated virus genome circularization and heterodimerization in muscle tissue. *Journal of Virology*, Vol.77, No.8, pp. 4751-4759, ISSN 0022-538X

Erles, K., Sebokova, P. & Schlehofer, J. R. (1999). Update on the prevalence of serum antibodies (igg and igm) to adeno-associated virus (aav). *Journal of Medical Virology*, Vol.59, No.3, pp. 406-411, ISSN 0146-6615

Erles, K., Rohde, V., Thaele, M., Roth, S., Edler, L. & Schlehofer, J. R. (2001). DNA of adeno-associated virus (aav) in testicular tissue and in abnormal semen samples. *Human Reproduction*, Vol.16, No.11, pp. 2333-2337, ISSN 0268-1161

Evans, J. D. & Hearing, P. (2005). Relocalization of the mre11-rad50-nbs1 complex by the adenovirus e4 orf3 protein is required for viral replication. *Journal of Virology*, Vol.79, No.10, pp. 6207-6215, ISSN 0022-538X

Excoffon, K. J., Koerber, J. T., Dickey, D. D., Murtha, M., Keshavjee, S., Kaspar, B. K., Zabner, J. & Schaffer, D. V. (2009). Directed evolution of adeno-associated virus to an infectious respiratory virus. *Proceedings of the National Academy of Sciences of the United States of America*, Vol.106, No.10, pp. 3865-3870, ISSN 1091-6490

Fattah, F. J., Lichter, N. F., Fattah, K. R., Oh, S. & Hendrickson, E. A. (2008). Ku70, an essential gene, modulates the frequency of raav-mediated gene targeting in human somatic cells. *Proceedings of the National Academy of Sciences of the United States of America*, Vol.105, No.25, pp. 8703-8708, ISSN 1091-6490

Ferrari, F. K., Samulski, T., Shenk, T. & Samulski, R. J. (1996). Second-strand synthesis is a rate-limiting step for efficient transduction by recombinant adeno-associated virus vectors. *Journal of Virology*, Vol.70, No.5, pp. 3227-3234, ISSN 0022-538X

Fisher, K. J., Gao, G. P., Weitzman, M. D., DeMatteo, R., Burda, J. F. & Wilson, J. M. (1996). Transduction with recombinant adeno-associated virus for gene therapy is limited by leading-strand synthesis. *Journal of Virology*, Vol.70, No.1, pp. 520-532, ISSN 0022-538X

Foust, K. D., Nurre, E., Montgomery, C. L., Hernandez, A., Chan, C. M. & Kaspar, B. K. (2009). Intravascular aav9 preferentially targets neonatal neurons and adult astrocytes. *Nature Biotechnology*, Vol.27, No.1, pp. 59-65, ISSN 1546-1696

Fragkos, M., Breuleux, M., Clement, N. & Beard, P. (2008). Recombinant adeno-associated viral vectors are deficient in provoking a DNA damage response. *Journal of Virology*, Vol.82, No.15, pp. 7379-7387, ISSN 1098-5514

Francois, A., Guilbaud, M., Awedikian, R., Chadeuf, G., Moullier, P. & Salvetti, A. (2005). The cellular tata binding protein is required for rep-dependent replication of a minimal adeno-associated virus type 2 p5 element. *Journal of Virology*, Vol.79, No.17, pp. 11082-11094, ISSN 0022-538X

Gao, G., Vandenberghe, L. H., Alvira, M. R., Lu, Y., Calcedo, R., Zhou, X. & Wilson, J. M. (2004). Clades of adeno-associated viruses are widely disseminated in human tissues. *Journal of Virology*, Vol.78, No.12, pp. 6381-6388, ISSN 0022-538X

The Role of DNA Repair Pathways in Adeno-Associated Virus Infection and Viral Genome
Replication / Recombination / Integration

95

Gao, G. P., Alvira, M. R., Wang, L., Calcedo, R., Johnston, J. & Wilson, J. M. (2002). Novel adeno-associated viruses from rhesus monkeys as vectors for human gene therapy. *Proc. Natl. Acad. Sci. U.S.A.*, Vol.99, No.18, pp. 11854-11859, ISSN 0027-8424

Garner, E., Martinon, F., Tschopp, J., Beard, P. & Raj, K. (2007). Cells with defective p53-p21-prb pathway are susceptible to apoptosis induced by p84n5 via caspase-6. *Cancer Research*, Vol.67, No.16, pp. 7631-7637, ISSN 0008-5472

Geoffroy, M. C. & Salvetti, A. (2005). Helper functions required for wild type and recombinant adeno-associated virus growth. *Current Gene Therapy*, Vol.5, No.3, pp. 265-271, ISSN 1566-5232

Ghosh, A., Yue, Y., Long, C., Bostick, B. & Duan, D. (2007). Efficient whole-body transduction with trans-splicing adeno-associated viral vectors. *Molecular Therapy*, Vol.15, No.4, pp. 750-755, ISSN 1525-0016

Harper, J. W. & Elledge, S. J. (2007). The DNA damage response: Ten years after. *Molecular Cell*, Vol.28, No.5, pp. 739-745, ISSN 1097-2765

Hauck, B., Zhao, W., High, K. & Xiao, W. (2004). Intracellular viral processing, not single-stranded DNA accumulation, is crucial for recombinant adeno-associated virus transduction. *Journal of Virology*, Vol.78, No.24, pp. 13678-13686, ISSN 0022-538X

Henckaerts, E. & Linden, R. M. (2010). Adeno-associated virus: A key to the human genome? *Future Virology*, Vol.5, No.5, pp. 555-574, ISSN 1746-0808

Hendrie, P. C., Hirata, R. K. & Russell, D. W. (2003). Chromosomal integration and homologous gene targeting by replication-incompetent vectors based on the autonomous parvovirus minute virus of mice. *Journal of Virology*, Vol.77, No.24, pp. 13136-13145, ISSN 0022-538X

Hendrie, P. C. & Russell, D. W. (2005). Gene targeting with viral vectors. *Molecular Therapy*, Vol.12, No.1, pp. 9-17, ISSN 1525-0016

Hermanns, J., Schulze, A., Jansen-Db1urr, P., Kleinschmidt, J. A., Schmidt, R. & zur Hausen, H. (1997). Infection of primary cells by adeno-associated virus type 2 results in a modulation of cell cycle-regulating proteins. *Journal of Virology*, Vol.71, No.8, pp. 6020-6027, ISSN 0022-538X

Hirata, R. K. & Russell, D. W. (2000). Design and packaging of adeno-associated virus gene targeting vectors. *Journal of Virology*, Vol.74, No.10, pp. 4612-4620, ISSN 0022-538X

Hirsch, M. L., Green, L., Porteus, M. H. & Samulski, R. J. (2010). Self-complementary aav mediates gene targeting and enhances endonuclease delivery for double-strand break repair. *Gene Therapy*, Vol.17, No.9, pp. 1175-1180, ISSN 1476-5462

Inagaki, K., Fuess, S., Storm, T. A., Gibson, G. A., McTiernan, C. F., Kay, M. A. & Nakai, H. (2006). Robust systemic transduction with aav9 vectors in mice: Efficient global cardiac gene transfer superior to that of aav8. *Molecular Therapy*, Vol.14, No.1, pp. 45-53, ISSN 1525-0016

Inagaki, K., Lewis, S. M., Wu, X., Ma, C., Munroe, D. J., Fuess, S., Storm, T. A., Kay, M. A. & Nakai, H. (2007a). DNA palindromes with a modest arm length of greater, similar 20 base pairs are a significant target for recombinant adeno-associated virus vector integration in the liver, muscles, and heart in mice. *Journal of Virology*, Vol.81, No.20, pp. 11290-11303, ISSN 0022-538X

Inagaki, K., Ma, C., Storm, T. A., Kay, M. A. & Nakai, H. (2007b). The role of DNA-pkcs and artemis in opening viral DNA hairpin termini in various tissues in mice. *Journal of Virology*, Vol.81, No.20, pp. 11304-11321, ISSN 0022-538X

Inagaki, K., Piao, C., Kotchey, N. M., Wu, X. & Nakai, H. (2008). Frequency and spectrum of genomic integration of recombinant adeno-associated virus serotype 8 vector in neonatal mouse liver. *Journal of Virology*, Vol.82, No.19, pp. 9513-9524, ISSN 1098-5514

Ingemarsdotter, C., Keller, D. & Beard, P. (2010). The DNA damage response to non-replicating adeno-associated virus: Centriole overduplication and mitotic catastrophe independent of the spindle checkpoint. *Virology*, Vol.400, No.2, pp. 271-286, ISSN 1096-0341

Jayaram, S., Gilson, T., Ehrlich, E. S., Yu, X. F., Ketner, G. & Hanakahi, L. (2008). E1b 55k-independent dissociation of the DNA ligase iv/xrcc4 complex by e4 34k during adenovirus infection. *Virology*, Vol.382, No.2, pp. 163-170, ISSN 1096-0341

Jurvansuu, J., Raj, K., Stasiak, A. & Beard, P. (2005). Viral transport of DNA damage that mimics a stalled replication fork. *Journal of Virology*, Vol.79, No.1, pp. 569-580, ISSN 0022-538X

Jurvansuu, J., Fragkos, M., Ingemarsdotter, C. & Beard, P. (2007). Chk1 instability is coupled to mitotic cell death of p53-deficient cells in response to virus-induced DNA damage signaling. *Journal of Molecular Biology*, Vol.372, No.2, pp. 397-406, ISSN 0022-2836

Khan, I. F., Hirata, R. K. & Russell, D. W. (2011). Aav-mediated gene targeting methods for human cells. *Nature Protocol*, Vol.6, No.4, pp. 482-501, ISSN 1750-2799

Koerber, J. T., Klimczak, R., Jang, J. H., Dalkara, D., Flannery, J. G. & Schaffer, D. V. (2009). Molecular evolution of adeno-associated virus for enhanced glial gene delivery. *Molecular Therapy*, Vol.17, No.12, pp. 2088-2095, ISSN 1525-0024

Kotin, R. M., Siniscalco, M., Samulski, R. J., Zhu, X. D., Hunter, L., Laughlin, C. A., McLaughlin, S., Muzyczka, N., Rocchi, M. & Berns, K. I. (1990). Site-specific integration by adeno-associated virus. *Proceedings of the National Academy of Sciences of the United States of America*, Vol.87, No.6, pp. 2211-2215, ISSN 0027-8424

Kotin, R. M., Linden, R. M. & Berns, K. I. (1992). Characterization of a preferred site on human chromosome 19q for integration of adeno-associated virus DNA by non-homologous recombination. EMBO Journal, Vol. 11, No. 13, pp. 5071-5078, ISSN 0261-4189

Kyostio, S. R., Owens, R. A., Weitzman, M. D., Antoni, B. A., Chejanovsky, N. & Carter, B. J. (1994). Analysis of adeno-associated virus (aav) wild-type and mutant rep proteins for their abilities to negatively regulate aav p5 and p19 mrna levels. *Journal of Virology*, Vol.68, No.5, pp. 2947-2957, ISSN 0022-538X

Li, L., Olvera, J. M., Yoder, K. E., Mitchell, R. S., Butler, S. L., Lieber, M., Martin, S. L. & Bushman, F. D. (2001). Role of the non-homologous DNA end joining pathway in the early steps of retroviral infection. *EMBO Journal*, Vol.20, No.12, pp. 3272-3281, ISSN 0261-4189

Lilley, C. E., Schwartz, R. A. & Weitzman, M. D. (2007). Using or abusing: Viruses and the cellular DNA damage response. *Trends in Microbiology*, Vol.15, No.3, pp. 119-126, ISSN 0966-842X

Linden, R. M., Ward, P., Giraud, C., Winocour, E. & Berns, K. I. (1996a). Site-specific integration by adeno-associated virus. *Proceedings of the National Academy of Sciences of the United States of America*, Vol.93, No.21, pp. 11288-11294, ISSN 0027-8424

Linden, R. M., Winocour, E. & Berns, K. I. (1996b). The recombination signals for adeno-associated virus site-specific integration. *Proceedings of the National Academy of Sciences of the United States of America*, Vol.93, No.15, pp. 7966-7972, ISSN 0027-8424

Liu, X., Yan, Z., Luo, M., Zak, R., Li, Z., Driskell, R. R., Huang, Y., Tran, N. & Engelhardt, J. F. (2004). Targeted correction of single-base-pair mutations with adeno-associated virus

The Role of DNA Repair Pathways in Adeno-Associated Virus Infection and Viral Genome
Replication / Recombination / Integration

97

vectors under nonselective conditions. *Journal of Virology*, Vol.78, No.8, pp. 4165-4175, ISSN 0022-538X

Ma, Y., Schwarz, K. & Lieber, M. R. (2005). The artemis:DNA-pkcs endonuclease cleaves DNA loops, flaps, and gaps. *DNA Repair*, Vol.4, No.7, pp. 845-851, ISSN 1568-7864

McCaffrey, A. P., Fawcett, P., Nakai, H., McCaffrey, R. L., Ehrhardt, A., Pham, T. T., Pandey, K., Xu, H., Feuss, S., Storm, T. A. & Kay, M. A. (2008). The host response to adenovirus, helper-dependent adenovirus, and adeno-associated virus in mouse liver. *Molecular Therapy*, Vol.16, No.5, pp. 931-941, ISSN 1525-0024

McCarty, D. M., Pereira, D. J., Zolotukhin, I., Zhou, X., Ryan, J. H. & Muzyczka, N. (1994). Identification of linear DNA sequences that specifically bind the adeno- associated virus rep protein. *Journal of Virology*, Vol.68, No.8, pp. 4988-4997, ISSN 0022-538X

McCarty, D. M., Fu, H., Monahan, P. E., Toulson, C. E., Naik, P. & Samulski, R. J. (2003). Adeno-associated virus terminal repeat (tr) mutant generates self-complementary vectors to overcome the rate-limiting step to transduction *in vivo*. *Gene Therapy*, Vol.10, No.26, pp. 2112-2118, ISSN 0969-7128

McCarty, D. M., Young, S. M., Jr. & Samulski, R. J. (2004). Integration of adeno-associated virus (aav) and recombinant aav vectors. *Annual Review of Genetics*, Vol.38, pp. 819-845, ISSN 0066-4197

McCarty, D. M. (2008). Self-complementary aav vectors; advances and applications. *Molecular Therapy*, Vol.16, No.10, pp. 1648-1656, ISSN 1525-0024

Miller, D. G., Petek, L. M. & Russell, D. W. (2003). Human gene targeting by adeno-associated virus vectors is enhanced by DNA double-strand breaks. *Molecular and Cellular Biology*, Vol.23, No.10, pp. 3550-3557, ISSN 0270-7306

Miller, D. G., Petek, L. M. & Russell, D. W. (2004). Adeno-associated virus vectors integrate at chromosome breakage sites. *Nature Genetics*, Vol.36, No.7, pp. 767-773, ISSN 1061-4036

Miller, D. G., Trobridge, G. D., Petek, L. M., Jacobs, M. A., Kaul, R. & Russell, D. W. (2005). Large-scale analysis of adeno-associated virus vector integration sites in normal human cells. *Journal of Virology*, Vol.79, No.17, pp. 11434-11442, ISSN 0022-538X

Mirzoeva, O. K. & Petrini, J. H. (2003). DNA replication-dependent nuclear dynamics of the mre11 complex. *Molecular Cancer Research*, Vol.1, No.3, pp. 207-218, ISSN 1541-7786

Nakai, H., Storm, T. A. & Kay, M. A. (2000). Recruitment of single-stranded recombinant adeno-associated virus vector genomes and intermolecular recombination are responsible for stable transduction of liver *in vivo*. *Journal of Virology*, Vol.74, No.20, pp. 9451-9463, ISSN 0022-538X

Nakai, H., Yant, S. R., Storm, T. A., Fuess, S., Meuse, L. & Kay, M. A. (2001). Extrachromosomal recombinant adeno-associated virus vector genomes are primarily responsible for stable liver transduction *in vivo*. *Journal of Virology*, Vol.75, No.15, pp. 6969-6976, ISSN 0022-538X

Nakai, H., Thomas, C. E., Storm, T. A., Fuess, S., Powell, S., Wright, J. F. & Kay, M. A. (2002). A limited number of transducible hepatocytes restricts a wide-range linear vector dose response in recombinant adeno-associated virus-mediated liver transduction. *Journal of Virology*, Vol.76, No.22, pp. 11343-11349, ISSN 0022-538X

Nakai, H., Montini, E., Fuess, S., Storm, T. A., Grompe, M. & Kay, M. A. (2003a). Aav serotype 2 vectors preferentially integrate into active genes in mice. *Nature Genetics*, Vol.34, No.3, pp. 297-302, ISSN 1061-4036

Nakai, H., Storm, T. A., Fuess, S. & Kay, M. A. (2003b). Pathways of removal of free DNA vector ends in normal and DNA-pkcs-deficient scid mouse hepatocytes transduced with raav vectors. *Human Gene Therapy*, Vol.14, No.9, pp. 871-881, ISSN 1043-0342

Nakai, H., Fuess, S., Storm, T. A., Muramatsu, S., Nara, Y. & Kay, M. A. (2005a). Unrestricted hepatocyte transduction with adeno-associated virus serotype 8 vectors in mice. *Journal of Virology*, Vol.79, No.1, pp. 214-224, ISSN 0022-538X

Nakai, H., Wu, X., Fuess, S., Storm, T. A., Munroe, D., Montini, E., Burgess, S. M., Grompe, M. & Kay, M. A. (2005b). Large-scale molecular characterization of adeno-associated virus vector integration in mouse liver. *Journal of Virology*, Vol.79, No.6, pp. 3606-3614, ISSN 0022-538X

Nash, K., Chen, W., McDonald, W. F., Zhou, X. & Muzyczka, N. (2007). Purification of host cell enzymes involved in adeno-associated virus DNA replication. *Journal of Virology*, Vol.81, No.11, pp. 5777-5787, ISSN 0022-538X

Nash, K., Chen, W., Salganik, M. & Muzyczka, N. (2009). Identification of cellular proteins that interact with the adeno-associated virus rep protein. *Journal of Virology*, Vol.83, No.1, pp. 454-469, ISSN 1098-5514

Nathwani, A. C., Rosales, C., McIntosh, J., Rastegarlari, G., Nathwani, D., Raj, D., Nawathe, S., Waddington, S. N., Bronson, R., Jackson, S., Donahue, R. E., High, K. A., Mingozzi, F., Ng, C. Y., Zhou, J., Spence, Y., McCarville, M. B., Valentine, M., Allay, J., Coleman, J., Sleep, S., Gray, J. T., Nienhuis, A. W. & Davidoff, A. M. (2011). Long-term safety and efficacy following systemic administration of a self-complementary aav vector encoding human fix pseudotyped with serotype 5 and 8 capsid proteins. *Molecular Therapy*, pp., ISSN 1525-0024

Nony, P., Tessier, J., Chadeuf, G., Ward, P., Giraud, A., Dugast, M., Linden, R. M., Moullier, P. & Salvetti, A. (2001). Novel cis-acting replication element in the adeno-associated virus type 2 genome is involved in amplification of integrated rep-cap sequences. *Journal of Virology*, Vol.75, No.20, pp. 9991-9994, ISSN 0022-538X

Penaud-Budloo, M., Le Guiner, C., Nowrouzi, A., Toromanoff, A., Cherel, Y., Chenuaud, P., Schmidt, M., von Kalle, C., Rolling, F., Moullier, P. & Snyder, R. O. (2008). Adeno-associated virus vector genomes persist as episomal chromatin in primate muscle. *Journal of Virology*, Vol.82, No.16, pp. 7875-7885, ISSN 1098-5514

Pereira, C. C., de Freitas, L. B., de Vargas, P. R., de Azevedo, M. L., do Nascimento, J. P. & Spano, L. C. (2010). Molecular detection of adeno-associated virus in cases of spontaneous and intentional human abortion. *Journal of Medical Virology*, Vol.82, No.10, pp. 1689-1693, ISSN 1096-9071

Petek, L. M., Russell, D. W. & Miller, D. G. (2010). Frequent endonuclease cleavage at off-target locations *in vivo*. *Molecular Therapy*, Vol.18, No.5, pp. 983-986, ISSN 1525-0024

Philpott, N. J., Gomos, J., Berns, K. I. & Falck-Pedersen, E. (2002). A p5 integration efficiency element mediates rep-dependent integration into aavs1 at chromosome 19. *Proceedings of the National Academy of Sciences of the United States of America*, Vol.99, No.19, pp. 12381-12385, ISSN 0027-8424

Porteus, M. H., Cathomen, T., Weitzman, M. D. & Baltimore, D. (2003). Efficient gene targeting mediated by adeno-associated virus and DNA double-strand breaks. *Molecular and Cellular Biology*, Vol.23, No.10, pp. 3558-3565, ISSN 0270-7306

Qing, K., Hansen, J., Weigel-Kelley, K. A., Tan, M., Zhou, S. & Srivastava, A. (2001). Adeno-associated virus type 2-mediated gene transfer: Role of cellular fkbp52 protein in

The Role of DNA Repair Pathways in Adeno-Associated Virus Infection and Viral Genome
Replication / Recombination / Integration

99

transgene expression. *Journal of Virology*, Vol.75, No.19, pp. 8968-8976, ISSN 0022-538X

Qing, K., Li, W., Zhong, L., Tan, M., Hansen, J., Weigel-Kelley, K. A., Chen, L., Yoder, M. C. & Srivastava, A. (2003). Adeno-associated virus type 2-mediated gene transfer: Role of cellular t-cell protein tyrosine phosphatase in transgene expression in established cell lines *in vitro* and transgenic mice *in vivo*. *Journal of Virology*, Vol.77, No.4, pp. 2741-2746, ISSN 0022-538X

Rabinowitz, J. E., Rolling, F., Li, C., Conrath, H., Xiao, W., Xiao, X. & Samulski, R. J. (2002). Cross-packaging of a single adeno-associated virus (aav) type 2 vector genome into multiple aav serotypes enables transduction with broad specificity. *Journal of Virology*, Vol.76, No.2, pp. 791-801, ISSN 0022-538X

Raj, K., Ogston, P. & Beard, P. (2001). Virus-mediated killing of cells that lack p53 activity. *Nature*, Vol.412, No.6850, pp. 914-917, ISSN 0028-0836

Rooney, S., Sekiguchi, J., Zhu, C., Cheng, H. L., Manis, J., Whitlow, S., DeVido, J., Foy, D., Chaudhuri, J., Lombard, D. & Alt, F. W. (2002). Leaky scid phenotype associated with defective v(d)j coding end processing in artemis-deficient mice. *Molecular Cell*, Vol.10, No.6, pp. 1379-1390, ISSN 1097-2765

Roth, D. B., Menetski, J. P., Nakajima, P. B., Bosma, M. J. & Gellert, M. (1992). V(d)j recombination: Broken DNA molecules with covalently sealed (hairpin) coding ends in scid mouse thymocytes. *Cell*, Vol.70, No.6, pp. 983-991, ISSN 0092-8674

Russell, D. W., Miller, A. D. & Alexander, I. E. (1994). Adeno-associated virus vectors preferentially transduce cells in s phase. *Proceedings of the National Academy of Sciences of the United States of America*, Vol.91, No.19, pp. 8915-8919, ISSN 0027-8424

Russell, D. W., Alexander, I. E. & Miller, A. D. (1995). DNA synthesis and topoisomerase inhibitors increase transduction by adeno-associated virus vectors. *Proceedings of the National Academy of Sciences of the United States of America*, Vol.92, No.12, pp. 5719-5723, ISSN 0027-8424

Russell, D. W. & Hirata, R. K. (1998). Human gene targeting by viral vectors [see comments]. *Nature Genetics*, Vol.18, No.4, pp. 325-330, ISSN 1061-4036

Samulski, R. J., Berns, K. I., Tan, M. & Muzyczka, N. (1982). Cloning of adeno-associated virus into pbr322: Rescue of intact virus from the recombinant plasmid in human cells. Proceedings of the National Academy of Sciences of the United States of America, Vol. 79, No. 6, pp. 2077-2081,ISSN 0027-8424

Samulski, R. J., Zhu, X., Xiao, X., Brook, J. D., Housman, D. E., Epstein, N. & Hunter, L. A. (1991). Targeted integration of adeno-associated virus (aav) into human chromosome 19 [published erratum appears in embo j 1992 mar;11(3):1228]. *EMBO Journal*, Vol.10, No.12, pp. 3941-3950, ISSN 0261-4189

Sanlioglu, S., Benson, P. & Engelhardt, J. F. (2000). Loss of atm function enhances recombinant adeno-associated virus transduction and integration through pathways similar to uv irradiation. *Virology*, Vol.268, No.1, pp. 68-78, ISSN 0042-6822

Sarkar, R., Mucci, M., Addya, S., Tetreault, R., Bellinger, D. A., Nichols, T. C. & Kazazian, H. H., Jr. (2006). Long-term efficacy of adeno-associated virus serotypes 8 and 9 in hemophilia a dogs and mice. *Human Gene Therapy*, Vol.17, No.4, pp. 427-439, ISSN 1043-0342

Saudan, P., Vlach, J. & Beard, P. (2000). Inhibition of s-phase progression by adeno-associated virus rep78 protein is mediated by hypophosphorylated prb. *EMBO Journal*, Vol.19, No.16, pp. 4351-4361, ISSN 0261-4189

Schnepp, B. C., Jensen, R. L., Chen, C. L., Johnson, P. R. & Clark, K. R. (2005). Characterization of adeno-associated virus genomes isolated from human tissues. *Journal of Virology,* Vol.79, No.23, pp. 14793-14803, ISSN 0022-538X

Schultz, B. R. & Chamberlain, J. S. (2008). Recombinant adeno-associated virus transduction and integration. *Molecular Therapy,* Vol.16, No.7, pp. 1189-1199, ISSN 1525-0024

Schwartz, R. A., Palacios, J. A., Cassell, G. D., Adam, S., Giacca, M. & Weitzman, M. D. (2007). The mre11/rad50/nbs1 complex limits adeno-associated virus transduction and replication. *Journal of Virology,* Vol.81, No.23, pp. 12936-12945, ISSN 1098-5514

Schwartz, R. A., Carson, C. T., Schuberth, C. & Weitzman, M. D. (2009). Adeno-associated virus replication induces a DNA damage response coordinated by DNA-dependent protein kinase. *Journal of Virology,* Vol.83, No.12, pp. 6269-6278, ISSN 1098-5514

Shiotani, B. & Zou, L. (2009). Atr signaling at a glance. *Journal of Cell Science,* Vol.122, No.Pt 3, pp. 301-304, ISSN 0021-9533

Smith, R. H. & Kotin, R. M. (2002). Adeno-associated virus, In: Mobile DNA II, N. L. Craig, R. Craigie, M. Gellert, A. M. Lambowitz (eds.), pp. 905-923, ASM press, ISBN 1-55581-209-0, Herndon, VA.

Song, S., Laipis, P. J., Berns, K. I. & Flotte, T. R. (2001). Effect of DNA-dependent protein kinase on the molecular fate of the raav2 genome in skeletal muscle. *Proceedings of the National Academy of Sciences of the United States of America,* Vol.98, No.7, pp. 4084-4088, ISSN 0027-8424

Song, S., Lu, Y., Choi, Y. K., Han, Y., Tang, Q., Zhao, G., Berns, K. I. & Flotte, T. R. (2004). DNA-dependent pk inhibits adeno-associated virus DNA integration. *Proceedings of the National Academy of Sciences of the United States of America,* Vol.101, No.7, pp. 2112-2116, ISSN 0027-8424

Sonntag, F., Schmidt, K. & Kleinschmidt, J. A. (2010). A viral assembly factor promotes aav2 capsid formation in the nucleolus. *Proceedings of the National Academy of Sciences of the United States of America,* Vol.107, No.22, pp. 10220-10225, ISSN 1091-6490

Stracker, T. H., Carson, C. T. & Weitzman, M. D. (2002). Adenovirus oncoproteins inactivate the mre11-rad50-nbs1 DNA repair complex. *Nature,* Vol.418, No.6895, pp. 348-352, ISSN 0028-0836

Strickler, H. D., Viscidi, R., Escoffery, C., Rattray, C., Kotloff, K. L., Goldberg, J., Manns, A., Rabkin, C., Daniel, R., Hanchard, B., Brown, C., Hutchinson, M., Zanizer, D., Palefsky, J., Burk, R. D., Cranston, B., Clayman, B. & Shah, K. V. (1999). Adeno-associated virus and development of cervical neoplasia. *Journal of Medical Virology,* Vol.59, No.1, pp. 60-65, ISSN 0146-6615

Su, P. F. & Wu, F. Y. (1996). Differential suppression of the tumorigenicity of hela and siha cells by adeno-associated virus. *British Journal of Cancer,* Vol.73, No.12, pp. 1533-1537, ISSN 0007-0920

Summerford, C. & Samulski, R. J. (1998). Membrane-associated heparan sulfate proteoglycan is a receptor for adeno-associated virus type 2 virions. *Journal of Virology,* Vol.72, No.2, pp. 1438-1445, ISSN 0022-538X

Sun, X., Yan, Z., Yi, Y., Li, Z., Lei, D., Rogers, C. S., Chen, J., Zhang, Y., Welsh, M. J., Leno, G. H. & Engelhardt, J. F. (2008). Adeno-associated virus-targeted disruption of the cftr gene in cloned ferrets. *Journal of Clinical Investigation,* Vol.118, No.4, pp. 1578-1583, ISSN 0021-9738

Tan, I., Ng, C. H., Lim, L. & Leung, T. (2001). Phosphorylation of a novel myosin binding subunit of protein phosphatase 1 reveals a conserved mechanism in the regulation of

The Role of DNA Repair Pathways in Adeno-Associated Virus Infection and Viral Genome
Replication / Recombination / Integration

101

actin cytoskeleton. *Journal of Biological Chemistry*, Vol.276, No.24, pp. 21209-21216, ISSN 0021-9258

Thomas, K. R. & Capecchi, M. R. (1987). Site-directed mutagenesis by gene targeting in mouse embryo-derived stem cells. *Cell*, Vol.51, No.3, pp. 503-512, ISSN 0092-8674

Torres-Ramos, C. A., Prakash, S. & Prakash, L. (1997). Requirement of yeast DNA polymerase delta in post-replicational repair of uv-damaged DNA. *Journal of Biological Chemistry*, Vol.272, No.41, pp. 25445-25448, ISSN 0021-9258

Trobridge, G., Hirata, R. K. & Russell, D. W. (2005). Gene targeting by adeno-associated virus vectors is cell-cycle dependent. *Human Gene Therapy*, Vol.16, No.4, pp. 522-526, ISSN 1043-0342

Tullis, G. E. & Shenk, T. (2000). Efficient replication of adeno-associated virus type 2 vectors: A cis-acting element outside of the terminal repeats and a minimal size. *Journal of Virology*, Vol.74, No.24, pp. 11511-11521, ISSN 0022-538X

Vakifahmetoglu, H., Olsson, M. & Zhivotovsky, B. (2008). Death through a tragedy: Mitotic catastrophe. *Cell Death and Differentiation*, Vol.15, No.7, pp. 1153-1162, ISSN 1350-9047

Vandendriessche, T., Thorrez, L., Acosta-Sanchez, A., Petrus, I., Wang, L., Ma, L., L, D. E. W., Iwasaki, Y., Gillijns, V., Wilson, J. M., Collen, D. & Chuah, M. K. (2007). Efficacy and safety of adeno-associated viral vectors based on serotype 8 and 9 vs. Lentiviral vectors for hemophilia b gene therapy. *Journal of Thrombosis Haemostasis*, Vol.5, No.1, pp. 16-24, ISSN 1538-7933

Vasileva, A. & Jessberger, R. (2005). Precise hit: Adeno-associated virus in gene targeting. *Nature Reviews: Microbiology*, Vol.3, No.11, pp. 837-847, ISSN 1740-1526

Vasileva, A., Linden, R. M. & Jessberger, R. (2006). Homologous recombination is required for aav-mediated gene targeting. *Nucleic Acids Res*, Vol.34, No.11, pp. 3345-3360, ISSN 1362-4962

Walz, C. & Schlehofer, J. R. (1992). Modification of some biological properties of hela cells containing adeno-associated virus DNA integrated into chromosome 17. *Journal of Virology*, Vol.66, No.5, pp. 2990-3002, ISSN 0022-538X

Wang, Z., Ma, H. I., Li, J., Sun, L., Zhang, J. & Xiao, X. (2003). Rapid and highly efficient transduction by double-stranded adeno-associated virus vectors *in vitro* and *in vivo*. *Gene Therapy*, Vol.10, No.26, pp. 2105-2111, ISSN 0969-7128

Wang, Z., Zhu, T., Qiao, C., Zhou, L., Wang, B., Zhang, J., Chen, C., Li, J. & Xiao, X. (2005). Adeno-associated virus serotype 8 efficiently delivers genes to muscle and heart. *Nature Biotechnology*, Vol.23, No.3, pp. 321-328, ISSN 1087-0156

Weitzman, M. D., Carson, C. T., Schwartz, R. A. & Lilley, C. E. (2004). Interactions of viruses with the cellular DNA repair machinery. *DNA Repair*, Vol.3, No.8-9, pp. 1165-1173, ISSN 1568-7864

Weitzman, M. D., Lilley, C. E. & Chaurushiya, M. S. (2010). Genomes in conflict: Maintaining genome integrity during virus infection. *Annual Review of Microbiology*, Vol.64, pp. 61-81, ISSN 1545-3251

Williams, G. J., Lees-Miller, S. P. & Tainer, J. A. (2010). Mre11-rad50-nbs1 conformations and the control of sensing, signaling, and effector responses at DNA double-strand breaks. *DNA Repair*, Vol.9, No.12, pp. 1299-1306, ISSN 1568-7856

Winocour, E., Callaham, M. F. & Huberman, E. (1988). Perturbation of the cell cycle by adeno-associated virus. *Virology*, Vol.167, No.2, pp. 393-399, ISSN 0042-6822

Xiao, X., Xiao, W., Li, J. & Samulski, R. J. (1997). A novel 165-base-pair terminal repeat sequence is the sole cis requirement for the adeno-associated virus life cycle. *Journal of Virology*, Vol.71, No.2, pp. 941-948, ISSN 0022-538X

Yakinoglu, A. O., Heilbronn, R., Burkle, A., Schlehofer, J. R. & zur Hausen, H. (1988). DNA amplification of adeno-associated virus as a response to cellular genotoxic stress. *Cancer Research*, Vol.48, No.11, pp. 3123-3129, ISSN 0008-5472

Yakobson, B., Koch, T. & Winocour, E. (1987). Replication of adeno-associated virus in synchronized cells without the addition of a helper virus. *Journal of Virology*, Vol.61, No.4, pp. 972-981, ISSN 0022-538X

Yakobson, B., Hrynko, T. A., Peak, M. J. & Winocour, E. (1989). Replication of adeno-associated virus in cells irradiated with uv light at 254 nm. *Journal of Virology*, Vol.63, No.3, pp. 1023-1030, ISSN 0022-538X

Yamamoto, N., Suzuki, M., Kawano, M. A., Inoue, T., Takahashi, R. U., Tsukamoto, H., Enomoto, T., Yamaguchi, Y., Wada, T. & Handa, H. (2007). Adeno-associated virus site-specific integration is regulated by trp-185. Journal of Virology, Vol. 81, No. 4, pp. 1990-2001, ISSN 0022-538X

Yan, Z., Lei-Butters, D. C., Zhang, Y., Zak, R. & Engelhardt, J. F. (2007). Hybrid adeno-associated virus bearing nonhomologous inverted terminal repeats enhances dual-vector reconstruction of minigenes *in vivo*. *Human Gene Therapy*, Vol.18, No.1, pp. 81-87, ISSN 1043-0342

Yang, L., Jiang, J., Drouin, L. M., Agbandje-McKenna, M., Chen, C., Qiao, C., Pu, D., Hu, X., Wang, D. Z., Li, J. & Xiao, X. (2009). A myocardium tropic adeno-associated virus (aav) evolved by DNA shuffling and *in vivo* selection. *Proceedings of the National Academy of Sciences of the United States of America*, Vol.106, No.10, pp. 3946-3951, ISSN 1091-6490

Yang, Q., Chen, F. & Trempe, J. P. (1994). Characterization of cell lines that inducibly express the adeno- associated virus rep proteins. *Journal of Virology*, Vol.68, No.8, pp. 4847-4856, ISSN 0022-538X

Zentilin, L., Marcello, A. & Giacca, M. (2001). Involvement of cellular double-stranded DNA break binding proteins in processing of the recombinant adeno-associated virus genome. *Journal of Virology*, Vol.75, No.24, pp. 12279-12287, ISSN 0022-538X

Zhong, L., Zhou, X., Li, Y., Qing, K., Xiao, X., Samulski, R. J. & Srivastava, A. (2008). Single-polarity recombinant adeno-associated virus 2 vector-mediated transgene expression *in vitro* and *in vivo*: Mechanism of transduction. *Molecular Therapy*, Vol.16, No.2, pp. 290-295, ISSN 1525-0024

Zhou, X., Zeng, X., Fan, Z., Li, C., McCown, T., Samulski, R. J. & Xiao, X. (2008). Adeno-associated virus of a single-polarity DNA genome is capable of transduction *in vivo*. *Molecular Therapy*, Vol.16, No.3, pp. 494-499, ISSN 1525-0024

6

Non-Steroidal Anti-Inflammatory Drugs, DNA Repair and Cancer

Harpreet K. Dibra, Chris J. Perry and Iain D. Nicholl
University of Wolverhampton
UK

1. Introduction

Colorectal cancer is the third most common cancer in women and fourth in men, with respect to incidence, and 529,000 deaths occurred worldwide in 2002 (Parkin *et al.*, 2005). Approximately 2 - 5% of cases of colorectal cancer are due to a genetic predisposition of which the most common is hereditary non-polyposis colorectal cancer (HNPCC). HNPCC is an autosomal dominant disorder with high penetrance and exhibits allelic and locus heterogeneity (Aarnio *et al.*, 1995; de la Chapelle, 2004; Dunlop *et al.*, 1997). In HNPCC there are heterozygous germline mutations in the DNA mismatch repair (MMR) genes MutS homologue 2 (*MSH2*), MutL homologue 1 (*MLH1*), MutS homologue 6 (*MSH6*), post-meiotic segregation increased 2 (*PMS2*) and post-meiotic segregation increased 1 (*PMS1*) (Bocker *et al.*, 1999; Buermeyer *et al.*, 1999; Jiricny, 1998; Jiricny & Marra, 2003; Lucci-Cordisco *et al.*, 2003; Mitchell *et al.*, 2002; Narayan & Roy, 2003; Nicolaides *et al.*, 1998; Plaschke *et al.*, 2004; Zabkiewicz & Clarke, 2004). Germline mutations in *hMLH1* and *hMSH2* are the most common with abnormalities in these genes found in more than 90% of HNPCC mutation carriers (Abdel-Rahman *et al.*, 2006; de la Chapelle, 2004; Hampel *et al.*, 2005; Lagerstedt Robinson *et al.*, 2007). The phenomenon of transmission of an epimutation in hMLH1 has also been reported (Hitchins *et al.*, 2007).

The DNA MMR system plays an essential role in identifying and correcting any replication errors and any additional errors which arise through physical or chemical damage. These errors may be base-base mismatches, short insertions/deletions and heteroduplexes, which can occur during DNA replication and recombination (Jiricny, 1998; Jiricny & Marra, 2003). The DNA MMR system therefore maintains genomic integrity and stability and in essence provides a tumour suppressor function. Deficiencies in DNA MMR lead to the accumulation of mutations in repetitive nucleotide regions, a phenomenon termed microsatellite instability (MSI) (Parsons *et al.*, 1993; Parsons *et al.*, 1995; Thibodeau *et al.*, 1993; Thibodeau *et al.*, 1998). Microsatellites are classically defined as simple tandem nucleotide sequence repeats of 1 – 6 base pairs in the genome (Hancock, 1999). Changes in the number of the repeat units due to defective DNA MMR are potentially cancer causing (Riccio *et al.*, 1999; Yamamoto *et al.*, 1998). The MSI phenotype or replication error positive (RER+) phenotype can be considered as an almost canonical feature of DNA MMR deficiency (Kinzler & Vogelstein, 1996; Parsons *et al.*, 1993). This MSI phenotype is observed in approximately 15% of all human colorectal cancer, gastric and endometrial carcinomas (Lothe *et al.*, 1993; Seruca *et al.*, 1995; Shibata, 1999; Umar *et al.*, 1994). Somatic inactivation of DNA MMR largely arises as a consequence of epigenetic silencing of *hMLH*1 (through hypermethylation of promoter CpG islands) rather than via classic mutational inactivation (Herman *et al.*, 1998; Jacinto & Esteller, 2007; Jones & Laird, 1999; Peltomaki, 2001; H. Yamamoto *et al.*, 1998). Genes particularly prone to MSI include *Bax*, *TGF-β receptor II*, *hMSH3* and *hMSH6* (Yamamoto *et al.*, 1998); other susceptible genes include the DNA glycosylase *MBD4* (Bader *et al.*, 2000; Bader *et al.*, 1999; Riccio *et al.*, 1999) and the epidermal growth factor receptor (EGFR) (Woerner *et al.*, 2010). Additionally, as a consequence of MSI, inactivation of proteins in the Wnt signalling pathway (eg TCF-4) has been reported (Shimizu *et al.*, 2002). Clinically defined MSI is where at least two of the loci tested in a panel out of five exhibit instability (Boland *et al.*, 1998). Mutation frequencies in cells defective in DNA MMR can be increased 100-1000 fold (Parsons *et al.*, 1993; Shibata, 1999).

The protective role of the DNA MMR system in suppressing the mutator phenotype in a range of common cancers is thus well established. The hypothesis that aspirin may potentially modulate this pathway to prevent carcinogenesis (Goel *et al.*, 2003) is of central interest, and has so far received relatively little attention and merits further investigation. The aim of this chapter will be to review the evidence that non-steroidal anti-inflammatory drugs (NSAIDS), including aspirin, celecoxib, sulindac and so on, affect DNA repair mechanisms and pathways and to further examine the consequences of this in relation to cancer development and progression. As NSAIDs are considered to be one of the most widely used over-the-counter drugs, we will also discuss the potential effect of NSAID use on cancer treatment. Aspirin and other NSAIDs may have the capacity to perturb DNA repair pathways and this may have important implications for the patient response to chemotherapeutic agents. It is also worth noting that inflammation – the 'seventh hallmark' of cancer (Colotta *et al.*, 2009) - can possibly repress (by epigenetic mechanisms) DNA mismatch repair.

2. Cancer and NSAIDs

From evidence adduced from epidemiological studies and clinical trials, it has been proposed that regular ingestion of aspirin and other non-steroidal anti-inflammatory drugs (NSAIDs) can promote colorectal tumour regression and reduce the relative risk of developing colorectal cancer (CRC) in the general population and in genetically susceptible individuals (for example see; (Baron *et al.*, 2003; Chan *et al.*, 2009; Cuzick *et al.*, 2009; Giovannucci, 1999; Imperiale, 2003; Logan *et al.*, 1993; Paganini-Hill, 1993; Sandler *et al.*, 2003; Thun *et al.*, 2002). NSAID use is also associated with a reduced risk of oesophageal adenocarcinoma particularly in patients with high risk molecular abnormalities, for example, with 17p LOH, 9p LOH, and DNA content abnormalities (Galipeau *et al.*, 2007). Recent meta-analyses of randomised clinical trials have strengthened the contention that aspirin has protective effects against CRC (Din *et al.*, 2010) and non-CRC related adenocarcinomas, including oesophageal and lung cancer (Rothwell *et al.*, 2011). Although such studies have now provided substantial evidence that regular use of aspirin based medication can reduce the risk of colorectal cancer (Bosetti *et al.*, 2002; Muscat *et al.*, 1994; Thun *et al.*, 1991) the molecular basis for the protective effect of aspirin *vis-à-vis* CRC and other cancers is rather controversial. A substantial number of theories are now in circulation. Whilst much of the focus in the recent past has understandably been on the intrinsic anti-inflammatory nature of the compounds in use, see for example, (Giovannucci, 1999; Keller & Giardiello, 2003), there are a number of intriguing findings which suggest that NSAIDs can impact upon genetic stability and it is these aspects which we wish to highlight in this chapter. However, the optimism that arises from the findings that NSAIDs may offer protection against cancer should be tempered: NSAID use can result in serious side effects (gastrointestinal disturbances and cardiovascular events) in susceptible individuals (Cuzick et al., 2009). This has lead to considerable debate amongst clinicians over recent years as to whether NSAIDs should be prescribed as chemopreventative agents, in particular, to those individuals at high risk of developing colorectal cancer, such as HNPCC or Familial Adenomatous Polyposis (FAP) patients.

Animal studies confirm that NSAIDs can protect against the development of colorectal neoplasia (Corpet & Pierre, 2003, 2005). For example, aspirin has been shown to suppress spontaneous intestinal adenoma formation and reduce incidence and volume of colon tumour induced by the carcinogen 1,2-dimethylhydrazine in rat models (Barnes & Lee, 1999). Continuous administration of a clinically relevant aspirin dosage was crucial in these studies in comparison to other studies where aspirin was administered at the start of carcinogenesis or one week after carcinogen exposure (Craven & DeRubertis, 1992). Taken together with findings from epidemiological studies in humans, there is thus the suggestion that long term, continuous usage of aspirin is required to gain any beneficial chemopreventative effects. Several studies carried out in the 1990s demonstrated inhibition of carcinogen induced tumour development by NSAIDs including aspirin and sulindac in rats (Rao et al., 1995; Reddy et al., 1993) and also in a murine model of FAP (Barnes & Lee, 1998; Chiu et al., 1997; Jacoby et al., 1996; Mahmoud et al., 1998; Oshima et al., 1996). Familial adenomatous polyposis (FAP) is a colorectal cancer syndrome inherited in humans in an autosomal dominant manner caused by an absence of a functional caretaker APC protein (Narayan & Roy, 2003). Lifetime administration of aspirin to a mouse model with germline defects in both the APC and Msh2 gens (APC Min/+ , Msh2 -/-) suppresses intestinal and mammary neoplasia formation (Sansom et al., 2001).

Epidemiological studies have identified environmental and dietary factors which alter the risk of developing colorectal cancer. Protective dietary factors include NSAIDs, fruit, vegetables, and folic acid and possibly calcium, whilst red and processed meat ingestion, alcohol use and obesity are perceived to increase risk (Forte et al., 2008; Key, 2011; La Vecchia et al., 2001; Ryan-Harshman & Aldoori, 2007; Scheier, 2001; Serrano et al., 2004). An assessment of chemopreventative measures, such as NSAID and micronutrient intake, for the general population and individuals with an increased risk for colorectal cancer based on family history, has recently been published (Cooper et al., 2010).

2.1 Inflammation and cancer

Debate has arisen with regards to the molecular mechanism of action of aspirin and other NSAIDs in reducing the incidence of certain cancers. Based on the anti-inflammatory effects of these agents, one obvious explanation is that inflammation can drive cancer development. Indeed, inflammation is becoming increasingly recognised as being critical to cancer formation, and building on the framework proposed by Hannahan and Weinberg (Hanahan & Weinberg, 2000), it has been proposed that inflammation should be considered the seventh hallmark of genetic instability (Colotta et al., 2009). It has been estimated that one in four cancers are linked to infection and chronic inflammation (Hussain & Harris, 2007). In an inflammatory microenvironment mutation frequency is increased (Bielas et al., 2006). There is strong evidence for an increased risk of cancer in individuals with chronic inflammatory states (inflammatory bowel disease, gastroesophageal reflux disease, asthma) with or without attendant bacterial or viral infection (eg *Helicobacter pylori*, hepatitis) (Grivennikov & Karin, 2010; Schetter *et al.*, 2010; Xie & Itzkowitz, 2008). The molecular drivers of cancer formation resulting from the interaction of pre-cancerous cells with activated immune cells and the surrounding stroma are complex. The host response to infection, injury and wound repair through production of reactive oxygen (ROS) and nitrogen oxide (RNOS) species, and pro-inflammatory cytokines (eg TNF-α, IL-1, IL-6) and chemokines (eg IL-8) (Wang *et al.*, 2009) is of central importance. Such 'micro-cytokine' storms can stimulate activation of transcriptions factors (eg Nuclear Factor-κB, AP-1, STAT3) fundamentally altering the expression profile of a cell and promoting cell survival, proliferation, angiogenesis, motility and invasion. It is clear that for individual transcription factors their activation can be context (eg tissue) dependent and they may not always promote tumour cell formation, and may indeed exhibit tumour suppressor activity (eg NF-κB in skin cancer) (Chaturvedi *et al.*, 2011; Ditsworth & Zong, 2004).

Microsatellite instability has been observed in non-neoplastic tissue in patients with chronic inflammatory conditions prior to the presence of dysplastic tissue, indicating that defects in DNA MMR can be an early event in inflammation-associated cancers (Brentnall *et al.*, 1995; Park *et al.*, 1998). There are tantalising findings which hint at the molecular basis for this MSI. Oxidative stress, in the guise of H_2O_2, increases frameshift mutations (Gasche *et al.*, 2001), and can inactivate the DNA MMR system (Chang *et al.*, 2002). Moreover, in a p53 and p21 dependent fashion, activated neutrophils induced replication errors and a G2/M arrest in colonic epithelial cells (Campregher *et al.*, 2008). In inflammatory bowel disease neoplasia, hypermethylation of the *hMLH1* gene and reduced hMLH1 protein expression occurs frequently (Fleisher *et al.*, 2000). In an animal model of colorectal cancer, inflammation and hypoxia were found to epigenetically silence hMLH1 expression: down-regulated expression of this DNA mismatch repair gene occurred as a consequence of decreased acetylation, which was reversible when the animals were treated with the HDAC inhibitor suberoylanilide hydroxamic acid (SAHA) (Edwards *et al.*, 2009). Decreased expression of hMLH1 can alter hPMS2 stability and consequently, genetic integrity. Moreover, hMLH1 and hPMS2 can have a role in activating cell-cycle checkpoints and promoting apoptosis (Cejka *et al.*, 2003; Davis *et al.*, 1998; Ding *et al.*, 2009; McDaid *et al.*, 2009; Sansom *et al.*, 2003; Yanamadala & Ljungman, 2003; Zhang *et al.*, 1999). Thus, a functional DNA mismatch repair system prohibits expansion of cells containing DNA damage (Carethers *et al.*, 1996; Papouli *et al.*, 2004). Dysregulated hMLH1/hPMS2 expression could conceivably impact on the survival of cells containing damaged DNA and promote cancer progression. hMLH1 expression has been reported to be altered by tobacco usage and inflammatory state in the epithelium of the oral mucosa (Fernandes *et al.*, 2007). Increased tissue specific hMLH1 hypermethylation has been observed in the progression of oesophageal cancer (Vasavi *et al.*, 2006); the authors also reported that patients with gastroesophageal reflux disease (GERD) exhibited a very significant degree of hMLH1 hypermethylation prompting the suggestion that reflux can promote hypermethylation. The relationship between acid reflux and inflammation in GERD has been recently reviewed (Orlando, 2010). The phenomenon of elevated microsatellite instability at selected nucleotide repeats (EMAST) is also seen in 60% of sporadic colon cancers, is more common in individuals of African-American origin and has been linked to reduced expression of the hMSH3 protein. Moreover, EMAST is also more prevalent in rectal cancer with immune cell infiltration (Devaraj *et al.*, 2010; Lee *et al.*, 2010). As MSI in CRC can result in products with potentially increased immunogenicity, it is possible that this further stimulates inflammation (Banerjea *et al.*, 2004). Tumour infiltrating lymphocytes in CRC with MSI are activated and cytotoxic (Phillips *et al.*, 2004). In a model of experimental colon carcinogenesis in rats, long-term, low-dose administration of aspirin significantly reduced cytokine and matrix metalloproteinase release (Bousserouel *et al.*, 2010). Based on the above findings, it would appear to be reasonable to suppose that research into the epigenetic modifying effects of NSAIDs, and inflammation itself (Maekawa & Watanabe, 2007), particularly with respect to alterations in DNA repair protein expression and MSI, should be a focus in the future.

Oxidative stress occurs as a consequence of the activation of the immune system, where oxidative bursts have a role in protecting the host against microbial invaders. Reactive oxide and nitrogen oxide species (ROS and RNOS) thus produced can ultimately cause DNA damage such as abasic sites, oxidised bases, DNA-intrastrand adducts, strand breaks, as well as RNA alkylation, and protein damage (Hussain *et al.*, 2003). Reaction with lipids produces extremely reactive peroxidation products, including malondialdehyde (MDA) and *trans*-4-hydroxynonenal (4-HNE). 4-HNE can form etheno adducts in DNA and has been found to preferentially form adducts in codon 249 of the human p53 gene (Federico *et al.*, 2007; Hu *et al.*, 2002). Mutations in the tumour suppressor p53 are found in inflamed tissue in ulcerative colitis (UC) patients (Hussain *et al.*, 2000). Accelerated telomere shortening, and DNA damage - as assessed by analysis of phosphorylated histone H2AX (γH2AX; a measure of DSBs) occurs in the bowel of UC patients (Risques *et al.*, 2008). ROS and RNOS - whilst generally perceived as having a negative impact on cell function - do have important roles as secondary messengers (Valko *et al.*, 2006). However, if the cellular defence mechanisms - anti-oxidant enzymes such as manganese superoxide dismutase and glutathione peroxidise, detoxification, and DNA repair systems - are overwhelmed, these reactive species are potentially mutagenic (Ferguson, 2010). The bystander effects from released cytokines and reactive signalling species may also occur some distance from the initial trauma. Redon *et al.* have shown that increased levels of DNA damage (measuring γH2AX levels) can occur systemically in mice implanted with a non-metastatic tumour (Redon *et al.*, 2010). Animal model studies confirm the role of RNOS and the inflammatory process in contributing to cancer development (Hussain *et al.*, 2003; Itzkowitz & Yio, 2004).

The base excision repair (BER) system is critically important for dealing with oxidative damage to DNA, such as removal of 8-oxo-G lesions (David *et al.*, 2007; Lindahl & Wood, 1999; McCullough *et al.*, 1999; Wood *et al.*, 2001). Increased expression of the BER proteins AAG (a 3-methyladenine DNA glycosylase) and APE1 (apurinic endonuclease1; Ref-1) is seen in inflamed tissue from UC patients. Paradoxically a positive correlation of MSI was noted with overexpression of AAG, and for MSI-high tissues with increased APE1 expression. In model systems this adaptive response was confirmed to positively correlate with an in increase in MSI in human cells and frameshift mutations in *S. cerevisiae* (Hofseth *et al.*, 2003). Dysregulated expression of BER proteins can generate a mutator phenotype (Glassner *et al.*, 1998) (as cited in Hofseth, 2003). In a mouse model of UC, expression of the Mutyh BER protein, which can recognise 8-oxoG:A mispairs and oxidised adenines was actually found to influence the inflammatory response to dextran sulphate sodium induced oxidative stress (Casorelli *et al.* 2010). The biomediator signalling molecule nitric oxide (NO·) formed during inflammation has the capacity to inhibit *in vitro* and *in vivo* the formamidopyrimidine-DNA glycosylase, which can recognise abasic sites and 8-oxoguanine lesions (Wink & Laval, 1994). Thus, oxidative stress can compromise genetic stability.

RNOS, and inflammatory cytokines and chemokines can activate the transcription factors activator protein-1 (AP-1), HIF-1 and NF-κB, the latter resulting in transcription of target genes including COX-2 and TNF-α (for example, see Olson & van der Vliet, 2011; Valko et al., 2006). DNA double strand breaks can also activate NF-κB (Rakoff-Nahoum, 2006), thus potentially creating a feedback loop where the inflammatory response is perpetuated. Persistent DNA damage can also trigger secretion of cytokines such as IL-6 (Rodier et al., 2009). There is evidence that NF-κB and cyclooxygenase activation and HIF-1 signalling are interlinked (Jung et al., 2003; Qiao et al., 2010). Hypoxia can induce MSI (Kondo et al., 2001): in human sporadic colon cancers HIF-1α over-expression is associated with loss of hMSH2 expression, and in vitro experiments confirm that in a p53 dependent manner HIF-1α can repress hMSH2 and hMSH6 (Koshiji et al., 2005; To et al., 2005). Recently HIF-1α has been suggested to regulate expression of an inhibitor of apoptosis protein, Survivin (Wu et al., 2010), which is notably present in CRC (Chen et al., 2004). There is increasing evidence that microRNAs (short, non coding RNAs that regulate translation) are mediators of the inflammatory process (Schetter et al., 2010). Two micro-RNAs, miR-210 and miR-373 are up regulated in an HIF-1α dependent manner in hypoxic cells: forced expression of mir-210 reduced expression of homologous recombination factor RAD52, whilst reduced mir-373 expression was found to suppress RAD52 and RAD23B (Crosby et al., 2009). Over-expression of another micro-RNA, miR-155 has been reported in colorectal cancer, and can regulate DNA MMR protein expression (Valeri et al., 2010). Inflammation can up-regulate miR-155 expression and increase mutation frequency two to threefold in spontaneous hypoxanthine phosphoribosyltransferase gene mutation assays (Tili et al., 2011). MiR-155 expression is associated with a poor prognosis in lung cancer (Yanaihara et al., 2006). The cyclooxygenase family of enzymes (COX-1: constitutively expressed; COX-2: induced in inflammation; COX-3: splice variant of COX-1) catalyse the conversion of arachidonic acid into prostanoids (prostaglandins and thromboxanes). Cyclooxygenase expression is increased in CRC (Kutchera et al., 1996). Prostaglandins promote epidermal growth factor receptor (EGFR) transactivation, increased cell proliferation, motility, invasion and angiogenesis (eg by altering vascular endothelial growth factor expression) and inhibit apoptosis, for example, by increasing Bcl-2 expression (Ghosh et al., 2010; Pai et al., 2003; Sheng et al., 1998; Wang & DuBois, 2008). To summarise: inflammation and hypoxia can result in genetic instability and suppression of apoptosis.

2.2 Mechanistic aspects of NSAID cytotoxicity

The mechanism by which NSAIDs protect the host from colorectal cancer development has been under investigation for decades, and as a consequence a plethora of hypotheses (some of which may be competing) have been proposed to explain this phenomenon. In addition to the evidence alluded to above of epidemiological studies and animal models examining the protective effect of NSAIDs, there also exists a substantive literature reporting that NSAIDs exhibit a degree of specific toxicity in vitro to colorectal cancer cell lines. Because of the intrinsic anti-inflammatory activity of NSAIDs a significant number of researchers have focused on this aspect as a protective mechanism. For example, aspirin can acetylate the cyclo-oxygenases (COX) significantly reducing arachidonic acid metabolism and prostaglandin production, thereby reducing inflammation (Elwood et al., 2009). Expression of the inducible COX, cyclooxygenase-2 is notably elevated in colorectal malignancies and in other cancers (Ferrandez et al., 2003; Kutchera et al., 1996; Soslow et al., 2000), and this overexpression has been actively implicated in the metastasic potential of tumours (Jang *et al.*, 2009; Tsujii *et al.*, 1997). These effects, however, may not be restricted only to colorectal cancer: a case control study has found that use of selective and non-selective COX-2 inhibitors (celecoxib, refecoxib and aspirin and ibuprofen) has utility in the chemoprevention of lung cancer (Harris *et al.*, 2007).

NSAIDs do not only affect cyclooxygenase activity: exposure to these drug can significantly alter gene expression and thus NSAIDs can be reasonably described as having pleiotropic effects, some of which may be relatively compound dependent. Chronic NSAID use can suppress CpG island hypermethylation of tumour suppressor genes [p14(Arf), p16(INK4a), E-cadherin] in the human gastric mucosa (Tahara *et al.*, 2009). Furthermore, NSAID toxicity may not be absolutely dependent on inhibition of COX activity: the proliferation of COX-2 negative cell lines can also be inhibited by NSAIDs (Lai *et al.*, 2008; Richter *et al.*, 2001) and the chemical precursor of aspirin - salicylate - which has weak anti-COX activity, can itself be anti-inflammatory (Amann & Peskar, 2002) and pro-apoptotic to CRC cells (Elder *et al.*, 1996). Additionally, whilst the NSAID sulindac sulfide and its sulfone derivative can both inhibit the HT-29 CRC cell line growth, sulindac sulfone is "devoid of prostaglandin inhibitory activity" (Piazza *et al.*, 1995). Additionally, aberrant crypt foci formation in a chemically induced rat model of CRC were suppressed by treatment with sulindac sulfone (Charalambous & O'Brien, 1996). Supporting these findings, a mechanism for NSAID toxicity (anti-proliferative and inducing apoptosis) – testing sulindac sulfide and piroxicam - toward a CRC line lacking cyclooxygenase activity (HCT-15) and thus independent of prostaglandin inhibition, has also been reported (Hanif *et al.*, 1996). Sulindac metabolites (sulphide and sulfone; see Fig.1) can inhibit the activation and expression of the EGF receptor (Pangburn *et al.*, 2005), with the down-regulated activity mediated by lysosomal and proteasomal degradation(Pangburn *et al.*, 2010). Rigas and others have cogently proposed that the anti-neoplastic activities of NSAIDs can be categorised as either being COX-dependent or COX-independent (Keller & Giardiello, 2003; Shiff & Rigas, 1999). This concept has been reviewed in some detail in (Ferrandez *et al.*, 2003). Smith *et al* examined the effects of NS-398 (a selective COX inhibitor), indomethacin (a non-selective COX inhibitor) and aspirin on the HT29Fu, HCA-7, SW480 and HCT116 CRC cell lines with respect to effects on cell proliferation, cell cycle arrest, apoptosis induction, β-catenin and COX-1 and COX-2 protein production. They concluded that NSAIDs act via COX-dependent and COX-independent mechanisms (Smith *et al.*, 2000). Indeed, acetylsalicylic acid regulates MMP-2 activity and inhibits colorectal invasion of B16F0 melanoma cells (Tsai *et al.*, 2009). Intriguingly, although medium conditioned by cultured colorectal cancer cell lines is capable of inducing endothelial cell (EC) tube formation (as a model for angiogenesis); aspirin and salicylate (both at 1mM) can reduce the ability of the conditioned medium from treated DLD-1, HT-29 and HCT116 CRC cell lines to promote EC tube formation (Shtivelband *et al.*, 2003).

Aspirin is principally metabolised to salicylate *in vivo* (Law *et al.*, 2000; Paterson & Lawrence, 2001*)*, with plasma salicylate concentrations of 0.95-1.9 mM achievable in patients receiving aspirin as an anti-inflammatory agent (Amann & Peskar, 2002; Urios *et al.*, 2007; Yin *et al.*, 1998). The effect of significantly higher concentrations than that achievable physiologically has been used by a number of investigators in a number of *in vitro* studies and one must interpret cautiously data produced from these analyses. To facilitate interpretation, we have incorporated the concentrations utilised in the relevant publications. We should also point out that whilst vegetables and fruits have been considered to be a natural source of salicylate, where it functions as a plant signalling molecule (Paterson & Lawrence, 2001; Schenk *et al.*, 2000, and refs therein), it has been reported that SA may be an endogenous compound, with SA found in the blood of carnivorous animals, for example in the burrowing owl (Paterson *et al.*, 1998; Paterson *et al* 2008).

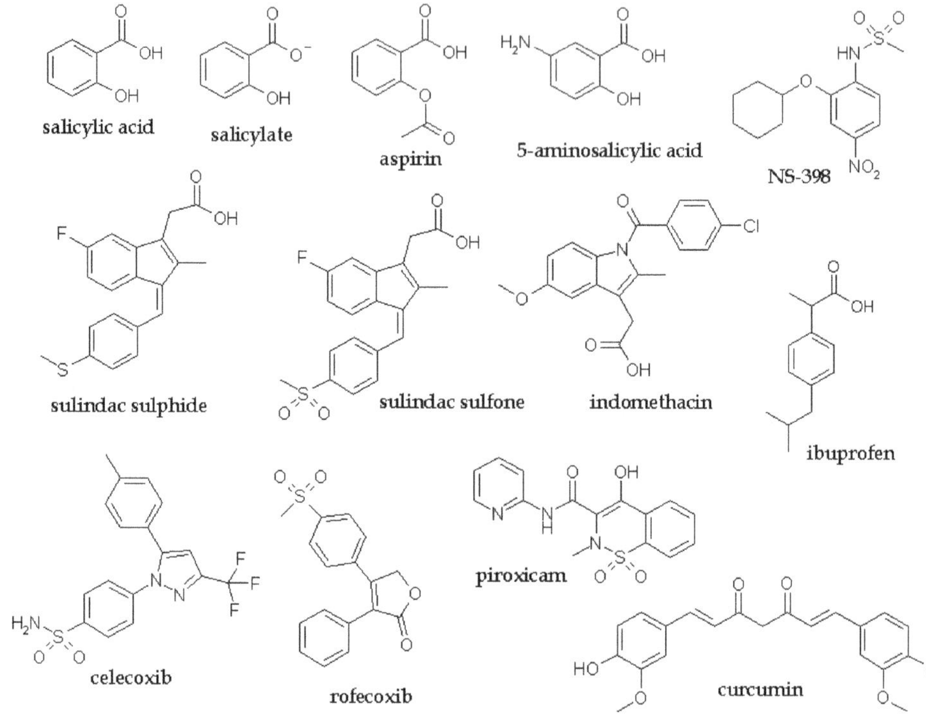

Fig. 1. The non-steroidal anti-inflammatory drugs (NSAIDS) referred to in this chapter can be sub-categorised into five groups. 1. Salicylates (salicylic acid/salicylate anion, aspirin, 5-aminosalicylic acid). 2 Acetic acid derivatives (indomethacin, sulindac sulphide, sulindac sulphone) 3. Propionic acid derivatives (ibuprofen). 4. Enolic acid derivatives or oxicams (piroxicam). 5. Selective COX-2 inhibitors (celecoxib, rofecoxib, NS-398). Curcumin has a dimeric structure with two identical phenolic moieties suggestive of salicylate-like character.

2.2.1 COX independent effects of NSAIDs

A substantial number of hypotheses regarding NSAID cytotoxicity not directly involving inhibition of COX activity exist (reviewed in: Goke, 2002; Watson, 2006). Much of the data is obtained from examining the effect of NSAIDs on cultured cell lines. For example, salicylate can cause cell cycle arrest: in a range of adenoma and carcinoma derived cell lines, incubation with 5 mM resulted in a decrease of cells in the S-phase with cells accumulating in the G_0-G_1 phase (Elder *et al.*, 1996). Activating mutations stabilizing the Wnt pathway and β-catenin are common in CRC (Behrens, 2005; Bienz & Clevers, 2000). In four CRC cell lines (SW948, SW480, HCT116, LoVo), aspirin (5 mM) and indomethacin (400 μM) downregulated cyclin D1 expression, and the authors proposed this was a consequence of reduced transcriptional activity of the β-catenin/TCF complex (Dihlmann *et al.*, 2001). Bos *et al* using reporter assays also showed that aspirin (up to 5 mM) can down-regulate APC-β-catenin-TCF4 signalling in the SW480 CRC cell line and increase the phosphorylation of protein phosphatase 2A (PP2A), resulting in decreased PP2A enzymatic activity. This alteration is stated to be essential for the observed effect on the Wnt/β-catenin pathway activity (Bos *et al.*, 2006). Mutations in the APC or β-catenin genes may also result in increased peroxisome proliferator-activated receptor δ (PPAR δ) activity; indeed, sulindac sulfide and indomethacin have been reported to suppress (by direct inhibition) in a dose-dependent fashion, PPARδ activity (He *et al.*, 1999). However, it should be noted that regulation of PPARδ by the APC/ β -catenin/TCF4 pathway and the effect of NSAIDs on PPAR function is a field not without some controversy; for example, Foreman *et al* recently reported not finding decreased PPARβ/δ expression following NSAID treatment in a number of human CRC cell lines (Foreman *et al.*, 2009).

2.2.2 NSAIDS, signalling pathways and apoptosis

Other transcriptional pathways affected by NSAID use include NF-κB signalling, which is critically involved in regulating immunity, inflammation and apoptosis and in cancer development (Nakano, 2004; Olivier *et al.*, 2006; Staudt, 2010). Aspirin and sodium salicylate can antagonise the NF-κB pathway (Kopp & Ghosh, 1994), via inhibition – by direct, but not covalent binding- of IκB kinase-B (IKK β kinase) (Yin *et al.*, 1998). Yamamoto *et al* extended this hypothesis by reporting that sulindac, sulindac sulfide and sulindac sulfone (but not indomethacin) also inhibits the NF-κB pathway by decreasing IKK β kinase activity (Yamamoto *et al.*, 1999). In HT-29 CRC cells, nitric oxide (NO)-donating aspirin inhibited NF-κB transcription more potently than aspirin as assessed by electrophoretic mobility shift assays (Williams *et al.*, 2003*).*

Zerbini *et al* reported that NF-κB can mediate the repression (assessed by RT-PCR analysis) of the growth arrest and DNA damage inducible (*GADD*) *45α* and *GADD45γ*genes and that this repression is both necessary and sufficient for cell survival, and that GADD45α and γ activity can contribute towards apoptosis of prostate cancer cells (assessed by transfection studies in DU145 and PC-3) (Zerbini *et al.*, 2004). The melanoma differentiation associated gene 8 (mda-7/IL-24) was induced by NSAIDs and affected growth arrest and apoptosis *in vitro*, in a manner dependent on GADD45α and γ expression affecting the p38/JNK pathway (Sarkar *et al.*, 2002; Zerbini *et al.*, 2006). However, it has been suggested that recombinant IL-24 lacks apoptosis inducing properties to melanoma cells (Kreis *et al.*, 2007). In a recent review, Siafakas and Richardson have suggested that the GADD family of proteins can be considered to be molecular targets for anti-tumour agents; indeed, commonly used NSAIDs can up-regulate GADD45α expression (Rosemary Siafakas & Richardson, 2009). GADD45α overexpression in NIH 3T3 cells has been shown to promote global DNA demethylation and loss of expression has been shown to induce DNA hypermethylation (including in *hMLH1*). Such findings led Barreto *et al* to conclude that GADD45α can relieve epigenetic silencing by promoting DNA repair (Barreto *et al.*, 2007). It is noteworthy that GADD45γ can be inactivated by epigenetic mechanisms in multiple tumours (Ying *et al.*, 2005).

In a review of the role of the NF-κB pathway in inflammation and cancer, the authors suggested that, '...constitutive NF-κB activation is likely involved in the enhanced growth properties seen in a variety of cancers' (Yamamoto & Gaynor, 2001). Specifically targeting the NF-κB pathway may thus have utility in cancer treatment (Olivier *et al.*, 2006): for example, attempts are ongoing to identify clinically useful and novel IKK-β inhibtors (for example see (Lauria *et al.*, 2010)), and inhibition of NF-κB (by siRNA) can enhance the chemosensitivity of HCT116 CRC cells to the DNA topoisomerase inhibitor, irinotecan (Guo *et al.*, 2004). In marked contrast however, Stark *et al*, have suggested that aspirin can activate NF-κB signalling *in vitro* (SW480, HRT-18, HCT116, CT26 cell lines) and has the capacity to induce apoptosis in *in vivo* (xenografts and APC Min+/-) models of CRC (Stark *et al.*, 2001; Stark *et al.*, 2007). Moreover, these effects are cell type specific to aspirin (for CRC cells): the induction of apoptosis was independent of COX-2 expression, APC and β-catenin mutation status, and DNA mismatch repair proficiency (Din *et al.*, 2004).

A number of other hypotheses have been invoked for the observed cytotoxicity of NSAIDs to CRC cell lines. Cytosolic phospholipase A_2 (cPLA2) expression is decreased in NIH 3T3 cells treated with either aspirin or sulindac (Yuan *et al.*, 2000) and in CRC cell lines (SW480, Colo320 and HT-29) when treated with low mM (2.5-10) concentrations of aspirin (Yu *et al.*, 2003). This observation is intriguing given that $cPLA_2$ expression has been proposed to participate in intestinal tumorigenesis (eg (Lim *et al.*, 2010) and refs therein). Law *et al* have indicated that (high mM concentrations of) salicylate (in Balb/MK cells) can inhibit the activity and phosphorylation of the mitogen activated protein kinase, $p70^{s6k}$ independent of p38 MAPK, with a concomitant reduction in DNA synthesis, cell proliferation and in expression of proliferation associated proteins such as c-MYC, cyclin D1, and PCNA and led the authors to conclude that salicylate may act via the mTOR pathway (Law *et al.*, 2000). In contrast, it has been suggested that salicylate-induced apoptosis in HCT116 CRC cells occurs through activation of p38 MAPK and p53; however, the concentration tested was - in our opinion - high (10mM), and thus casts doubt on the utility of the findings (Lee *et al.*, 2003). NO-donating aspirin has also been reported to activate p38 and JNK MAP kinase pathways in HT-29 colorectal cancer cells (Hundley & Rigas, 2006). Using subtractive hybridization, Baek *et al* identified an increase in the expression of the NSAID activated gene (NAG-1) – a member of the TGF-β superfamily, with pro-apoptotic properties - in indomethacin treated HCT116 cells. A range of NSAIDs including sulindac sulfide and aspirin also increased NAG-1 expression (Baek *et al.*, 2001). NCX-4040 (*para*-NO-aspirin), an NO donating aspirin derivative can also induce NAG-1 expression and it was confirmed that NAG-1 has a pro-apoptotic role (Tesei *et al.*, 2008, and refs therein). Another nitro-derivative of aspirin, NCX-4016 inhibited EGFR and STAT3 signalling in cisplatin-resistant human ovarian cancer cells (Selvendiran *et al.*, 2008). NSAIDs can also up-regulate 15-lipoxygenase-1 (15-LOX-1) in CRC cells: NS-398 and sulindac sulfone both induced expression in the DLD-1 (COX-1 and COX-2 negative) cell line; significantly, inhibiting 15-LOX-1 blocked the induction of apoptosis (Shureiqi *et al.*, 2000).

With respect to characterisation of the pathway by which NSAID toxicity occurs, reports have been rather contradictory: *in vitro* studies have suggested that whilst aspirin and other NSAIDs can cause cell cycle arrest and inhibit CRC proliferation, this may, (Din *et al.*, 2004; Elder *et al.*, 1996; Piazza *et al.*, 1995; Yu *et al.*, 2002; Yu *et al.*, 2003) or may not (Shiff *et al.*, 1996; Smith *et al.*, 2000) occur with the induction of apoptosis, or may occur as consequence a combination of activation of both apoptotic and necrotic 'pathways' (Lai *et al.*, 2008). Notwithstanding the apparently contradictory reports, an absence of Bax expression in CRC cells has been found to abolish the apoptotic response to NSAIDs (Zhang *et al.*, 2000). These authors reported finding Bax mutations in indomethacin resistant cells. Bax and BCl-2 expression can be up and down-regulated respectively, in a dose-dependent fashion, (up to 10 mM) in SW480 cells incubated with aspirin (Lai *et al.*, 2008). BCL-2 expression can be reduced by aspirin in SW480 cells (Yu *et al.*, 2002) and can also suppress apoptosis in CRC cells (Jiang & Milner, 2003). Pretreating LNCap (human prostate) and CX-01 (colorectal carcinoma) cell lines with aspirin was found to enhance the capacity of tumour necrosis factor-related apoptosis-inducing ligand (TRAIL) to intiate apoptosis, an effect – according to the authors - related to down regulation of *BCL-2* gene expression resulting from the inhibition of NF-κB (of which BCL-2 is a known target) (K.M.Kim *et al.*, 2005). HeLa cells incubated with aspirin undergo apoptosis as assessed by cleavage of procaspase 3, PARP and PKC-δ, and annexin V staining. Moreover, the caspase inhibitor zVAD-fmk suppressed cell death, Bax was noted to translocate from the cytosol to mitochondria, and cytochrome c release from mitochondria was seen using time-lapse confocal microscopy (Zimmermann *et al.*, 2000). Sulindac sulfide (up to 500 μM tested) can inhibit growth of NIH3T3 and SAOS cells: an inhibtion of ras mediated proliferation and transformation was noted (Herrmann *et al.*, 1998). Hughes *et al.*, (2003) showed that NSAID treatment of colorectal cancer cell lines caused a decrease in intracellular polyamine content and was cytotoxic. Polyamines are growth factors, and involved in protein synthesis. An increase in intracellular polyamine concentration is observed in the early stages of carcinogenesis. When polyamines were re-introduced to NSAID treated cells, apoptosis was inhibited suggesting that the polyamine pathway is affected by NSAID treatment in CRC cell, and that modulation of this pathway may explain the chemoprotective effects of NSAIDs (Hughes *et al.*, 2003). Dikshit *et al.*, reported that aspirin disrupted proteasome and mitochondrial function in mouse Neuro 2a cells (Dikshit *et al.*, 2006). Hardwick *et al.*, (2004) analysed changes to gene expression employing DNA microarray in the colorectal cancer cell line HT-29 upon aspirin treatment, and found a significant increase in *Rac1* gene and protein expression in a time and concentration dependant manner. Rac1 is involved in intestinal epithelial cell differentiation (Stappenbeck & Gordon, 2000) proliferation, motility and resistance to apoptosis (Parri & Chiarugi, 2010). Spitz *et al* report that aspirin and salicylate can inhibit purified phosphofructokinase (PFK) in a dose-dependent manner: as cancer cells utilise glycolysis for energy production in which PFK is the rate limiting step, the authors suggest that these NSAIDs may be pro-apoptotic through disturbing the glycolytic pathway (Spitz *et al.*, 2009). We have recently identified novel derivatives of di-aspirin (bis-carboxyphenol succinate) to have potential as anti-colorectal cancer agents (Deb *et al.*, 2011).

2.3 NSAIDS and DNA repair

A relatively unexplored area of research is that the anti-tumour mechanism of action of aspirin may be via 'interaction' with the DNA repair systems. This is of key interest particularly in the context of hereditary and sporadic colorectal cancer where DNA repair defects can be a causative factor. It has been shown that the MSI mutator phenotype is suppressed by aspirin. For example, treatment of the colorectal cancer cell line HCT116 - which is DNA MMR deficient with a defect in *hMLH1* - reduced the MSI phenotype and induced apoptosis (Ruschoff *et al.*, 1998). It is speculated that aspirin exposure resulted in genetic selection against cells with MSI and that MSI unstable cells were weeded out by apoptosis (Ruschoff *et al.*, 1998). This observation is important as MSI resulting from a genetic mutation in *hMLH1*, accounts for 5 - 10% of colonic tumours. Nitric oxide releasing NSAIDS (NO-NSAIDS) suppressed MSI in DNA mismatch repair deficient colorectal cancer cells (McIlhatton *et al.*, 2007), and the authors suggested that since these NO containing derivatives of aspirin are more effective than aspirin itself, they should be considered for use in chemopreventitive trials in patients at high risk of developing CRC. Recently, in a mouse model of HNPCC, McIlhatton *et al.*, reported that aspirin and low dose NO-aspirin increased life span. However, though the intestinal tumours in aspirin treated animals showed less microsatellite instability, low dose NO-aspirin had 'minimal effect on MSI status' and high dose NO-aspirin decreased life span and increased MSI (McIlhatton *et al.*, 2011). In addition to the phenomenon of aspirin selecting for microsatellite stability in colorectal cancer cells (Ruschoff *et al.*, 1998), aspirin *in vitro* can inhibit CRC growth and increase the level of the DNA MMR proteins hMLH1, hMSH2, hMSH6 and hPMS2 in DNA MMR proficient cells (Goel *et al.*, 2003). Increased DNA MMR levels could conceivably facilitate programmed cell death. This is a highly significant observation as defects in DNA MMR proteins are ultimately responsible for HNPCC and this study speculates in particular on the involvement of MLH1 function in the chemoprotective effect of aspirin. In addition to this, recent evidence has shown that although MLH1 expression is decreased in cases of sporadic colorectal adenoma, MLH1 expression was found to be increased in cases of sporadic colorectal adenomas with regular aspirin use (Sidelnikov *et al.*, 2009). Aspirin is not alone in having the capacity to select for microsatellite stability: the NSAID mesalazine (5-aminosalicylic acid), used to treat patients with inflammatory bowel disease (IBD), experimentally reduced frameshift mutations in cultured CRC cells (HCT116 and HCT116+chr 3) independent of DNA mismatch repair proficiency (Gasche *et al.*, 2005). *In vitro*, mesalazine inhibits the growth of HCT116 and HT-29 cells, a result reported a consequence of the compound inhibiting CDC25A, a cell cycle protein (Stolfi *et al.*, 2008). Studies have also implicated cell-cycle arrest as a cellular response to aspirin exposure (Lai *et al.*, 2008; Ricchi *et al.*, 1997). Decreased transcription of CCNB1 (Cyclin B1) which regulates cell-cycle progression at the G_2/M phase by sulindac treatment has been observed (Iizaka *et al.*, 2002). To summarise: NSAIDs can select for microsatellite stability and cause cell-cycle arrest.

2.3.1 NSAIDs and DNA repair protein expression

Microarray analysis has been extensively utilised to examine alterations in gene expression in response to NSAID exposure in a number of colon cancer cell lines (Germann *et al.*, 2003; Hardwick *et al.*, 2004; Huang *et al.*, 2006; Iizaka *et al.*, 2002; Yin *et al.*, 2006). Hardwick *et al.*, (2004) reported that cell-cycle related genes and NF-κB were repressed upon aspirin treatment. Iizaka *et al.*, (2002) reported an increase in *GADD45α* upon treatment with the NSAID sulindac. However, although, microarray analysis has been previously carried out to determine the effects of aspirin on colorectal cancer (Hardwick *et al.*, 2004; Iizaka *et al.*, 2002) these studies have not looked specifically at DNA damage signalling pathways. In addition, Hardwick *et al.*, (2004) and also Yin *et al.*, (2006) have shown that notably different gene expression patterns are seen when different concentrations of NSAID are used. Both studies showed that at low concentrations (1 mM) aspirin elicited activation of a different set of genes in the colorectal cancer cell line HT-29, compared to cells incubated with 5 mM aspirin. There is a lack of consistency in the literature regarding dosages utilised for both clinical and experimental studies. Intriguingly, clinical trials have shown that low dose aspirin (81mg) is more protective against colorectal cancer than 'high' dose aspirin (325mg) (Baron *et al.*, 2003). The variation in experimental design, especially with regards to what dose is clinically relevant makes it problematic when deciding on appropriate drug concentrations for experimental work.

In addition to the report by Iizaka *et al.*, (2002), a number of other studies have also shown NSAID regulation of growth arrest and DNA damage (GADD) gene expression. Germann *et al* (2003) analysed gene expression of CC531 colorectal cancer cells treated with 4.5mM Butyrate or 3mM aspirin and showed that *GADD153* is up-regulated upon aspirin treatment. *GADD153* expression has also been shown to be induced by celecoxib treatment in cervical cancer cells (Kim *et al.*, 2007). Microarray analysis of the colorectal cancer cell line HT-29 treated with 1mM and 5mM aspirin showed an up-regulation of *GADD45α* (Yin *et al.*, 2006). Further to this, microarray analysis also shows *GADD45* gene expression to be up-regulated by NS-398 (Huang *et al.*, 2006) and celecoxib (Fatima *et al.*, 2008) in colorectal cancer cells and by ibuprofen in human gastric adenocarcinoma cell line (Bonelli *et al.*, 2010). Suppression of *GADD45α* expression confers resistance to sulindac and indomethacin induced gastric mucosal injury and apoptosis (Chiou *et al.*, 2010) .

Other genes involved in DNA repair have also been shown to be regulated by NSAIDs. High concentrations of NS-398, ibuprofen, and RNAi mediated inhibition of COX-2 in human prostate carcinoma cells affected genes involved in DNA replication, recombination and repair (John-Aryankalayil *et al.*, 2009). *PCNA* gene expression has been shown to be up-regulated by ibuprofen treatment of a human gastric adenocarcinoma cell line (Bonelli *et al.*, 2010), and also in the human hepatocellular carcinoma cell line HepG2 treated with 25mM vanillin (Cheng *et al.*, 2007). In contrast, down-regulation of *PCNA* gene expression has been reported in colorectal cancer cell lines treated with celecoxib suggesting that these compounds may modulate cell cycle regulation in these model (Fatima *et al.*, 2008). Interestingly, *FADD* gene expression is down-regulated by NS-398 but up-regulated by indomethacin in the colorectal cancer cell line Caco-2 (Huang *et al.*, 2006). Sulindac has been reported to down-regulate *XRCC5*, *ERCC5* and *UNG* gene expression in colorectal cancer cell lines (Iizaka *et al.*, 2002). Celecoxib up-regulated *ATM*, *MAP3K2*, *CDKN1A* and *Bax* gene expression in the colorectal cancer cell line HCA-7; in contrast, *Bax* gene expression was down-regulated in the HCT116 cell line upon celecoxib treatment (Fatima *et al.*, 2008) suggesting that there may be variation in response from cell line to cell line to NSAID exposure.

We have recently reported finding that XRCC3 protein expression in SW480 cells was increased upon 1 mM aspirin treatment for 48 hours (Dibra *et al.*, 2010). The altered expression of *XRCC3* upon aspirin exposure may have implications to the sensitivity of cells to chemotherapeutic agents. Indeed, previous research in the breast cancer cell line MCF7 demonstrated that over-expression of XRCC3 induced cisplatin resistance (Xu *et al.*, 2005). Studies have shown that in contrast to XRCC3 over-expression and cisplatin resistance, *XRCC3* deficient HCT116 cells have increased sensitivity to cisplatin and also mitomycin C (Yoshihara *et al.*, 2004). Depletion of XRCC3 by siRNA in MCF7 cells inhibited cell proliferation, leading to accumulation of DNA breaks and triggering activation of p53-dependant cell death (Loignon *et al.*, 2007). Although some studies have shown no association between polymorphisms in *XRCC3* and colorectal cancer risk (Mort *et al.*, 2003; Yeh *et al.*, 2005; Tranah *et al.*, 2004; Skjelbred *et al.*, 2006) some studies have (Improta *et al.*, 2008), and in *XRCC3* polymorphisms have also been associated with breast and lung cancer susceptibility (Smith *et al.*, 2003; Jacobsen *et al.*, 2004). One essential point to note is that there is a lack of information in current literature about the effects of NSAIDs on normal human colonocytes. The information that we have relates to cell lines/*in vitro* studies and murine models. There is a need to understand the effects of these compounds on normal, healthy colon cells and how these effects prevent carcinogenesis in these cells. With the majority of the models used in studies already established as cancerous, it is difficult to separate the effects of these compounds on normal cells rather than cells which are already cancerous and subject to pathway dysregulation. In addition to NSAIDs, flavonoids have also been associated with anti−carcinogenic properties. It is interesting to note that a recent study has shown that these compounds, which occur naturally in fruits and vegetables, not only have a protective effect against oxidative DNA damage but also increase repair activity *in vitro* (Ramos *et al.*, 2010). To summarise: NSAIDs can alter the expression of DNA repair, and pro- and anti-apoptotic proteins.

2.3.2 Curcumin and DNA repair

Curcumin is a naturally occurring turmeric derivative with anti-inflammatory properties and apoptotic, anti-proliferative, anti-oxidant and anti-angiogenic effects (Shehzad *et al.*, 2010). *In vivo* studies have shown that curcumin decreased intestinal polyp formation in the APC$^{min/+}$ mouse model (Murphy *et al.*, 2010). Curcumin is considered an attractive compound for chemopreventative use and there are at present clinical trials ongoing testing the effectiveness of the compound against different types of cancer (Shehzad *et al.*, 2010). However, as with aspirin, a known mechanism of action of curcumin is yet to be elucidated with a range of molecular targets proposed (as reviewed in Shehzad *et al.*, 2010 and Ravindran *et al.*, 2009). As discussed in a recent review (Burgos-Moron *et al.*, 2010), although curcumin is widely regarded as a potential chemopreventative drug its safety and efficiency is yet to be fully elucidated and results from studies, clinical or otherwise, should be interpreted with this in mind. Curcumin has been shown to affect DNA damage and repair. Curcumin has been found to induce DNA damage in mouse-rat hybrid retina ganglion cells (Lu *et al.*, 2009). The study reported that curcumin decreased expression of the DNA repair genes *ATR, ATM, BRCA1, DNA-PK* and *MGMT*. Curcumin has also been seen to cause DNA damage, as tested in the Comet Assay, in gastric mucosa cells and human peripheral blood lymphocytes (Blasiak *et al.*, 1999). Curcumin has been shown to induce DNA single strand breaks (Scott & Loo, 2004) and induce the expression of the pro-apoptotic gene *GADD153* in HCT116 colonocytes. It is suggested that the up-regulation of GADD153 is a direct response to DNA damage caused by curcumin, ultimately resulting in the induction of apoptosis (Scott & Loo, 2004). Microarray analysis of human lung cancer cells after curcumin treatment saw an upregulation of GADD45 and GADD153 gene expression (Saha *et al.*, 2010) and microarray analysis has also shown an up-regulation of GADD45 by curcumin treatment in a human breast cancer cell line (Ramachandran *et al.*, 2005). It has recently been proposed that DNA MMR may play a role in the cellular response to curcumin (Jiang *et al.*, 2010): DNA MMR proficient cells showed a greater accumulation of double strand breaks (DSB) upon curcumin treatment compared to MMR deficient cells suggesting that DSB formation induced by curcumin is primarily a DNA MMR-dependent process; further to this, curcumin was reported to activate ATM/Chk1 and cause cell-cycle arrest and apoptosis in human pancreatic cancer cells. DNA MMR proficient cells showed activation of Chk1 and induction of the G(2)-M cell cycle checkpoint (Jiang *et al.*, 2010) suggesting that the curcumin induced checkpoint response may be a DNA MMR dependent mechanism. Interestingly, microarray analysis of gene expression of invasive lung adenocarcinoma (CL1-5) cells exposed to curcumin found an induction in MLH1 gene expression and reduction in MMP expression (Chen *et al.*, 2004). Curcumin is also reported to affect the Fanconi anemia (FA)/BRCA pathway. Curcumin sensitises ovarian and breast cancer cells with a functional FA/BRCA pathway to cisplatin

(Chirnomas *et al.*, 2006). This is a clinically significant finding as resistance to chemotherapeutic drugs such as cisplatin is common and monoketone analogs of curcumin are now being developed as a new class of FA pathway inhibitors (Landais *et al.*, 2009). Recently, curcumin inhibition of the FA/BRCA pathway has also been suggested to be a mechanism for the reversal of multiple resistance in a multiple myeloma cell line (Xiao *et al.*, 2010). In a recent phase IIa clinical trial report, curcumin reduced aberrant crypt foci formation (Carroll *et al.*, 2011).

2.3.3 Interaction of NSAIDs with anti-cancer treatments

The capacity for specific cyclooxygenase inhibitors and NSAIDs to enhance the cellular response to chemotherapeutic and radiotherapeutic agents has been examined. Additive, synergistic and antagonistic effects have been reported. For example, the effect of a selective COX-2 inhibitor SC-236 (4-[5-(4-chlorophenyl)-3-trifluoromethyl)-1H-pyrazol-1-yl) benzene sulphonamide) was tested on cells derived from a murine sarcoma in the absence and presence of γ-ray irradiation, and a clonogenic cell survival assay confirmed that the compound significantly enhanced cell radiosensitivity (Raju *et al.*, 2002). In the human hepatocellular carcinoma cell line HepG2, indomethacin and SC-236 enhanced doxorubicin toxicity reportedly via inhibiting P-glycoprotein and the multidrug resistance-associated protein 1 (MRP1) (Ye *et al.*, 2011). Exogenous prostaglandin E2 addition failed to reverse the cellular accumulation and retention of doxorubicin and the authors concluded that the action of the drugs was via a COX-independent mechanism. Synergistic cell death characterised as being apoptotic based on Bax expression, DNA fragmentation and TUNEL assay, was observed in HT-29 cells co-treated with aspirin and 5-fluorouracil (Ashktorab *et al.*, 2005). In marked contrast to the above findings, an antagonistic activity of celecoxib and SC-236 to cytotoxicity mediated by cisplatin to human esophageal squamous cell carcinoma cells has been observed; mechanistic analysis indicated that the compounds decrease cisplatin accumulation and DNA platination, in a COX-2 independent manner (Yu *et al.*, 2011). As previously intimated, there is evidence that NSAIDs can affect double strand break repair pathways. It is known that the homologous recombination protein Rad51 is overexpressed in chemo-radioresistent carcinomas. A study by *Ko et al.*, (2009) showed that celecoxib enhanced gefitinib induced cytotoxicity in NSCLC cells: combined celecoxib/gefitinib treatment resulted in the reduction of Rad51 protein levels. Degradation of Rad51 occurred via a 26S proteasome-dependent pathway. Celecoxib has been shown to inhibit growth of head and neck carcinoma cells and enhance radiosensitivity in a dose-dependent manner: celecoxib downregulated Ku70 protein expression and inhibited DNA-PKcs kinase activity which is known to be involved in DSB repair (Raju *et al.*, 2005). Further to this, sodium salicylate has been shown to inhibit the kinase activity of ATM and DNA-PK which suppresses their DNA damage response (Fan *et al.*, 2010). A recent study in prostate cancer demonstrated that treatment of the prostate cancer cell line PC-3 with NO-sulindac increased the rate of single strand DNA breaks and that there was slower repair of these lesions (Stewart *et al.*, 2011). We thus suggest that caution is exercised in situations where patients are prescribed NSAIDs when undergoing chemotherapy or radiotherapy as unexpected additive or antagonistic reactions may arise, and thus potentially compromise treatment effectiveness. However, there is also the promise that NSAIDs (either known or novel) may significantly synergise and enhance responses to chemotherapeutic, biologic, or radiotherapeutic modalities.

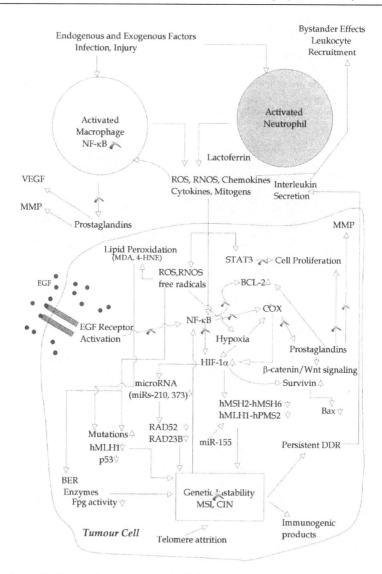

Fig. 2. A schematic illustration (composite) of the possible interconnections of the molecules and activities cited in the text. Where NSAIDs can potentially act is illustrated with **X**. Abbreviations: BER, base excision repair; CIN, chromosomal instability; COX, cyclooxygenase; DDR, DNA damage response; EGF, epidermal growth factor; Fpg, formamidopyrimidine-DNA glycosylase; 4-HNE, trans-4-hydroxynonenal; HIF-1α, hypoxia inducible factor-1α; MDA, malondialdehyde; MIN, microsatellite instability; MMP, matrix metalloproteinase; miR, micro RNA; NF-κB, nuclear factor kappa B; RNOS, reactive nitrogen oxide species; ROS, reactive oxygen species; STAT3, signal transducer and activator of transcription 3; VEGF, vascular endothelial growth factor. For reasons of clarity, chemokine and cytokine receptor interactions are not shown.

3. Conclusion

The accumulated findings from a significant body of research indicates that NSAIDs – including aspirin- act via multiple mechanisms in reducing the morbidity and mortality of cancer, and that aspirin and other NSAIDs reduce inflammation via COX-dependent *and* COX-independent pathways. NSAIDs can select for DNA mismatch repair competency and microsatellite stable cells thus inhibiting at least one well recognised pathway of colorectal cancer progression; furthermore, *in vitro* data suggest that NSAIDs exhibit 'direct' and relatively specific and rapid toxicity to colorectal cancer cells, with evidence suggesting that this may (but almost certainly not exclusively) involve DNA repair pathways. There is a paucity of information regarding the effect of NSAIDS on gene expression in non-transformed cell lines, including colonocytes and stromal cells and stem cells. Epidemiological evidence strongly indicates that NSAIDs are particularly protective against adenocarcinoma formation. Given the potential as chemopreventative agents, significant effort should be directed into producing novel NSAID derivatives that do not produce the adverse gastrointestinal and cardiovascular effects but retain the multiple and potent protective actions that are involved in suppressing adenocarcinoma formation.

We feel that the following questions need to be addressed:

a. What is the mechanism by which aspirin selects for microsatellite stability?
b. What is the mechanism by which aspirin and other NSAIDs show their relatively specific toxicity to colorectal cancer cells?
c. Does long term usage of aspirin and other NSAIDs preferentially reprogram the colonic epithelium via epigenetic mechanisms *eg* altering histone deacetylase and DNA methyltransferase activities?
d. How do NSAIDS affect gene expression in non-transformed cells, including colonic stem cells? Do NSAIDs affect epithelial miRNA profiles?

4. Acknowledgement

We wish to thank Dr Paul Hooley for helpful discussions and comments during the preparation of this chapter.

5. References

Aarnio, M., Mecklin, J. P., Aaltonen, L. A., Nystrom-Lahti, M., & Jarvinen, H. J. (1995). Lifetime risk of different cancers in hereditary non-polyposis colorectal cancer (HNPCC) syndrome. *Int J Cancer*, 64, pp.430-433.

Abdel-Rahman, W. M., Mecklin, J. P., & Peltomaki, P. (2006). The genetics of HNPCC: Application to diagnosis and screening. *Crit Rev Oncol Hematol*, 58, pp.208-220.

Amann, R., & Peskar, B. A. (2002). Anti-inflammatory effects of aspirin and sodium salicylate. *Eur J Pharmacol*, 447, pp.1-9.

Ashktorab, H., Dawkins, F. W., Mohamed, R., Larbi, D., & Smoot, D. T. (2005). Apoptosis induced by aspirin and 5-fluorouracil in human colonic adenocarcinoma cells. *Dig Dis Sci*, 50, pp.1025-1032.

Bader, S., Walker, M., & Harrison, D. (2000). Most microsatellite unstable sporadic colorectal carcinomas carry mbd4 mutations. *Br J Cancer*, 83, pp.1646-1649.

Bader, S., Walker, M., Hendrich, B., Bird, A., Bird, C., Hooper, M., et al. (1999). Somatic frameshift mutations in the MBD4 gene of sporadic colon cancers with mismatch repair deficiency. *Oncogene*, 18, pp.8044-8047.

Baek, S. J., Kim, K. S., Nixon, J. B., Wilson, L. C., & Eling, T. E. (2001). Cyclooxygenase inhibitors regulate the expression of a tgf-beta superfamily member that has proapoptotic and antitumorigenic activities. *Mol Pharmacol*, 59, pp.901-908.

Banerjea, A., Ahmed, S., Hands, R. E., Huang, F., Han, X., Shaw, P. M., et al. (2004). Colorectal cancers with microsatellite instability display mRNA expression signatures characteristic of increased immunogenicity. *Mol Cancer*, 3, pp.21.

Barnes, C. J., & Lee, M. (1998). Chemoprevention of spontaneous intestinal adenomas in the adenomatous polyposis coli min mouse model with aspirin. *Gastroenterology*, 114, pp.873-877.

Barnes, C. J., & Lee, M. (1999). Determination of an optimal dosing regimen for aspirin chemoprevention of 1,2-dimethylhydrazine-induced colon tumours in rats. *Br J Cancer*, 79, pp.1646-1650.

Baron, J. A., Cole, B. F., Sandler, R. S., Haile, R. W., Ahnen, D., Bresalier, R., et al. (2003). A randomized trial of aspirin to prevent colorectal adenomas. *N Engl J Med*, 348, pp.891-899.

Barreto, G., Schafer, A., Marhold, J., Stach, D., Swaminathan, S. K., Handa, V., et al. (2007). Gadd45α promotes epigenetic gene activation by repair-mediated DNA demethylation. *Nature*, 445, pp.671-675.

Behrens, J. (2005). The role of the wnt signalling pathway in colorectal tumorigenesis. *Biochem Soc Trans*, 33, pp.672-675.

Bielas, J. H., Loeb, K. R., Rubin, B. P., True, L. D., & Loeb, L. A. (2006). Human cancers express a mutator phenotype. *Proc Natl Acad Sci U S A*, 103, pp.18238-18242.

Bienz, M., & Clevers, H. (2000). Linking colorectal cancer to wnt signaling. *Cell*, 103, pp.311-320.

Blasiak, J., Trzeciak, A, and Kowalik, J. (1999) Curcumin damages DNA in human gastric mucosa cells and lymphocytes. *J Environ Pathol Toxicol Oncol.* 18, pp.271-6.

Bocker, T., Ruschoff, J., & Fishel, R. (1999). Molecular diagnostics of cancer predisposition: Hereditary non- polyposis colorectal carcinoma and mismatch repair defects. *Biochim Biophys Acta*, 1423, 3. pp.O1-O10.

Boland, C. R., Thibodeau, S. N., Hamilton, S. R., Sidransky, D., Eshleman, J. R., Burt, R. W., et al. (1998). A national cancer institute workshop on microsatellite instability for cancer detection and familial predisposition: Development of international criteria for the determination of microsatellite instability in colorectal cancer. *Cancer Res*, 58, pp.5248-5257.

Bonelli, P., Tuccillo, F. M., Calemma, R., Pezzetti, F., Borrelli, A., Martinelli, R., et al. (2010). Changes in the gene expression profile of gastric cancer cells in response to ibuprofen: A gene pathway analysis. *Pharmacogenomics J*,June 15.

Bos, C. L., Kodach, L. L., van den Brink, G. R., Diks, S. H., van Santen, M. M., Richel, D. J., et al. (2006). Effect of aspirin on the wnt/beta-catenin pathway is mediated via protein phosphatase 2a. *Oncogene*, 25, pp.6447-6456.

Bosetti, C., Gallus, S., & La Vecchia, C. (2002). Aspirin and cancer risk: An update to 2001. *Eur J Cancer Prev*, 11, pp.535-542.

Bousserouel, S., Gosse, F., Bouhadjar, M., Soler, L., Marescaux, J., & Raul, F.(2010). Long-term administration of aspirin inhibits tumour formation and triggers antineoplastic molecular changes in a pre-clinical model of colon carcinogenesis. *Oncol Rep*, 23, pp.511-517.

Brentnall, T. A., Chen, R., Lee, J. G., Kimmey, M. B., Bronner, M. P., Haggitt, R. C., *et al.* (1995). Microsatellite instability and k-ras mutations associated with pancreatic adenocarcinoma and pancreatitis. *Cancer Res*, 55, pp.4264-4267.

Buermeyer, A. B., Wilson-Van Patten, C., Baker, S. M., & Liskay, R. M. (1999). The human MLH1 cDNA complements DNA mismatch repair defects in mlh1-deficient mouse embryonic fibroblasts. *Cancer Res*, 59, pp.538-541.

Burgos-Morón, E., Calderón-Montaño, J. M., Salvador, J., Robles, A, and López-Lázaro, M. (2010) The dark side of curcumin. *Int J Cancer*. 126, pp.1771-5.

Campregher, C., Luciani, M. G., & Gasche, C. (2008). Activated neutrophils induce an hMSH2-dependent G2/M checkpoint arrest and replication errors at a (CA)13-repeat in colon epithelial cells. *Gut*, 57, pp.780-787.

Carethers, J. M., Hawn, M. T., Chauhan, D. P., Luce, M. C., Marra, G., Koi, M., *et al.* (1996). Competency in mismatch repair prohibits clonal expansion of cancer cells treated with n-methyl-n'-nitro-n-nitrosoguanidine. *J Clin Invest*, 98, pp.199-206.

Carroll, R. E., Benya, R. V., Turgeon, D. K., Vareed, S., Neuman, M., Rodriguez, L., *et al.* (2011). Phase IIa clinical trial of curcumin for the prevention of colorectal neoplasia. *Cancer Prev Res (Phila)*, 4, pp.354-364.

Casorelli, I., Pannellini, T., De Luca, G., Degan, P., Chiera, F., Iavarone, I., et al. The Mutyh base excision repair gene influences the inflammatory response in a mouse model of ulcerative colitis. *PLoS ONE*, 5, e12070.

Cejka, P., Stojic, L., Mojas, N., Russell, A. M., Heinimann, K., Cannavo, E., *et al.* (2003). Methylation-induced G(2)/M arrest requires a full complement of the mismatch repair protein hMLH1. *EMBO J*, 22, pp.2245-2254.

Chan, A. T., Ogino, S., & Fuchs, C. S. (2009). Aspirin use and survival after diagnosis of colorectal cancer. *Jama*, 302, pp.649-658.

Chang, C. L., Marra, G., Chauhan, D. P., Ha, H. T., Chang, D. K., Ricciardiello, L., *et al.* (2002). Oxidative stress inactivates the human DNA mismatch repair system. *Am J Physiol Cell Physiol*, 283, pp.C148-154.

Charalambous, D., & O'Brien, P. E. (1996). Inhibition of colon cancer precursors in the rat by sulindac sulphone is not dependent on inhibition of prostaglandin synthesis. *J Gastroenterol Hepatol*, 11, pp.307-310.

Chaturvedi, M. M., Sung, B., Yadav, V. R., Kannappan, R., & Aggarwal, B. B. (2011). NF-κB addiction and its role in cancer: 'one size does not fit all'. *Oncogene*, 30, pp.1615-1630.

Chen, H. W., Yu, S. L., Chen, J. J., Li, H. N., Lin, Y. C., Yao, P. L., *et al.* (2004). Anti-invasive gene expression profile of curcumin in lung adenocarcinoma based on a high throughput microarray analysis. *Mol Pharmacol*, 65, pp.99-110.

Chen, W. C., Liu, Q., Fu, J. X., & Kang, S. Y. (2004). Expression of survivin and its significance in colorectal cancer. *World J Gastroenterol*, 10, 2886-2889.

Cheng, W. Y., Hsiang, C. Y., Bau, D. T., Chen, J. C., Shen, W. S., Li, C. C., *et al.* (2007). Microarray analysis of vanillin-regulated gene expression profile in human hepatocarcinoma cells. *Pharmacol Res*, 56, pp.474-482.

Chiou, S. K., Hodges, A., & Hoa, N. (2010). Suppression of growth arrest and DNA damage-inducible 45alpha expression confers resistance to sulindac and indomethacin-induced gastric mucosal injury. *J Pharmacol Exp Ther*, 334, pp.693-702.

Chirnomas, D., Taniguchi, T., de la Vega, M., Vaidya, A. P., Vasserman, M., Hartman, A. R., Kennedy, R., Foster, R., Mahoney, J., Seiden, M. V, and D'Andrea, A. D. (2006) Chemosensitization to cisplatin by inhibitors of the Fanconi anemia/BRCA pathway. *Mol Cancer Ther.* 5, pp.952-61.

Chiu, C. H., McEntee, M. F., & Whelan, J. (1997). Sulindac causes rapid regression of preexisting tumors in min/+ mice independent of prostaglandin biosynthesis. *Cancer Res*, 57, pp.4267-4273.

Colotta, F., Allavena, P., Sica, A., Garlanda, C., & Mantovani, A. (2009). Cancer-related inflammation, the seventh hallmark of cancer: Links to genetic instability. *Carcinogenesis*, 30, pp.1073-1081.

Cooper, K., Squires, H., Carroll, C., Papaioannou, D., Booth, A., Logan, R. F., *et al.* (2010). Chemoprevention of colorectal cancer: Systematic review and economic evaluation. *Health Technol Assess*, 14, pp.1-206.

Corpet, D. E., & Pierre, F. (2003). Point: From animal models to prevention of colon cancer. Systematic review of chemoprevention in min mice and choice of the model system. *Cancer Epidemiol Biomarkers Prev*, 12, pp.391-400.

Corpet, D. E., & Pierre, F. (2005). How good are rodent models of carcinogenesis in predicting efficacy in humans? A systematic review and meta-analysis of colon chemoprevention in rats, mice and men. *Eur J Cancer*, 41, pp.1911-1922.

Craven, P. A., & DeRubertis, F. R. (1992). Effects of aspirin on 1,2-dimethylhydrazine-induced colonic carcinogenesis. *Carcinogenesis*, 13, pp.541-546.

Crosby, M. E., Kulshreshtha, R., Ivan, M., & Glazer, P. M. (2009). MicroRNA regulation of DNA repair gene expression in hypoxic stress. *Cancer Res*, 69, pp.1221-1229.

Cuzick, J., Otto, F., Baron, J. A., Brown, P. H., Burn, J., Greenwald, P., *et al.* (2009). Aspirin and non-steroidal anti-inflammatory drugs for cancer prevention: An international consensus statement. *Lancet Oncol*, 10, pp.501-507.

David, S. S., O'Shea, V. L., & Kundu, S. (2007). Base-excision repair of oxidative DNA damage. *Nature*, 447, pp.941-950.

Davis, T. W., Wilson-Van, P. C., Meyers, M., Kunugi, K. A., Cuthill, S., Reznikoff, C., *et al.* (1998). Defective expression of the DNA mismatch repair protein, MLH1, alters G2-M cell cycle checkpoint arrest following ionizing radiation. *Cancer Res*, 58, 767-778.

de la Chapelle, A. (2004). Genetic predisposition to colorectal cancer. *Nat Rev Cancer*, 4, pp.769-780.

Deb, J., Dibra, H., Shan, S., Rajan, S., Manneh, J., Kankipati, C.S., Perry, C.J., & Nicholl, I.D. (2011). Activity of aspirin analogues and vanillin in a human colorectal cancer cell line. *Oncol Rep* (in press).

Devaraj, B., Lee, A., Cabrera, B. L., Miyai, K., Luo, L., Ramamoorthy, S., *et al.* (2010). Relationship of emast and microsatellite instability among patients with rectal cancer. *J Gastrointest Surg*, 14, pp.1521-1528.

Dibra, H.K., Brown, J.E., Hooley, P. & Nicholl, I.D. (2010). Aspirin and alterations in DNA repair proteins in the SW480 colorectal cancer cell line. *Oncol Rep*, 24:37-46.

Dihlmann, S., Siermann, A., & von Knebel Doeberitz, M. (2001). The nonsteroidal anti-inflammatory drugs aspirin and indomethacin attenuate beta-catenin/tcf-4 signaling. *Oncogene*, 20, 645-653.

Dikshit, P., Chatterjee, M., Goswami, A., Mishra, A., & Jana, N. R. (2006). Aspirin induces apoptosis through the inhibition of proteasome function. *J Biol Chem*, 281, pp.29228-29235.

Din, F. V., Dunlop, M. G., & Stark, L. A. (2004). Evidence for colorectal cancer cell specificity of aspirin effects on NFκB signalling and apoptosis. *Br J Cancer*, 91, 381-388.

Din, F. V., Theodoratou, E., Farrington, S. M., Tenesa, A., Barnetson, R. A., Cetnarskyj, R., *et al.* (2010). Effect of aspirin and nsaids on risk and survival from colorectal cancer. *Gut*, 59, 1670-1679.

Ding, X., Mohd, A. B., Huang, Z., Baba, T., Bernardini, M. Q., Lyerly, H. K., *et al.* (2009). Mlh1 expression sensitises ovarian cancer cells to cell death mediated by xiap inhibition. *Br J Cancer*, 101, pp.269-277.

Ditsworth, D., & Zong, W. X. (2004). NF-κB: Key mediator of inflammation-associated cancer. *Cancer Biol Ther*, 3, 1214-1216.

Dunlop, M. G., Farrington, S. M., Carothers, A. D., Wyllie, A. H., Sharp, L., Burn, J., *et al.* (1997). Cancer risk associated with germline DNA mismatch repair gene mutations. *Hum Mol Genet*, 6, pp.105-110.

Edwards, R. A., Witherspoon, M., Wang, K., Afrasiabi, K., Pham, T., Birnbaumer, L., *et al.* (2009). Epigenetic repression of DNA mismatch repair by inflammation and hypoxia in inflammatory bowel disease-associated colorectal cancer. *Cancer Res*, 69, pp.6423-6429.

Elder, D. J., Hague, A., Hicks, D. J., & Paraskeva, C. (1996). Differential growth inhibition by the aspirin metabolite salicylate in human colorectal tumor cell lines: Enhanced apoptosis in carcinoma and in vitro-transformed adenoma relative to adenoma relative to adenoma cell lines. *Cancer Res*, 56, pp.2273-2276.

Elwood, P. C., Gallagher, A. M., Duthie, G. G., Mur, L. A., & Morgan, G. (2009). Aspirin, salicylates, and cancer. *Lancet*, 373, 1301-1309.

Fan, J. R., Huang, T. H., Wen, C. Y., Shen, T. L., & Li, T. K. (2010). Sodium salicylate acts through direct inhibition of phosphoinositide 3-kinase-like kinases to modulate topoisomerase-mediated DNA damage responses. *Eur J Pharmacol*, 638, pp.13-20.

Fatima, N., Yi, M., Ajaz, S., Stephens, R. M., Stauffer, S., Greenwald, P., *et al.* (2008). Altered gene expression profiles define pathways in colorectal cancer cell lines affected by celecoxib. *Cancer Epidemiol Biomarkers Prev*, 17, 3051-3061.

Federico, A., Morgillo, F., Tuccillo, C., Ciardiello, F., & Loguercio, C. (2007). Chronic inflammation and oxidative stress in human carcinogenesis. *Int J Cancer*, 121, pp.2381-2386.

Ferguson, L. R. (2010). Chronic inflammation and mutagenesis. *Mutat Res*, 690, 3-11.

Fernandes, A. M., De Souza, V. R., Springer, C. R., Cardoso, S. V., Loyola, A. M., Mesquita, R. A., *et al.* (2007). Tobacco and inflammation effects in immunoexpression of hMSH2 and hMLH1 in epithelium of oral mucosa. *Anticancer Res*, 27, pp.2433-2437.

Ferrandez, A., Prescott, S., & Burt, R. W. (2003). Cox-2 and colorectal cancer. *Curr Pharm Des*, 9, pp.2229-2251.

Fleisher, A. S., Esteller, M., Harpaz, N., Leytin, A., Rashid, A., Xu, Y., *et al.* (2000). Microsatellite instability in inflammatory bowel disease-associated neoplastic lesions is associated with hypermethylation and diminished expression of the DNA mismatch repair gene, hMLH1. *Cancer Res*, 60, 4864-4868.

Foreman, J. E., Sorg, J. M., McGinnis, K. S., Rigas, B., Williams, J. L., Clapper, M. L., *et al.* (2009). Regulation of peroxisome proliferator-activated receptor-beta/delta by the apc/beta-catenin pathway and nonsteroidal antiinflammatory drugs. *Mol Carcinog*, 48, pp.942-952.

Forte, A., De Sanctis, R., Leonetti, G., Manfredelli, S., Urbano, V., & Bezzi, M. (2008). Dietary chemoprevention of colorectal cancer. *Ann Ital Chir*, 79, pp.261-267.

Galipeau, P. C., Li, X., Blount, P. L., Maley, C. C., Sanchez, C. A., Odze, R. D., *et al.* (2007). NSAIDS modulate CDKN2A, TP53, and DNA content risk for progression to esophageal adenocarcinoma. *PLoS Med*, 4, e67.

Gasche, C., Chang, C. L., Rhees, J., Goel, A., & Boland, C. R. (2001). Oxidative stress increases frameshift mutations in human colorectal cancer cells. *Cancer Res*, 61, pp.7444-7448.

Gasche, C., Goel, A., Natarajan, L., & Boland, C. R. (2005). Mesalazine improves replication fidelity in cultured colorectal cells. *Cancer Res*, 65, 3993-3997.

Germann, A., Dihlmann, S., Hergenhahn, M., Doeberitz, M. K., & Koesters, R. (2003). Expression profiling of cc531 colon carcinoma cells reveals similar regulation of beta-catenin target genes by both butyrate and aspirin. *Int J Cancer*, 106, pp. 187-197.

Ghosh, N., Chaki, R., Mandal, V., & Mandal, S. C. (2010). Cox-2 as a target for cancer chemotherapy. *Pharmacol Rep*, 62, pp.233-244.

Giovannucci, E. (1999). The prevention of colorectal cancer by aspirin use. *Biomed Pharmacother*, 53, pp.303-308.

Glassner, B. J., Rasmussen, L. J., Najarian, M. T., Posnick, L. M., & Samson, L. D. (1998). Generation of a strong mutator phenotype in yeast by imbalanced base excision repair. *Proc Natl Acad Sci U S A*, 95, pp.9997-10002.

Goel, A., Chang, D. K., Ricciardiello, L., Gasche, C., & Boland, C. R. (2003). A novel mechanism for aspirin-mediated growth inhibition of human colon cancer cells. *Clin Cancer Res*, 9, pp.383-390.

Goke, M. N. (2002). Cox-2-independent antiproliferative action of acetylsalicylic acid in human colon cancer cells. *Eur J Clin Invest*, 32, pp.793-794.

Grivennikov, S. I., & Karin, M. (2010). Inflammation and oncogenesis: A vicious connection. *Curr Opin Genet Dev*, 20, 65-71.

Guo, J., Verma, U. N., Gaynor, R. B., Frenkel, E. P., & Becerra, C. R. (2004). Enhanced chemosensitivity to irinotecan by rna interference-mediated down-regulation of the nuclear factor-kappab p65 subunit. *Clin Cancer Res*, 10, pp.3333-3341.

Hampel, H., Frankel, W. L., Martin, E., Arnold, M., Khanduja, K., Kuebler, P., *et al.* (2005). Screening for the Lynch syndrome (hereditary nonpolyposis colorectal cancer). *N Engl J Med*, 352, pp.1851-1860.

Hanahan, D., & Weinberg, R. A. (2000). The hallmarks of cancer. *Cell*, 100, 57-70.

Hancock, J. M. 1999. Microsatellites and other simple sequences: Genomic context and mutational mechanisms. *In* D. B. Goldstein & C. Schlotterer (Eds) *Microsatellites evolution and applications* pp. 1-9). Oxford: Oxford University Press. ISBN 978-0198504078.

Hanif, R., Pittas, A., Feng, Y., Koutsos, M. I., Qiao, L., Staiano-Coico, L., *et al.* (1996). Effects of nonsteroidal anti-inflammatory drugs on proliferation and on induction of apoptosis in colon cancer cells by a prostaglandin-independent pathway. *Biochem Pharmacol*, 52, pp.237-245.

Hardwick, J. C., van Santen, M., van den Brink, G. R., van Deventer, S. J., & Peppelenbosch, M. P. (2004). DNA array analysis of the effects of aspirin on colon cancer cells: Involvement of rac1. *Carcinogenesis*, 25, 1293-1298.

Harris, R. E., Beebe-Donk, J., & Alshafie, G. A. (2007). Reduced risk of human lung cancer by selective cyclooxygenase 2 (cox-2) blockade: Results of a case control study. *Int J Biol Sci*, 3, pp.328-334.

He, T. C., Chan, T. A., Vogelstein, B., & Kinzler, K. W. (1999). PPARδ is an APC-regulated target of nonsteroidal anti-inflammatory drugs. *Cell*, 99, pp.335-345.

Herman, J. G., Umar, A., Polyak, K., Graff, J. R., Ahuja, N., Issa, J. P., *et al.* (1998). Incidence and functional consequences of hmlh1 promoter hypermethylation in colorectal carcinoma. *Proc Natl Acad Sci U S A*, 95, pp.6870-6875.

Herrmann, C., Block, C., Geisen, C., Haas, K., Weber, C., Winde, G., et al. (1998). Sulindac sulfide inhibits ras signaling. *Oncogene*, 17, pp.1769-1776.

Hitchins, M. P., Wong, J. J., Suthers, G., Suter, C. M., Martin, D. I., Hawkins, N. J., *et al.* (2007). Inheritance of a cancer-associated MLH1 germ-line epimutation. *N Engl J Med*, 356, pp.697-705.

Hofseth, L. J., Khan, M. A., Ambrose, M., Nikolayeva, O., Xu-Welliver, M., Kartalou, M., *et al.* (2003). The adaptive imbalance in base excision-repair enzymes generates microsatellite instability in chronic inflammation. *J Clin Invest*, 112, pp.1887-1894.

Hu, W., Feng, Z., Eveleigh, J., Iyer, G., Pan, J., Amin, S., *et al.* (2002). The major lipid peroxidation product, trans-4-hydroxy-2-nonenal, preferentially forms DNA adducts at codon 249 of human p53 gene, a unique mutational hotspot in hepatocellular carcinoma. *Carcinogenesis*, 23, pp.1781-1789.

Huang, R. H., Chai, J., & Tarnawski, A. S. (2006). Identification of specific genes and pathways involved in nsaids-induced apoptosis of human colon cancer cells. *World J Gastroenterol*, 12, pp.6446-6452.

Hughes, A., Smith, N. I., & Wallace, H. M. (2003). Polyamines reverse non-steroidal anti-inflammatory drug-induced toxicity in human colorectal cancer cells. *Biochem J*, 374, pp.481-488.

Hundley, T. R., & Rigas, B. (2006). Nitric oxide-donating aspirin inhibits colon cancer cell growth via mitogen-activated protein kinase activation. *J Pharmacol Exp Ther*, 316, pp.25-34.

Hussain, S. P., Amstad, P., Raja, K., Ambs, S., Nagashima, M., Bennett, W. P., *et al.* (2000). Increased p53 mutation load in noncancerous colon tissue from ulcerative colitis: A cancer-prone chronic inflammatory disease. *Cancer Res*, 60, pp.3333-3337.

Hussain, S. P., & Harris, C. C. (2007). Inflammation and cancer: An ancient link with novel potentials. *Int J Cancer*, 121, pp.2373-2380.

Hussain, S. P., Hofseth, L. J., & Harris, C. C. (2003). Radical causes of cancer. *Nat Rev Cancer*, 3, pp.276-285.

Iizaka, M., Furukawa, Y., Tsunoda, T., Akashi, H., Ogawa, M., & Nakamura, Y. (2002). Expression profile analysis of colon cancer cells in response to sulindac or aspirin. *Biochem Biophys Res Commun.*, 292, pp.498-512.

Imperiale, T. F. (2003). Aspirin and the prevention of colorectal cancer. *N Engl J Med*, 348, 879-880.

Improta, G., Sgambato, A., Bianchino, G., Zupa, A., Grieco, V., La Torre, G., Traficante, A. and Cittadini, A. (2008) Polymorphisms of the DNA repair genes XRCC1 and XRCC3 and risk of lung and colorectal cancer: a case-control study in a Southern Italian population. *Anticancer Res*, 28, pp.2941-2946.

Itzkowitz, S. H., & Yio, X. (2004). Inflammation and cancer iv. Colorectal cancer in inflammatory bowel disease: The role of inflammation. *Am J Physiol Gastrointest Liver Physiol*, 287, G7-17.

Jacinto, F. V., & Esteller, M. (2007). Mutator pathways unleashed by epigenetic silencing in human cancer. *Mutagenesis*, 22, pp.247-253.

Jacobsen, N. R., Raaschou-Nielsen, O., Nexo, B., Wallin, H., Overvad, K., Tjonneland, A. and Vogel, U. (2004) XRCC3 polymorphisms and risk of lung cancer. *Cancer Lett*, 213, pp.67-72.

Jacoby, R. F., Marshall, D. J., Newton, M. A., Novakovic, K., Tutsch, K., Cole, C. E., *et al.* (1996). Chemoprevention of spontaneous intestinal adenomas in the apc min mouse model by the nonsteroidal anti-inflammatory drug piroxicam. *Cancer Res*, 56, pp.710-714.

Jang, T. J., Jeon, K. H., & Jung, K. H. (2009). Cyclooxygenase-2 expression is related to the epithelial-to-mesenchymal transition in human colon cancers. *Yonsei Med J*, 50, pp.818-824.

Jiang, M., & Milner, J. (2003). Bcl-2 constitutively suppresses p53-dependent apoptosis in colorectal cancer cells. *Genes Dev*, 17, 832-837.

Jiang, Z., Jin, S., Yalowich, J. C., Brown, K. D, and Rajasekaran, B. (2010) The mismatch repair system modulates curcumin sensitivity through induction of DNA strand breaks and activation of G2-M checkpoint. *Mol Cancer Ther.* 9, pp.558-68.

Jiricny, J. (1998). Replication errors: Cha(lle)nging the genome. *EMBO J*, 17, pp.6427-6436.

Jiricny, J., & Marra, G. (2003). DNA repair defects in colon cancer. *Curr Opin Genet Dev.*, 13, pp.61-69.

John-Aryankalayil, M., Palayoor, S. T., Cerna, D., Falduto, M. T., Magnuson, S. R., & Coleman, C. N. (2009). NS-398, ibuprofen, and cyclooxygenase-2 RNA interference produce significantly different gene expression profiles in prostate cancer cells. *Mol Cancer Ther*, 8, pp.261-273.

Jones, P. A., & Laird, P. W. (1999). Cancer epigenetics comes of age. *Nat Gene*, 21, 163-167.

Jung, Y. J., Isaacs, J. S., Lee, S., Trepel, J., & Neckers, L. (2003). Il-1β-mediated up-regulation of HIF-1α via an NFκB/COX-2 pathway identifies HIF-1 as a critical link between inflammation and oncogenesis. *Faseb J*, 17, pp.2115-2117.

Keller, J. J., & Giardiello, F. M. (2003). Chemoprevention strategies using NSAIDs and COX-2 inhibitors. *Cancer Biol Ther*, 2, S140-149.

Key, T. J. (2011). Fruit and vegetables and cancer risk. *Br J Cancer*, 104, pp.6-11.

Kim, K. M., Song, J. J., An, J. Y., Kwon, Y. T., & Lee, Y. J. (2005). Pretreatment of acetylsalicylic acid promotes tumor necrosis factor-related apoptosis-inducing ligand-induced apoptosis by down-regulating BCL-2 gene expression. *J Biol Chem*, 280, pp.41047-41056.

Kim, S. H., Hwang, C. I., Juhnn, Y. S., Lee, J. H., Park, W. Y., & Song, Y. S. (2007). GADD153 mediates celecoxib-induced apoptosis in cervical cancer cells. *Carcinogenesis*, 28, pp.223-231.

Kinzler, K. W., & Vogelstein, B. (1996). Lessons from hereditary colorectal cancer. *Cell*, 87, pp.159-170.

Ko, J. C., Wang, L. H., Jhan, J. Y., Ciou, S. C., Hong, J. H., Lin, S. T., *et al.* (2009). The role of celecoxib in Rad51 expression and cell survival affected by gefitinib in human non-small cell lung cancer cells. *Lung Cancer*, 65, pp.290-298.

Kondo, A., Safaei, R., Mishima, M., Niedner, H., Lin, X., & Howell, S. B. (2001). Hypoxia-induced enrichment and mutagenesis of cells that have lost DNA mismatch repair. *Cancer Res*, 61, pp.7603-7607.

Kopp, E., & Ghosh, S. (1994). Inhibition of NF-κB by sodium salicylate and aspirin. *Science*, 265, 956-959.

Koshiji, M., To, K. K., Hammer, S., Kumamoto, K., Harris, A. L., Modrich, P., *et al.* (2005). HIF-1α induces genetic instability by transcriptionally downregulating mutsalpha expression. *Mol Cell*, 17, pp.793-803.

Kreis, S., Philippidou, D., Margue, C., Rolvering, C., Haan, C., Dumoutier, L., *et al.* (2007). Recombinant interleukin-24 lacks apoptosis-inducing properties in melanoma cells. *PLoS ONE*, 2, e1300.

Kutchera, W., Jones, D. A., Matsunami, N., Groden, J., McIntyre, T. M., Zimmerman, G. A., *et al.* (1996). Prostaglandin h synthase 2 is expressed abnormally in human colon cancer: Evidence for a transcriptional effect. *Proc Natl Acad Sci U S A*, 93, pp.4816-4820.

La Vecchia, C., Altieri, A., & Tavani, A. (2001). Vegetables, fruit, antioxidants and cancer: A review of Italian studies. *Eur J Nutr*, 40, pp.261-267.

Lagerstedt Robinson, K., Liu, T., Vandrovcova, J., Halvarsson, B., Clendenning, M., Frebourg, T., *et al.* (2007). Lynch syndrome (hereditary nonpolyposis colorectal cancer) diagnostics. *J Natl Cancer Inst*, 99, pp.291-299.

Lai, M. Y., Huang, J. A., Liang, Z. H., Jiang, H. X., & Tang, G. D. (2008). Mechanisms underlying aspirin-mediated growth inhibition and apoptosis induction of cyclooxygenase-2 negative colon cancer cell line SW480. *World J Gastroenterol*, 14, pp.4227-4233.

Lauria, A., Ippolito, M., Fazzari, M., Tutone, M., Di Blasi, F., Mingoia, F., et al. (2010). Ikk-β inhibitors: An analysis of drug-receptor interaction by using molecular docking and pharmacophore 3d-qsar approaches. *J Mol Graph Model*, 29, pp.72-81.

Law, B. K., Waltner-Law, M. E., Entingh, A. J., Chytil, A., Aakre, M. E., Norgaard, P., *et al.* (2000). Salicylate-induced growth arrest is associated with inhibition of p70[s6k] and down-regulation of c-Myc, Cyclin D1, Cyclin A, and Proliferating Cell Nuclear Antigen. *J Biol Chem*, 275, pp.38261-38267.

Lee, E. J., Park, H. G., & Kang, H. S. (2003). Sodium salicylate induces apoptosis in HCT116 colorectal cancer cells through activation of p38MAPK. *Int J Oncol*, 23, pp.503-508.

Lee, S. Y., Chung, H., Devaraj, B., Iwaizumi, M., Han, H. S., Hwang, D. Y., *et al.* (2010). Microsatellite alterations at selected tetranucleotide repeats are associated with morphologies of colorectal neoplasias. *Gastroenterology*, 139, pp.1519-1525.

Lim, S. C., Cho, H., Lee, T. B., Choi, C. H., Min, Y. D., Kim, S. S., et al. (2010). Impacts of cytosolic phospholipase A2, 15-prostaglandin dehydrogenase, and cyclooxygenase-2 expressions on tumor progression in colorectal cancer. *Yonsei Med J*, 51, pp.692-699.

Lindahl, T., & Wood, R. D. (1999). Quality control by DNA repair. *Science*, 286, 1897-1905.

Logan, R. F., Little, J., Hawtin, P. G., & Hardcastle, J. D. (1993). Effect of aspirin and non-steroidal anti-inflammatory drugs on colorectal adenomas: Case-control study of subjects participating in the nottingham faecal occult blood screening programme. *BMJ*, 307, 285-289.

Loignon, M., Amrein, L., Dunn, M., & Aloyz, R. (2007). Xrcc3 depletion induces spontaneous DNA breaks and p53-dependent cell death. *Cell Cycle*, 6, pp.606-611.

Lothe, R. A., Peltomaki, P., Meling, G. I., Aaltonen, L. A., Nystrom-Lahti, M., Pylkkanen, L., *et al.* (1993). Genomic instability in colorectal cancer: Relationship to clinicopathological variables and family history. *Cancer Res*, 53, pp.5849-5852.

Lu, H. F., Lai, K. C., Hsu, S. C., Lin, H. J., Yang, M. D., Chen, Y. L., Fan, M.J., Yang, J.S., Cheng, P.Y., Kuo, C. L, and Chung, J. G. (2009) Curcumin induces apoptosis through FAS and FADD, in caspase-3-dependent and -independent pathways in the N18 mouse-rat hybrid retina ganglion cells. *Oncol Rep.* 22, pp.97-104.

Lucci-Cordisco, E., Zito, I., Gensini, F., & Genuardi, M. (2003). Hereditary nonpolyposis colorectal cancer and related conditions. *Am J Med Genet*, 122A, pp.325-334.

Maekawa, M., & Watanabe, Y. (2007). Epigenetics: Relations to disease and laboratory findings. *Curr Med Chem*, 14, pp.2642-2653.

Mahmoud, N. N., Boolbol, S. K., Dannenberg, A. J., Mestre, J. R., Bilinski, R. T., Martucci, C., *et al.* (1998). The sulfide metabolite of sulindac prevents tumors and restores enterocyte apoptosis in a murine model of familial adenomatous polyposis. *Carcinogenesis*, 19, pp.87-91.

McCullough, A. K., Dodson, M. L., & Lloyd, R. S. (1999). Initiation of base excision repair: Glycosylase mechanisms and structures. *Annu Rev Biochem* 68, pp.255-285.

McDaid, J. R., Loughery, J., Dunne, P., Boyer, J. C., Downes, C. S., Farber, R. A., *et al.* (2009). Mlh1 mediates parp-dependent cell death in response to the methylating agent n-methyl-n-nitrosourea. *Br J Cancer*, 101, pp.441-451.

McIlhatton, M. A., Tyler, J., Burkholder, S., Ruschoff, J., Rigas, B., Kopelovich, L., *et al.* (2007). Nitric oxide-donating aspirin derivatives suppress microsatellite instability in mismatch repair-deficient and hereditary nonpolyposis colorectal cancer cells. *Cancer Res*, 67, pp.10966-10975.

McIlhatton, M. A., Tyler, J., Kerepesi, L. A., Bocker Edmonston, T., Kucherlapati, M. H., Edelmann, W., et al. (2011). Aspirin and low dose nitric oxide-donating aspirin increase life span in a lynch syndrome mouse model. *Cancer Prev Res (Phila)*, 4, pp.684-693.

Landais, I., Hiddingh, S., McCarroll, M., Yang, C., Sun, A., Turker, M. S., Snyder, J.P, and Hoatlin, M. E. (2009) Monoketone analogs of curcumin, a new class of Fanconi anemia pathway inhibitors. *Mol Cancer.*, pp.133.

Mitchell, R. J., Farrington, S. M., Dunlop, M. G., & Campbell, H. (2002). Mismatch repair genes hmlh1 and hmsh2 and colorectal cancer: A huge review. *Am J Epidemiol*, 156, pp.885-902.

Mort, R., Mo, L., McEwan, C. and Melton, D. W. (2003) Lack of involvement of nucleotide excision repair gene polymorphisms in colorectal cancer. *Br J Cancer*, 89, pp.333-337.

Murphy, E. A., Davis, J. M., McClellan, J. L., Gordon, B. T, and Carmichael, M. D. (2011) Curcumin's effect on intestinal inflammation and tumorigenesis in the ApcMin/+ mouse. *J Interferon Cytokine Res.* 31, pp.219-26.

Muscat, J. E., Stellman, S. D., & Wynder, E. L. (1994). Nonsteroidal antiinflammatory drugs and colorectal cancer. *Cancer*, 74, pp.1847-1854.

Nakano, H. (2004). Signaling crosstalk between NF-κB and jnk. *Trends Immunol*, 25, pp.402-405.

Narayan, S., & Roy, D. (2003). Role of apc and DNA mismatch repair genes in the development of colorectal cancers. *Mol Cancer* 2, pp.41.

Nicolaides, N. C., Littman, S. J., Modrich, P., Kinzler, K. W., & Vogelstein, B. (1998). A naturally occurring hpms2 mutation can confer a dominant negative mutator phenotype. *Mol Cell Biol*, 18, pp.1635-1641.

Olivier, S., Robe, P., & Bours, V. (2006). Can NF-κB be a target for novel and efficient anti-cancer agents? *Biochem Pharmacol*, 72, pp.1054-1068.

Olson, N., & van der Vliet, A. (2011). Interactions between nitric oxide and hypoxia-inducible factor signaling pathways in inflammatory disease. *Nitric Oxide*. In Press.

Orlando, R. C. (2010). The integrity of the esophageal mucosa. Balance between offensive and defensive mechanisms. *Best Pract Res Clin Gastroenterol*, 24, pp.873-882.

Oshima, M., Dinchuk, J. E., Kargman, S. L., Oshima, H., Hancock, B., Kwong, E., *et al.* (1996). Suppression of intestinal polyposis in APC$^{\Delta 716}$ knockout mice by inhibition of cyclooxygenase 2 (COX-2). *Cell*, 87, pp.803-809.

Paganini-Hill, A. (1993). Aspirin and colorectal cancer. *BMJ*, 307, pp.278-279.

Pai, R., Nakamura, T., Moon, W. S., & Tarnawski, A. S. (2003). Prostaglandins promote colon cancer cell invasion; signaling by cross-talk between two distinct growth factor receptors. *Faseb J*, 17, pp.1640-1647.

Pangburn, H. A., Ahnen, D. J., & Rice, P. L. (2010). Sulindac metabolites induce proteosomal and lysosomal degradation of the epidermal growth factor receptor. *Cancer Prev Res (Phila)*, 3, pp.560-572.

Pangburn, H. A., Kraus, H., Ahnen, D. J., & Rice, P. L. (2005). Sulindac metabolites inhibit epidermal growth factor receptor activation and expression. *J Carcinog*, 4, pp.16.

Papouli, E., Cejka, P., & Jiricny, J. (2004). Dependence of the cytotoxicity of DNA-damaging agents on the mismatch repair status of human cells. *Cancer Res*, 64, pp.3391-3394.

Park, W. S., Pham, T., Wang, C., Pack, S., Mueller, E., Mueller, J., *et al.* (1998). Loss of heterozygosity and microsatellite instability in non-neoplastic mucosa from patients with chronic ulcerative colitis. *Int J Mol Med*, 2, pp.221-224.

Parkin, D. M., Bray, F., Ferlay, J., & Pisani, P. (2005). Global cancer statistics, 2002. *CA Cancer J Clin*, 55, pp.74-108.

Parri, M., & Chiarugi, P. (2010). Rac and rho gtpases in cancer cell motility control. *Cell Commun Signal*, 8, pp.23.

Parsons, R., Li, G. M., Longley, M. J., Fang, W. H., Papadopoulos, N., Jen, J., *et al.* (1993). Hypermutability and mismatch repair deficiency in rer+ tumor cells. *Cell*, 75, pp.1227-1236.

Parsons, R., Myeroff, L. L., Liu, B., Willson, J. K., Markowitz, S. D., Kinzler, K. W., *et al.* (1995). Microsatellite instability and mutations of the transforming growth factor beta type ii receptor gene in colorectal cancer. *Cancer Res*, 55, pp.5548-5550.

Paterson, J. R., Baxter, G., Dreyer, J.S., Halket, J.M., Flynn, R., Lawrence, J.R. (2008). Salicylic acid sans aspirin in animals and man: Persistence in fasting and biosynthesis from benzoic acid. *J Agric Food Chem*, 56, pp.11648-11652.

Paterson, J. R., Blacklock, C., Campbell, G., Wiles, D., & Lawrence, J. R. (1998). The identification of salicylates as normal constituents of serum: A link between diet and health? *J Clin Pathol*, 51, pp.502-505.

Paterson, J. R., & Lawrence, J. R. (2001). Salicylic acid: A link between aspirin, diet and the prevention of colorectal cancer. *Qjm*, 94, pp.445-448.

Peltomaki, P. (2001). Deficient DNA mismatch repair: A common etiologic factor for colon cancer. *Hum Mol Genet*, 10, pp.735-740.

Phillips, S. M., Banerjea, A., Feakins, R., Li, S. R., Bustin, S. A., & Dorudi, S. (2004). Tumour-infiltrating lymphocytes in colorectal cancer with microsatellite instability are activated and cytotoxic. *Br J Surg*, 91, pp.469-475.

Piazza, G. A., Rahm, A. L., Krutzsch, M., Sperl, G., Paranka, N. S., Gross, P. H., et al. (1995). Antineoplastic drugs sulindac sulfide and sulfone inhibit cell growth by inducing apoptosis. *Cancer Res*, 55, pp.3110-3116.

Plaschke, J., Kruger, S., Jeske, B., Theissig, F., Kreuz, F. R., Pistorius, S., *et al.* (2004). Loss of MSH3 protein expression is frequent in MLH1-deficient colorectal cancer and is associated with disease progression. *Cancer Res*, 64, pp.864-870.

Qiao, Q., Nozaki, Y., Sakoe, K., Komatsu, N., & Kirito, K. (2010). NF-κB mediates aberrant activation of hif-1 in malignant lymphoma. *Exp Hematol*, 38, pp.1199-1208.

Ramos, A. A., Azqueta, A., Pereira-Wilson C. and Collins, A. R. (2010) Polyphenolic compounds from Salvia species protect cellular DNA from oxidation and stimulate DNA repair in cultured human cells. *J Agric Food Chem*, 58, pp.7465-71.

Raju, U., Ariga, H., Dittmann, K., Nakata, E., Ang, K. K., & Milas, L. (2005). Inhibition of DNA repair as a mechanism of enhanced radioresponse of head and neck carcinoma cells by a selective cyclooxygenase-2 inhibitor, celecoxib. *Int J Radiat Oncol Biol Phys*, 63, pp.520-528.

Raju, U., Nakata, E., Yang, P., Newman, R. A., Ang, K. K., & Milas, L. (2002). In vitro enhancement of tumor cell radiosensitivity by a selective inhibitor of cyclooxygenase-2 enzyme: Mechanistic considerations. *Int J Radiat Oncol Biol Phys*, 54, pp.886-894.

Rakoff-Nahoum, S. (2006). Why cancer and inflammation? *Yale J Biol Med*, 79, pp.123-130.

Ravindran, J., Prasad, S, and Aggarwal, B. B. (2009) Curcumin and cancer cells: how many ways can curry kill tumor cells selectively? *AAPS J.* 11, pp.495-510.

Ramachandran, C., Rodriguez, S., Ramachandran, R., Raveendran Nair, P. K., Fonseca, H., Khatib, Z., Escalon, E, and Melnick, S. J. (2005) Expression profiles of apoptotic genes induced by curcumin in human breast cancer and mammary epithelial cell lines. *Anticancer Res.* 25, pp.3293-302.

Rao, C. V., Rivenson, A., Simi, B., Zang, E., Kelloff, G., Steele, V., *et al.* (1995). Chemoprevention of colon carcinogenesis by sulindac, a nonsteroidal anti-inflammatory agent. *Cancer Res*, 55, pp.1464-1472.

Reddy, B. S., Rao, C. V., Rivenson, A., & Kelloff, G. (1993). Inhibitory effect of aspirin on azoxymethane-induced colon carcinogenesis in f344 rats. *Carcinogenesis*, 14, pp.1493-1497.

Redon, C. E., Dickey, J. S., Nakamura, A. J., Kareva, I. G., Naf, D., Nowsheen, S., *et al.* (2010). Tumors induce complex DNA damage in distant proliferative tissues in vivo. *Proc Natl Acad Sci U S A*, 107, pp.17992-17997.

Ricchi, P., Pignata, S., Di Popolo, A., Memoli, A., Apicella, A., Zarrilli, R., *et al.* (1997). Effect of aspirin on cell proliferation and differentiation of colon adenocarcinoma caco-2 cells. *Int J Cancer*, 73, pp.880-884.

Riccio, A., Aaltonen, L. A., Godwin, A. K., Loukola, A., Percesepe, A., Salovaara, R., et al. (1999). The DNA repair gene mbd4 (med1) is mutated in human carcinomas with microsatellite instability. *Nat Genet*, 23, pp.266-268.

Richter, M., Weiss, M., Weinberger, I., Furstenberger, G., & Marian, B. (2001). Growth inhibition and induction of apoptosis in colorectal tumor cells by cyclooxygenase inhibitors. *Carcinogenesis*, 22, pp.17-25.

Risques, R. A., Lai, L. A., Brentnall, T. A., Li, L., Feng, Z., Gallaher, J., *et al.* (2008). Ulcerative colitis is a disease of accelerated colon aging: Evidence from telomere attrition and DNA damage. *Gastroenterology*, 135, pp.410-418.

Rodier, F., Coppe, J. P., Patil, C. K., Hoeijmakers, W. A., Munoz, D. P., Raza, S. R., *et al.* (2009). Persistent DNA damage signalling triggers senescence-associated inflammatory cytokine secretion. *Nat Cell Biol*, 11, pp.973-979.

Rosemary Siafakas, A., & Richardson, D. R. (2009). Growth arrest and DNA damage-45 alpha (Gadd45α). *Int J Biochem Cell Biol*, 41, pp.986-989.

Rothwell, P. M., Fowkes, F. G., Belch, J. F., Ogawa, H., Warlow, C. P., & Meade, T. W. (2011). Effect of daily aspirin on long-term risk of death due to cancer: Analysis of individual patient data from randomised trials. *Lancet*, 377, 31-41.

Ruschoff, J., Wallinger, S., Dietmaier, W., Bocker, T., Brockhoff, G., Hofstadter, F., *et al.* (1998). Aspirin suppresses the mutator phenotype associated with hereditary nonpolyposis colorectal cancer by genetic selection. *Proc Natl Acad Sci U S A*, 95, pp.11301-11306.

Ryan-Harshman, M., & Aldoori, W. (2007). Diet and colorectal cancer: Review of the evidence. *Can Fam Physician*, 53, pp.1913-1920.

Saha, A., Kuzuhara, T., Echigo, N., Fujii, A., Suganuma, M, and Fujiki, H. (2010). Apoptosis of human lung cancer cells by curcumin mediated through up-regulation of "growth arrest and DNA damage inducible genes 45 and 153". Biol Pharm Bull. 33, pp.1291-9.

Sandler, R. S., Halabi, S., Baron, J. A., Budinger, S., Paskett, E., Keresztes, R., et al. (2003). A randomized trial of aspirin to prevent colorectal adenomas in patients with previous colorectal cancer. *N Engl J Med*, 348, pp.883-890.

Sansom, O. J., Bishop, S. M., Court, H., Dudley, S., Liskay, R. M., & Clarke, A. R. (2003). Apoptosis and mutation in the murine small intestine: Loss of Mlh1- and Pms2-dependent apoptosis leads to increased mutation in vivo. *DNA Repair (Amst)*, 2, pp.1029-1039.

Sansom, O. J., Stark, L. A., Dunlop, M. G., & Clarke, A. R. (2001). Suppression of intestinal and mammary neoplasia by lifetime administration of aspirin in apc(min/+) and apc(min/+), msh2(-/-) mice. *Cancer Res*, 61, pp.7060-7064.

Sarkar, D., Su, Z. Z., Lebedeva, I. V., Sauane, M., Gopalkrishnan, R. V., Valerie, K., *et al.* (2002). *mda-7* (Il-24) mediates selective apoptosis in human melanoma cells by inducing the coordinated overexpression of the GADD family of genes by means of p38 MAPK. *Proc Natl Acad Sci U S A*, 99, pp.10054-10059.

Scheier, L. (2001). Salicylic acid: One more reason to eat your fruits and vegetables. *J Am Diet Assoc*, 101, pp.1406-1408.

Schenk, P. M., Kazan, K., Wilson, I., Anderson, J. P., Richmond, T., Somerville, S. C., *et al.* (2000). Coordinated plant defense responses in arabidopsis revealed by microarray analysis. *Proc Natl Acad Sci U S A*, 97, 11655-11660.

Schetter, A. J., Heegaard, N. H., & Harris, C. C. (2010). Inflammation and cancer: Interweaving microRNA, free radical, cytokine and p53 pathways. *Carcinogenesis*, 31, pp.37-49.

Scott, D. W, and Loo, G. (2004) Curcumin-induced GADD153 gene up-regulation in human colon cancer cells. *Carcinogenesis*. 25, pp.2155-64.

Selvendiran, K., Bratasz, A., Tong, L., Ignarro, L. J., & Kuppusamy, P. (2008). Ncx-4016, a nitro-derivative of aspirin, inhibits egfr and stat3 signaling and modulates bcl-2 proteins in cisplatin-resistant human ovarian cancer cells and xenografts. *Cell Cycle*, 7, pp.81-88.

Serrano, D., Lazzeroni, M., & Decensi, A. (2004). Chemoprevention of colorectal cancer: An update. *Tech Coloproctol*, 8 Suppl 2, s248-252.

Seruca, R., Santos, N. R., David, L., Constancia, M., Barroca, H., Carneiro, F., *et al.* (1995). Sporadic gastric carcinomas with microsatellite instability display a particular clinicopathologic profile. *Int J Cancer*, 64, pp.32-36.

Shehzad, A., Wahid, F. and Lee, Y. S. (2010) Curcumin in cancer chemoprevention: molecular targets, pharmacokinetics, bioavailability, and clinical trials. *Arch Pharm (Weinheim)*, 343, pp.489-99.

Sheng, H., Shao, J., Morrow, J. D., Beauchamp, R. D., & DuBois, R. N. (1998). Modulation of apoptosis and BCL-2 expression by prostaglandin E2 in human colon cancer cells. *Cancer Res*, 58, 362-366.

Shibata, D. 1999. Microsatellite analysis of human tumours. *In* D. B. S. Goldstein, C. (Ed) *Microsatellites evolution and applications* pp. 266-273). Oxford: Oxford University Press. ISBN 978-0198504078.

Shiff, S. J., Koutsos, M. I., Qiao, L., & Rigas, B. (1996). Nonsteroidal antiinflammatory drugs inhibit the proliferation of colon adenocarcinoma cells: Effects on cell cycle and apoptosis. *Exp Cell Res*, 222, pp.179-188.

Shiff, S. J., & Rigas, B. (1999). The role of cyclooxygenase inhibition in the antineoplastic effects of nonsteroidal antiinflammatory drugs (nsaids). *J Exp Med*, 190, 445-450.

Shimizu, Y., Ikeda, S., Fujimori, M., Kodama, S., Nakahara, M., Okajima, M., *et al.* (2002). Frequent alterations in the wnt signaling pathway in colorectal cancer with microsatellite instability. *Genes Chromosomes Cancer*, 33, pp.73-81.

Shtivelband, M. I., Juneja, H. S., Lee, S., & Wu, K. K. (2003). Aspirin and salicylate inhibit colon cancer medium- and vegf-induced endothelial tube formation: Correlation with suppression of cyclooxygenase-2 expression. *J Thromb Haemost*, 1, pp.2225-2233.

Shureiqi, I., Chen, D., Lotan, R., Yang, P., Newman, R. A., Fischer, S. M., *et al.* (2000). 15-lipoxygenase-1 mediates nonsteroidal anti-inflammatory drug-induced apoptosis independently of cyclooxygenase-2 in colon cancer cells. *Cancer Res*, 60, pp.6846-6850.

Sidelnikov, E., Bostick, R. M., Flanders, W. D., Long, Q., Cohen, V. L., Dash, C., *et al.* (2009). Mutl-homolog 1 expression and risk of incident, sporadic colorectal adenoma: Search for prospective biomarkers of risk for colorectal cancer. *Cancer Epidemiol Biomarkers Prev*, 18, pp.1599-1609.

Skjelbred, C. F., Saebo, M., Wallin, H., *et al.* (2006) Polymorphisms of the XRCC1, XRCC3 and XPD genes and risk of colorectal adenoma and carcinoma, in a Norwegian cohort: a case control study. *BMC Cancer*, 6, pp. 67.

Smith, T. R., Miller, M. S., Lohman, L., Lange, E. M., Case, L. D., Mohrenweiser, H. W. and Hu, J. J. (2003) Polymorphisms of XRCC1 and XRCC3 genes and susceptibility to breast cancer. *Cancer Lett*, 190, pp.183-90.

Smith, M. L., Hawcroft, G., & Hull, M. A. (2000). The effect of non-steroidal anti-inflammatory drugs on human colorectal cancer cells: Evidence of different mechanisms of action. *Eur J Cancer* 36, pp.664-674.

Soslow, R. A., Dannenberg, A. J., Rush, D., Woerner, B. M., Khan, K. N., Masferrer, J., *et al.* (2000). Cox-2 is expressed in human pulmonary, colonic, and mammary tumors. *Cancer*, 89, pp.2637-2645.

Spitz, G. A., Furtado, C. M., Sola-Penna, M., & Zancan, P. (2009). Acetylsalicylic acid and salicylic acid decrease tumor cell viability and glucose metabolism modulating 6-phosphofructo-1-kinase structure and activity. *Biochem Pharmacol*, 77, pp.46-53.

Stappenbeck, T. S., & Gordon, J. I. (2000). Rac1 mutations produce aberrant epithelial differentiation in the developing and adult mouse small intestine. *Development*, 127, pp.2629-2642.

Stark, L. A., Din, F. V., Zwacka, R. M., & Dunlop, M. G. (2001). Aspirin-induced activation of the NF-κB signaling pathway: A novel mechanism for aspirin-mediated apoptosis in colon cancer cells. *Faseb J*, 15, pp.1273-1275.

Stark, L. A., Reid, K., Sansom, O. J., Din, F. V., Guichard, S., Mayer, I., *et al.* (2007). Aspirin activates the NF-κB signalling pathway and induces apoptosis in intestinal neoplasia in two in vivo models of human colorectal cancer. *Carcinogenesis*, 28, pp.968-976.

Staudt, L. M. (2010). Oncogenic activation of NF-κB. *Cold Spring Harb Perspect Biol*, 2, (6):a000109.

Stewart, G. D., Nanda, J., Katz, E., Bowman, K. J., Christie, J. G., Brown, D. J., *et al.* (2011). DNA strand breaks and hypoxia response inhibition mediate the radiosensitisation effect of nitric oxide donors on prostate cancer under varying oxygen conditions. *Biochem Pharmacol*, 81, pp.203-210.

Stolfi, C., Fina, D., Caruso, R., Caprioli, F., Fantini, M. C., Rizzo, A., *et al.* (2008). Mesalazine negatively regulates CDC25A protein expression and promotes accumulation of colon cancer cells in S phase. *Carcinogenesis*, 29, pp.1258-1266.

Tahara, T., Shibata, T., Yamashita, H., Nakamura, M., Yoshioka, D., Okubo, M., *et al.* (2009). Chronic nonsteroidal anti-inflammatory drug (nsaid) use suppresses multiple cpg islands hyper methylation (cihm) of tumor suppressor genes in the human gastric mucosa. *Cancer Sci*, 100, pp.1192-1197.

Tranah, G. J., Giovannucci, E., Ma, J., Fuchs, C., Hankinson, S. E. and Hunter, D. J. (2004) XRCC2 and XRCC3 polymorphisms are not associated with risk of colorectal adenoma. *Cancer Epidemiol Biomarkers Prev*, 13, pp.1090-1091.

Tesei, A., Zoli, W., Fabbri, F., Leonetti, C., Rosetti, M., Bolla, M., *et al.* (2008). Ncx 4040, an no-donating acetylsalicylic acid derivative: Efficacy and mechanisms of action in cancer cells. *Nitric Oxide*, 19, pp.225-236.

Thibodeau, S. N., Bren, G., & Schaid, D. (1993). Microsatellite instability in cancer of the proximal colon. *Science*, 260, 816-819.

Thibodeau, S. N., French, A. J., Cunningham, J. M., Tester, D., Burgart, L. J., Roche, P. C., *et al.* (1998). Microsatellite instability in colorectal cancer: Different mutator phenotypes and the principal involvement of hMLH1. *Cancer Res*, 58, pp.1713-1718.

Thun, M. J., Henley, S. J., & Patrono, C. (2002). Nonsteroidal anti-inflammatory drugs as anticancer agents: Mechanistic, pharmacologic, and clinical issues. *J Natl Cancer Inst*, 94, pp.252-266.

Thun, M. J., Namboodiri, M. M., & Heath, C. W., Jr. (1991). Aspirin use and reduced risk of fatal colon cancer. *N Engl J Med*, 325, 1593-1596.

Tili, E., Michaille, J. J., Wernicke, D., Alder, H., Costinean, S., Volinia, S., et al. (2011). Mutator activity induced by microRNA-155 (mir-155) links inflammation and cancer. Proc Natl Acad Sci U S A, 108, pp.4908-4913.

To, K. K., Koshiji, M., Hammer, S., & Huang, L. E. (2005). Genetic instability: The dark side of the hypoxic response. Cell Cycle, 4, pp.881-882.

Tsai, C. S., Luo, S. F., Ning, C. C., Lin, C. L., Jiang, M. C., & Liao, C. F. (2009). Acetylsalicylic acid regulates mmp-2 activity and inhibits colorectal invasion of murine b16f0 melanoma cells in c57bl/6j mice: Effects of prostaglandin f(2)alpha. Biomed Pharmacother, 63, pp.522-527.

Tsujii, M., Kawano, S., & DuBois, R. N. (1997). Cyclooxygenase-2 expression in human colon cancer cells increases metastatic potential. Proc Natl Acad Sci U S A, 94, pp.3336-3340.

Umar, A., Boyer, J. C., Thomas, D. C., Nguyen, D. C., Risinger, J. I., Boyd, J., et al. (1994). Defective mismatch repair in extracts of colorectal and endometrial cancer cell lines exhibiting microsatellite instability. J Biol Chem, 269, pp.14367-14370.

Urios, P., Grigorova-Borsos, A. M., & Sternberg, M. (2007). Aspirin inhibits the formation of pentosidine, a cross-linking advanced glycation end product, in collagen. Diabetes Res Clin Pract, 77, pp.337-340.

Valeri, N., Gasparini, P., Fabbri, M., Braconi, C., Veronese, A., Lovat, F., et al. (2010). Modulation of mismatch repair and genomic stability by mir-155. Proc Natl Acad Sci U S A, 107, pp.6982-6987.

Valko, M., Rhodes, C. J., Moncol, J., Izakovic, M., & Mazur, M. (2006). Free radicals, metals and antioxidants in oxidative stress-induced cancer. Chem Biol Interact, 160, pp.1-40.

Vasavi, M., Ponnala, S., Gujjari, K., Boddu, P., Bharatula, R. S., Prasad, R., et al. (2006). DNA methylation in esophageal diseases including cancer: Special reference to hMLH1 gene promoter status. Tumori, 92, pp.155-162.

Wang, D., & DuBois, R. N. (2008). Pro-inflammatory prostaglandins and progression of colorectal cancer. Cancer Lett, 267, pp.197-203.

Wang, D., Dubois, R. N., & Richmond, A. (2009). The role of chemokines in intestinal inflammation and cancer. Curr Opin Pharmacol, 9, pp.688-696.

Watson, A. J. (2006). An overview of apoptosis and the prevention of colorectal cancer. Crit Rev Oncol Hematol, 57, pp.107-121.

Williams, J. L., Nath, N., Chen, J., Hundley, T. R., Gao, J., Kopelovich, L., et al. (2003). Growth inhibition of human colon cancer cells by nitric oxide (NO)-donating aspirin is associated with Cyclooxygenase-2 induction and β-catenin/T-cell factor signaling, Nuclear Factor-κB, and NO Synthase 2 inhibition: implications for chemoprevention. Cancer Res, 63, pp.7613-7618.

Wink, D. A., & Laval, J. (1994). The fpg protein, a DNA repair enzyme, is inhibited by the biomediator nitric oxide in vitro and in vivo. Carcinogenesis, 15, pp.2125-2129.

Woerner, S. M., Yuan, Y. P., Benner, A., Korff, S., von Knebel Doeberitz, M., & Bork, P. (2010). SelTarbase, a database of human mononucleotide-microsatellite mutations and their potential impact to tumorigenesis and immunology. Nucleic Acids Res, 38, D682-689.

Wood, R. D., Mitchell, M., Sgouros, J., & Lindahl, T. (2001). Human DNA repair genes. Science, 291, 1284-1289.

Wu, X. Y., Fu, Z. X., & Wang, X. H. (2010). Effect of hypoxia-inducible factor 1-α on survivin in colorectal cancer. Mol Med Report, 3, pp.409-415.

Xu, Z. Y., Loignon, M., Han, F. Y., Panasci, L. and Aloyz (2005) XRCC3 induces cisplatin resistance by stimulation of Rad51-related recombinational repair, S-phase checkpoint activation, and reduced apoptosis. *J Pharmacol Exp Ther*, 314, pp.495-505.

Xiao, H., Xiao, Q., Zhang, K., Zuo, X., & Shrestha, U. K. (2010). Reversal of multidrug resistance by curcumin through fa/brca pathway in multiple myeloma cell line molp-2/r. *Ann Hematol*, 89, pp.399-404.

Xie, J., & Itzkowitz, S. H. (2008). Cancer in inflammatory bowel disease. *World J Gastroenterol*, 14, pp.378-389.

Yamamoto, H., Sawai, H., Weber, T. K., Rodriguez-Bigas, M. A., & Perucho, M. (1998). Somatic frameshift mutations in DNA mismatch repair and proapoptosis genes in hereditary nonpolyposis colorectal cancer. *Cancer Res*, 58, pp.997-1003.

Yamamoto, Y., & Gaynor, R. B. (2001). Therapeutic potential of inhibition of the NF-κB pathway in the treatment of inflammation and cancer. *J Clin Invest*, 107, pp.135-142.

Yamamoto, Y., Yin, M. J., Lin, K. M., & Gaynor, R. B. (1999). Sulindac inhibits activation of the NF-κB pathway. *J Biol Chem*, 274, pp.27307-27314.

Yanaihara, N., Caplen, N., Bowman, E., Seike, M., Kumamoto, K., Yi, M., et al. (2006). Unique microRNA molecular profiles in lung cancer diagnosis and prognosis. *Cancer Cell*, 9, pp.189-198.

Yanamadala, S., & Ljungman, M. (2003). Potential role of MLH1 in the induction of p53 and apoptosis by blocking transcription on damaged DNA templates. *Mol Cancer Res*, 1, pp.747-754.

Ye, C. G., Wu, W. K., Yeung, J. H., Li, H. T., Li, Z. J., Wong, C. C., et al. (2011). Indomethacin and SC236 enhance the cytotoxicity of doxorubicin in human hepatocellular carcinoma cells via inhibiting P-glycoprotein and MRP1 expression. *Cancer Lett*, 304, pp.90-96.

Yeh, C. C., Sung, F. C., Tang, R., Chang-Chieh, C. R. and Hsieh, L. L. (2005) Polymorphisms of the XRCC1, XRCC3, & XPD genes, and colorectal cancer risk: a case-control study in Taiwan. *BMC Cancer*, 5, pp.183-193.

Yin, H., Xu, H., Zhao, Y., Yang, W., Cheng, J., & Zhou, Y. (2006). Cyclooxygenase-independent effects of aspirin on HT-29 human colon cancer cells, revealed by oligonucleotide microarrays. *Biotechnol Lett*, 28, pp.1263-1270.

Yin, M. J., Yamamoto, Y., & Gaynor, R. B. (1998). The anti-inflammatory agents aspirin and salicylate inhibit the activity of IκB kinase-β. *Nature*, 396, pp.77-80.

Ying, J., Srivastava, G., Hsieh, W. S., Gao, Z., Murray, P., Liao, S. K., et al. (2005). The stress-responsive gene *GADD45G* is a functional tumor suppressor, with its response to environmental stresses frequently disrupted epigenetically in multiple tumors. *Clin Cancer Res*, 11, pp.6442-6449.

Yoshihara, T., Ishida, M., Kinomura, A., Katsura, M., Tsuruga, T., Tashiro, S., Asahara, T. and Miyagawa, K. (2004) XRCC3 deficiency results in a defect in recombination and increased endoreduplication in human cells. *EMBO J*, 23, pp.670-680.

Yu, H. G., Huang, J. A., Yang, Y. N., Huang, H., Luo, H. S., Yu, J. P., et al. (2002). The effects of acetylsalicylic acid on proliferation, apoptosis, and invasion of cyclooxygenase-2 negative colon cancer cells. *Eur J Clin Invest*, 32, pp.838-846.

Yu, H. G., Huang, J. A., Yang, Y. N., Luo, H. S., Yu, J. P., Meier, J. J., et al. (2003). Inhibition of cytosolic phospholipase A2 mRNA expression: A novel mechanism for acetylsalicylic acid-mediated growth inhibition and apoptosis in colon cancer cells. *Regul Pept*, 114, pp.101-107.

Yu, L., Chen, M., Li, Z., Wen, J., Fu, J., Guo, D., *et al.* (2011). Celecoxib antagonizes the cytotoxicity of cisplatin in human esophageal squamous cell carcinoma cells by reducing intracellular cisplatin accumulation. *Mol Pharmacol*, 79, pp.608-617.

Yuan, C. J., Mandal, A. K., Zhang, Z., & Mukherjee, A. B. (2000). Transcriptional regulation of cyclooxygenase-2 gene expression: Novel effects of nonsteroidal anti-inflammatory drugs. *Cancer Res*, 60, 1084-1091.

Zabkiewicz, J., & Clarke, A. R. (2004). DNA damage-induced apoptosis: Insights from the mouse. *Biochim Biophys Acta*, 1705, pp.17-25.

Zerbini, L. F., Czibere, A., Wang, Y., Correa, R. G., Otu, H., Joseph, M., *et al.* (2006). A novel pathway involving melanoma differentiation associated gene-7/interleukin-24 mediates nonsteroidal anti-inflammatory drug-induced apoptosis and growth arrest of cancer cells. *Cancer Res*, 66, pp.11922-11931.

Zerbini, L. F., Wang, Y., Czibere, A., Correa, R. G., Cho, J. Y., Ijiri, K., *et al.* (2004). NF-κB-mediated repression of growth arrest- and DNA-damage-inducible proteins 45α and γ is essential for cancer cell survival. *Proc Natl Acad Sci U S A*, 101, pp.13618-13623.

Zhang, H., Richards, B., Wilson, T., Lloyd, M., Cranston, A., Thorburn, A., *et al.* (1999). Apoptosis induced by overexpression of hMSH2 or hMLH1. *Cancer Res*, 59, pp.3021-3027.

Zhang, L., Yu, J., Park, B. H., Kinzler, K. W., & Vogelstein, B. (2000). Role of bax in the apoptotic response to anticancer agents. *Science*, 290, pp.989-992.

Zimmermann, K. C., Waterhouse, N. J., Goldstein, J. C., Schuler, M., & Green, D. R. (2000). Aspirin induces apoptosis through release of cytochrome c from mitochondria. *Neoplasia*, 2, pp.505-513.

7

Integration of the DNA Damage Response with Innate Immune Pathways

Gordon M. Xiong and Stephan Gasser
Department of Microbiology, National University of Singapore
Singapore

1. Introduction

Genotoxic or replicative stress triggers a DNA damage response (DDR) that induces cell cycle arrest, DNA repair or – if the damage is too severe – apoptosis. The DDR has been suggested to represent a barrier against tumorigenesis by preventing the uncontrolled proliferation of cells with genomic instability or harmful mutations. Recent studies have uncovered novel links of the DDR to innate immune signaling pathways. The activation of NF-κB in response to DNA damage is mediated by ATM (ataxia telangiectasia mutated)-dependent phosphorylation of NEMO, resulting in the induction of the classical NF-κB pathways. Furthermore links between the DDR and various members of the type I interferon (IFN) pathway have been uncovered. The DDR also increases the sensitivity of cells to immune cell-mediated killing by inducing the expression of surface ligands for activating immune receptors. Here, we review how the DDR links to innate immune pathways and the potential role of these interactions in cancer and viral infection.

2. The DNA damage response (DDR)

The genome integrity is constantly challenged by environmental genotoxic agents (chemicals, ultra-violet, viral infection etc.) and endogenous genotoxic stress (replication, oxidative stress, etc.) (Lindahl, 1993; Nyberg et al., 2002; Kunkel, 2004). DNA damage may also be caused by reactive oxygen species and nitrogen compounds produced by neutrophils and macrophages at sites of inflammation (deRojas-Walker T et al., 1995; Kawanishi et al., 2006). These DNA lesions or aberrations can block transcription and genome replication, and if not repaired, lead to mutations or large-scale genome aberrations that threaten the survival of the individual cells and the whole organism (Jackson & Bartek, 2009). To cope with genomic DNA damage, organisms have evolved a repertoire of surveillance and repair mechanisms to detect and combat the deleterious effects of damaged DNA (Zhou & Elledge, 2000). The DDR is composed of sensor protein kinases that are recruited to the sites of DNA damage, the signal transducer proteins that propagate the signal downstream, and the effector proteins which activate the appropriate responses such as DNA repair, cell cycle arrest and apoptosis (Gasser et al., 2007) (Figure 1).

2.1 ATM and ATR
The diversity in the types of DNA lesions necessitates specific protein complexes to detect and initiate the correct repair programme. Studies on the biochemistry of specific DNA

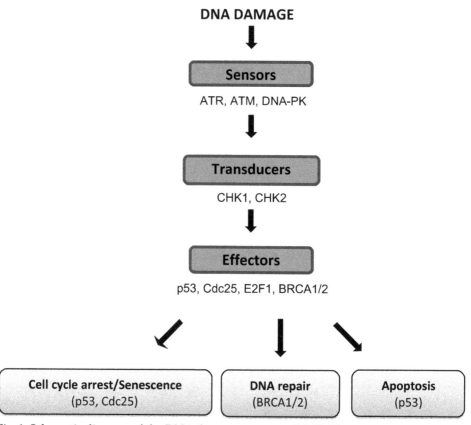

Fig. 1. Schematic diagram of the DNA damage response (DDR). The DDR is initiated by the sensors ATM and/or ATR depending of the nature of the DNA damage inducing cell cycle arrest and DNA repair or apoptosis if the damage is beyond repair.

lesions are complicated by the fact that the DNA damaging agents or ionizing radiation may each generate multiple types of DNA damage, and possibly recruiting several DNA damage sensors (Zhou & Elledge, 2000). The chemotherapeutic drug doxorubicin, for example, is a DNA topoisomerase II inhibitor that not only creates DNA strand-breaks, but also forms doxorubicin-DNA adducts, which induce torsional stress in the DNA structure (Swift et al., 2006). The different types of DNA damage eventually induce the activation of the phosphoinositide-3-kinase (PI3K)-related protein kinases (PIKKs) ATM and ATR (ATM- and Rad3-related) (Yang et al., 2003). Single-stranded DNA resulting from various types of genotoxic stress is bound by ssDNA-binding proteins such as RPA (replication protein A) (Wold, 1997). ATR and the ATR-interacting protein (ATRIP) then localizes to the RPA-coated ssDNA (Zou & Elledge, 2003). ATR also responds to stalled DNA replication forks in humans and mice (Cortez et al., 2001; Brown & Baltimore, 2000). On the other hand, ATM is recruited by double-stranded (ds) DNA breaks resulting primarily from ionizing radiation and oxidative stress (Zhou & Elledge, 2000; Shiloh, 2003). ATM is also activated by programmed dsDNA breaks during V(D)J recombination, an important process in the generation of the diverse repertoire of immunoglobulins and T-cell receptors in B and T lymphocytes (Perkins et al., 2002; Dujka et al., 2009). It is currently not clear how ATM and ATR initiate the correct repair programmes for the wide variety of DNA lesions. Most likely different types of DNA damage recruit specific proteins (e.g. BRCA-1, H2AX, Nbs1, 53BP1 etc.) that interact with ATM and ATR thereby initiating a DNA damage-specific repair programme (Yang et al., 2003; Matsuoka et al., 2007).

2.2 DNA-PK

The DNA-dependent protein kinase (DNA-PK), a member of the PI3K superfamily, is a nuclear serine/threonine kinase composed of the catalytic subunit (DNA-PKcs) and the DNA-binding Ku70/80 subunit (Carter et al., 1990; Kurimasa et al., 1999). Similar to ATM, DNA-PK is involved in the detection of dsDNA breaks and is activated by DNA damage following ionizing radiation, UV radiation and V(D)J recombination events (Kurimasa et al., 1999; Yang et al., 2003). The binding of Ku70/Ku80 to dsDNA breaks is required for the activation of DNA-PKcs and the subsequent ligation of the double-stranded DNA ends by other protein components of the NHEJ (non-homologous end-joining) machinery (Kurimasa et al., 1999; Walker et al., 2001). Recent data suggest that DNA-PK and ATM are partially redundant in their function (Stiff et al., 2004). DNA-PK has been reported to be able to phosphorylate H2AX in ATM-deficient cells after treatment with ionizing radiation (Stiff et al., 2004). Furthermore, association of ATR and DNA-PK is observed during UV irradiation and the activation of DNA-PK is impaired when ATR is inhibited (Yajima et al., 2006). Taken together, DNA-PK appears to co-operate with ATM and ATR to initiate the DDR.

2.3 CHK1 and CHK2

ATM and ATR partially coordinate the DDR through the signal transducers CHK1 and CHK2 (Zhou & Elledge, 2000; Gasser 2007). CHK1 and CHK2 contain conserved kinase domains but differ in their function and structure (reviewed in Bartek et al., 2001; McGowan 2002). The main functions of CHK1 and CHK2 are to reinforce signals from ATM and ATR (Matsuoka et al., 1998; Abraham, 2001; Shiloh, 2003). CHK1 is an unstable protein that is specifically expressed during the S and G2 phases of cell cycle (Lukas et al., 2001). Interestingly, while CHK1 is expressed and activated in unperturbed cell cycles, stalled replication forks and ssDNA breaks enhance its activity further (Kaneko et al., 1999; Zhao et al., 2002; Sørensen et al., 2003). In contrast, CHK2 is expressed throughout the cell cycle (Lukas et al., 2001) but is activated specifically in response to dsDNA breaks. Similar to ATM, CHK2 activation depends on its dimerization and autophosphorylation (Cai et al., 2009). Historically, it was thought that ATR specifically activates CHK1, while CHK2 activation depends on ATM, but recent data suggests that a certain degree of redundancy exists in the ability of ATR and ATM to activate the signal transducers. For example it was reported that the phosphorylation of CHK1 in response to ionizing radiation depends on ATM (Gatei et al., 2003; Sørensen et al., 2003). CHK1 and CHK2 share many overlapping substrates and are therefore often found to be functionally redundant (Bartek et al., 2001; McGowan, 2002). The targets of CHK1 and CHK2 regulate many fundamental cellular functions such as cell cycle, DNA repair and apoptosis (Figure 1). For example, both CHK2 and CHK1 reduce the activity of cyclin-dependent kinases (CDKs) such as CDK2 and CDK1. The resulting inhibition of these G1/S- and G2/M-promoting CDKs results in cell cycle delays (Falck et al, 2001; Zhao & Piwnica-Worms, 2001). Despite their functional redundancy, mouse studies have revealed striking differences for CHK1 and CHK2 during development (Liu et al., 2000; Takai et al., 2000). CHK1-deficient mice are embryonic lethal in contrast to CHK2-deficient mice (Liu et al., 2000; Takai et al., 2000; Hirao et al., 2000; Takai et al., 2002). CHK2 is required for radiation-induced, p53-dependent apoptosis and the stability of p53 is reduced in mice lacking CHK2 (Hirao et al., 2000; Takai et al., 2002). Nevertheless both CHK1 and CHK2 have been shown to be able to phosphorylate p53 on several sites in response to DNA damage (Hirao et al., 2000; Shieh et al., 2000; Ou et al., 2005).

2.4 p53

Whether the DNA repair machinery or cellular apoptosis is initiated as a consequence of DNA damage is a crucial decision of the DDR. Although not fully understood, a large body of evidence hints at p53 playing a critical role in this important decision (reviewed in Vousden & Lu, 2002; Das et al., 2008). Depending on the nature of the DNA damage, p53 is phosphorylated on several serine residues by ATM (Banin et al., 1998; Khanna et al., 1998), ATR (Tibbetts et al., 1999) or DNA-PK (Shieh et al., 1997; Achanta et al., 2001). In addition the signal transducers CHK1 and CHK2 directly bind and phosphorylate p53 (Hirao et al., 2000; Ou et al., 2005, Dumaz & Meek, 1999). The phosphorylation of p53 at Ser20 is known to be important for destabilizing the interaction of p53 with its inhibitor MDM2 (Shieh et al., 1997; Unger et al., 1999). In addition, studies have demonstrated that p53 function is modulated by acetylation in response to DNA damage (Ou et al., 2005). These posttranslational modifications allow p53 to induce the expression of its target genes such as p21, a CDK2 inhibitor implicated in G1/S transition (Wade Harper et al., 1993; Chen et al., 1995). In case of irreparable DNA damage, p53 induces a differential set of target genes leading to the activation of both the mitochondrial and CD95-FasL apoptotic pathways (Kastan et al., 1991; Lowe et al., 1993b; Bennett et al., 1998; Chipuk et al., 2003; Mihara et al., 2003).

Recent studies demonstrated that p53 is activated early in tumorigenesis as a result of oncogene expression. Oncogene activation is thought to induce "replication stress" leading to the collapse of DNA replication forks and the formation of dsDNA breaks (Halazonetis et al., 2008). It has been suggested that p53 acts as an anti-cancer barrier in precancerous lesions. In support of this hypothesis, functional inactivation of p53 has been observed in 50% of all human cancers (Hanahan & Weinberg, 2000). Thus, oncogene-induced DNA damage may explain two key features of cancer: the high frequency of p53 mutations and the resulting genomic instability, which is often observed in cells lacking p53 (reviewed in Jackson & Bartek, 2009).

3. DDR and the immune system

As early as the 19th century it was recognized that some tumors are infiltrated by innate and adaptive immune cells (reviewed in Dvorak, 1986). In recent years new data suggests that DDR can initiate an immune response. As discussed below in more detail, the DDR directly activates a variety of transcription factors such as NF-κB and interferon regulatory factors (IRFs). These transcription factors induce the expression of various immune genes, including inflammatory cytokines and chemokines. In addition, the DDR and oxidative stress induce the expression of a number of ligands for activating immune receptors such as NKG2D and DNAM-1, which are mainly expressed by cytotoxic immune cells such as T cells and NK cells.

3.1 NF-κB

Transcription factors belonging to the NF-κB family are mostly nuclear proteins that were initially reported to bind to the promoter of the κ immunoglobulin gene in B cells upon lipopolysaccharide (LPS) stimulation (Sen & Baltimore, 1986). It is now recognized that these transcription factors regulate many key aspects of innate immune signaling (Baeuerle & Henkel, 1994; Pahl, 1999). The NF-κB subunits are usually sequestered in the cytoplasm through their interactions with inhibitory IκB proteins. Phosphorylation of IκB proteins by the IκB kinase (IKK) complex, consisting of IKKα, IKKβ and the scaffold protein NEMO/IKKγ, leads to the degradation of IκB (Scheidereit 2006). Upon IκB degradation, NF-κB subunits subunits translocate to the nucleus (Scheidereit 2006) and modulate the expression of NF-κB target genes such as IL-6 (Libermann & Baltimore, 1990), IL-8 (Kunsch et al., 1994), and IL-1β (Cogswell et al., 199). The picture is complicated by the fact that NF-κB complexes consist of homodimers or heterodimers of five NF-κB family proteins: p65 (Rel-A), Rel-B, c-Rel, p50 and p52 (Hayden & Ghosh, 2008). The Rel subfamily of NF-κB proteins possess C-terminal transactivation domains (TADs) that promote target gene expression when bound to κB sites as heterodimers with either p50 or p52 (Ghosh et al., 1998). The p50/p65 heterodimer is the main activating NF-κB dimer in many cells, and the combinatorial diversity of heterodimers confers specificity in gene activation under specific physiological conditions (Ghosh et al., 1998). In contrast, the p52 and p50 homodimers inhibit transcription (Ghosh & Karin, 2002).

NF-κB is also activated in response to DNA damage (Brach et al., 1991; Simon et al., 1994). In ATM-deficient mice, NF-κB activation is impaired after irradiation (Li et al., 2001). Similarly, in DNA-PK-deficient cells, the activation of NF-κB was impaired upon irradiation (Basu et al., 1998). The activation of NF-κB following DNA damage mainly results in survival signals (Wang et al., 1998; Wang et al., 1999) that could provide a time window for cells to repair damaged DNA (Beg & Baltimore, 1996; Wang et al., 1996).

3.1.1 NEMO

Recent insights into the molecular mechansims leading to NF-κB activation in response to DNA damage indicate an important role for NEMO (Huang et al., 2000; Huang et al., 2002; Huang et al., 2003). The reconstitution of NEMO-deficient cells with wild-type NEMO restored NF-κB activation in response to DNA damage (Huang et al., 2002). The dsDNA breaks promote the SUMO (small ubiquitin-like modifier) modification of nuclear NEMO, which prevents its nuclear export (Huang et al., 2003; Janssens et al., 2005). At the same time, activated ATM phosphorylates SUMOylated NEMO leading to the removal of SUMO and the attachment of ubiquitin (Wu et al., 2006). These modifications allow NEMO to enter in a complex with ATM to be exported to the cytoplasm, where ATM mediates K63-linked polyubiquitination of ELKS and TRAF6 (Hinz et al., 2010; Wu et al., 2010). In addition NEMO is monoubiquitinated on lysine 285 via cIAP1 (Hinz et al., 2010). The polyubiquitinated complex activates IKKε in a TAK1-dependent manner. Activated IKKε then phosphorylates IκBα leading to K48-linked polyubiquitination and the subsequent degradation of IκBα by the proteasome (Figure 2 and Scheidereit 2006). The free NF-κB (p50/p65) dimer undergoes nuclear translocation and induces the transcription of pro-survival genes (Beg & Baltimore, 1996; Wang et al., 1998).

The activation of NF-κB in tumor cells in response to constitutive genotoxic stress has been suggested to be tumor- promoting (Annunziata et al., 2007; Grosjean-Raillard et al., 2009;

Meylan et al., 2009). The ATM-NEMO-NF-κB pathway is constitutively activated in acute myeloid leukemia (AML) cell lines, samples from high-risk myelodysplastic syndrome (MDS) and AML patients (Grosjean-Raillard et al., 2009), multiple myeloma (Annunziata et al., 2007) and lung adenocarcinomas (Meylan et al., 2009). The pharmacological inhibition or knockdown of ATM in AML cell lines ablated ATM-NEMO interactions, downregulated NF-κB and induced apoptosis (Grosjean-Raillard et al., 2009). In summary, the constitutive activation of the DDR in early cancer not only induces cell cycle arrest, thereby establishing a barrier to cancer progression, but also promotes the survival of cancer cells by the activation of NF-κB (Bartkova et al., 2005; Gorgoulis et al., 2005).

Apart from promoting tumorigenesis, DDR-mediated NF-κB activation also plays an important role in lymphocyte development and survival (Bredemeyer et al., 2008). DsDNA breaks are generated as result of recombinase activating gene (RAG) expression during V(D)J recombination in pre-B cells. The subsequent activation of the ATM-NEMO-NF-κB pathway is critical for the expression of genes involved in lymphocyte development, survival and function (Bredermeyer et al., 2008).

3.2 Interferon regulatory factors

IRFs are a class of transcription factors that have diverse roles in immune responses (Honda & Taniguchi, 2006). There are nine members in the mammalian IRF family. Each IRF contains a well-conserved DNA-binding domain, which recognizes a consensus DNA sequence known as the IFN-stimulated response element (ISRE) (Honda & Taniguichi, 2006). ISRE sequences are found on the promoter regions of type I interferons (IFN-α and IFN-β and other pro-inflammatory genes, thus making IRFs the essential mediators of IFN-α/β and other pro-inflammatory cytokines (Tanaka et al., 1993; Taniguchi et al., 2001). IRFs are well known to be activated upon binding of invariant microbial motifs, often referred to as pattern-associated molecular patterns (PAMPs), to pattern recognition receptors (PRRs) such as Toll-like receptors (TLRs), NOD-like receptors (NLRs) and RIG-I-like receptors (RLRs) (Akira et al., 2006; Creagh & O'Neill, 2006; Kanneganti et al., 2007; Yoneyama and Fujita, 2007). However, some IRFs are also activated in response to genotoxic stress as discussed below in more detail (Taniguchi et al., 2001).

3.2.1 IRF-1 and IRF-2

The link between IRFs and the DDR was first shown for IRF-1. IRF-1 was found to be essential for the apoptosis of T lymphocytes and embryonic fibroblasts in response to ionizing radiation or chemotherapeutic agents (Tanaka et al., 1994; Tamura et al., 1995). Recent studies have shown that the overexpression of IRF-1 results in the apoptosis of cancer cells through both cell intrinsic mitochondrial and extrinsic death ligand pathways (Strang et al., 2007; Gao et al., 2010). Furthermore, ATM-deficient cells derived from patients with ataxia telagienctasia (AT) fail to induce IRF-1 mRNA transcription in response to DNA damage (Pamment et al., 2002). The reconstitution of ATM restored IRF-1 induction in response to radiation (Pamment et al., 2002). These findings suggest that IRF-1 participates in DDR-mediated cell cycle arrest, although the precise molecular mechanisms still need to be established in more details (Tanaka et al., 1996).

3.2.2 IRF-3

IRF-3 interacts with CREB-binding protein (CBP)/p300 co-activators to form a dsDNA-activated transcription factor 1 (DRAF-1) complex which binds to the ISRE of type 1 interferons and other interferon-stimulated genes (ISGs) (Weaver et al., 1998). In contrast to other IRF members, IRF-3 is constitutively expressed in the cytoplasm of most cells (Kumar et al., 2000). IRF-3 is activated through phosphorylation by TANK-binding kinase 1 (TBK1) and/or IKKε leading to its dimerization and translocation to the nucleus (Kim et al., 1999; Fitzgerald et al., 2003). It was later discovered that IRF-3 is also a direct target of DNA-PK (Karporva et al., 2002). Our own data suggest that IRF-3 phosphorylation and activation in response to DNA damaging agents Ara-C or aphidicolin critically depends on ATM and ATR (Lam et al., submitted). Interestingly, IRF-3 may also participate in the DDR-mediated anti-cancer barrier. A dominant negative mutant of IRF-3 promoted the transformation of NIH3T3 cells and tumorigenesis *in vivo* (Kim et al., 2003). The overexpression of IRF-3 inhibited the proliferation of fibroblasts and astrocytes. Interestingly, the IRF-3 induced cell cycle arrest depended on p53 (Kim et al., 2006). Similarly, over-expression of IRF-3 in B16 melanoma cells resulted in growth suppression *in vivo* (Duguay et al., 2002). Recent evidence suggests that IRF-3 also induces apoptosis under certain circumstances such as in response to Sendai virus and NDV virus infection (Heylbroeck et al., 2000; Weaver et al., 2001). The molecular mechanisms of IRF-3-induced apoptosis are not well understood, but may in part rely on the ISRE promoter element present in TNF-related apoptosis-inducing ligand (TRAIL), an important member of the apoptotic machinery (Kirschner et al., 2005). In summary, it is possible that IRF-3 acts as a tumor suppressor gene that partially depends on p53 for its function.

3.2.3 IRF-5

IRF-5 is constitutively expressed in cytoplasm of a variety of cell types, particularly, in cells of lymphoid origins (Barnes et al., 2001; Yanai et al., 2007). IRF-5 is a direct target of p53 (Mori et al., 2002) and IRF-5 transcript levels further increase in response to DNA damage (Barnes et al., 2003; Hu et al., 2005). However, the induction of p53 target genes was not impaired in IRF5-deficient cells (Hu et al., 2005). Overexpression of IRF-5 rendered cells more susceptible to DNA damage-induced apoptosis even in p53-deficient cancer cell lines (Hu et al., 2005). In response to TLR agonists or DNA damage, IRF-5 is activated, possibly by phosphorylation, and translocates to the nucleus. Similar to other IRFs it promotes gene transcription by binding to target ISRE sequences in the regulatory region of target genes (Barnes et al., 2001), such as the interleukin-12b gene (Takaoka et al., 2005). In summary IRF-5 is a type I IFN-responsive p53 target gene that induces the expression of target genes distinct from those of p53.

3.2.4 Type I IFNs

Type I IFNs belong to a multigene family that includes IFN-α and IFN-β. Type I IFNs are expressed rapidly in response to many viral infections (Tanaka et al., 1998). They are best known to induce the expression of genes that increase the resistance of cells to virus infection (Taniguchi & Takaoka, 2002). In addition, type I IFNs were shown to modulate other cellular functions, such as proliferation and apoptosis (reviewed in Chawla et al., 2003). The increased sensitivity of cells to apoptosis in the presence of type I IFNs depends in part on their ability to increase p53 protein levels (Takaoka et al., 2003). Binding of type I IFNs to the IFN receptor activates the receptor-associated kinases Jak1 and Tyk2 leading to phosphorylation of the STAT1 and STAT2 proteins. The activated STAT proteins bind the IFN-regulatory factor 9 (IRF-9) to form the trimeric IFN-stimulated gene factor 3 (ISGF-3) complex. The ISGF-3 complex translocates to the nucleus and binds to ISREs sites present in the mouse and human p53 genes thereby activating p53 transcription (Takaoka et al., 2003). However, type I IFN treatment is not sufficient to activate p53. It rather enhances the p53 response, thereby rendering cells more sensitive to the DDR (Takaoka et al., 2003; Yuan et al., 2007). In clinical trials type I IFNs have been successfully utilized for both first-line and salvage therapy for a variety of cancers such as human papilloma virus (HPV)-associated cervical cancer, hepatic cancer and leukemias (Parmar & Platanias, 2003; Wang et al., 2011).

3.3 NKG2D ligands

One of the best-characterized NK cell-activating receptor in the context of cancer is the NKG2D receptor (reviewed in Raulet, 2003). All NK cells constitutively express the NKG2D receptor. In humans its cell surface expression requires association with the adaptor protein DAP10. Engagement of NKG2D leads to cytokine secretion and cytotoxicity (Billadeau et al., 2003; Upshaw et al., 2006). NKG2D recognizes MHC class I chain-related (MIC) A and B proteins and RAET1 (retinoic acid early transcript 1) gene family members in humans (Raulet, 2003, Cosman et al., 2001). No MIC homologs have been found in the mouse genome so far. The mouse Raet1 genes can be further divided into Rae1, H60 and Mult1 subfamilies that share little homology but are structurally similar. The Rae1 subfamily consists of highly related isoforms Rae1α - Rae1ε encoded by different genes (Diefenbach et al., 2000; Cerwenka et al., 2000; Raulet, 2003). NKG2D ligand expression has been observed on tumors of many origins, in particular in solid tumors, lymphomas and myeloid leukemia (Groh et al., 1999; Pende et al., 2002; Rohner et al., 2007). NKG2D was shown to be critical for the immunosurveillance of carcinoma, epithelial and lymphoid tumors in mouse models of de novo tumorigenesis. We and others have demonstrated that NKG2D ligand expression can be induced by DNA damage and oxidative stress (Gasser et al., 2005; Peraldi et al., 2009). The upregulation of NKG2D ligands in response to DNA damage critically depends on ATR or ATM, depending on the nature of the DNA damage (Gasser et al., 2005). On tumour cells that constitutively express NKG2D ligands, inhibition of the DDR decreased ligand cell surface expression (Gasser et al, 2005), suggesting that persistent DNA damage in the tumour cells at least partially maintains constitutive NKG2D ligand expression. An important question is if the p53- and the NKG2D-mediated tumor surveillance are linked or provide independent protection against the development of malignant cells. In favor of the latter idea, we found that NKG2D ligands could be induced in cells that lacked p53. While p53 is not required for the expression of NKG2D ligands in tumor cell lines or in cells with DNA damage, it is possible that other p53 family members, along with p53, function in a partially redundant fashion to induce NKG2D ligand expression. Intriguingly, the loss of p53 is implicated in the loss of genomic stability. It is therefore plausible that the resulting genomic lesions may further increase the DDR and upregulate the expression of NKG2D ligands on tumor cells.

3.4 DNAM-1 ligands

Although NKG2D is a major receptor implicated in recognition of cells with damaged DNA, NKG2D blocking experiments suggested that additional immunomodulatory molecules are required (Gasser et al., data not shown). A recent study showed that the DDR also upregulates the expression of DNAM-1 ligands (Soriani et al., 2009). DNAM-1 ligands include CD155 (also called poliovirus receptor, tumor associated antigen 4 and necl-5) and

CD112 (Nectin-2) (Bottino et al., 2003). CD112 and CD155 are ubiquitously expressed on most normal cells of neuronal, epithelial endothelial and fibroblast origin, however their expression levels are significantly enhanced in tumor cells including acute myeloid leukemias, neuroblastomas, melanomas and colorectal carcinomas (Castriconi et al., 2004; Carlsten et al., 2007; El-Sherbiny et al., 2007). DNAM-1 is a member of the immunoglobulin superfamily and is constitutively expressed on most immune cells including T cells, NK cells, a subset of B cells and monocytes/macrophages (Shibuya et al., 1996). DNAM-1 is physically and functionally associated with LFA-1, a receptor for ICAM-1 which is also upregulated in response to DNA damage (see below). The expression of CD112 or CD155 on tumor cells induces NK cell- and CD8+ T cell-mediated cytotoxicity and cytokine secretion (Bottino et al., 2003). Strikingly, DNAM-1-deficient mice injected with carcinogen-induced tumor cells developed tumors faster and showed higher mortality (Iguchi-Manaka et al., 2008). CD155 is also recognized by CD96, a stimulatory receptor expressed by NK cells and other immune cells (Fuchs et al., 2004). The existence of a dual receptor system recognizing CD155 further suggests an important role of this ligand in NK cell-mediated recognition of tumor cells. In addition to its activating functions, CD155 has recently also been shown to suppress immune cell activation through a third receptor called TIGIT/ VSTM/WUCAM, primarily expressed on T cells and on NK cells (Stanietsky et al., 2009). Moreover, the binding of CD155 to TIGIT on DCs leads to the secretion of IL-10 and inhibition of pro-inflammatory cytokine secretion (Yu et al., 2009). CD155 has higher affinity for TIGIT than DNAM-1. In contrast CD112 preferentially binds to DNAM-1 (Bottino et al., 2003). Hence the over-all avidity of cells for DNAM-1 over TIGIT may ultimately determine if an immune response is initiated or inhibited by DNAM-1 ligands.

3.5 ICAM-1

Intercellular adhesion molecule-1 (ICAM-1, also called CD54) is a cell adhesion molecule, which is expressed by fibroblasts, epithelial, endothelial and immune cells such as lymphocytes and macrophages (Dustin et al., 1986; Rothlein et al., 1986). Binding of ICAM-1 to its receptors LFA-1 and macrophage-1 antigen (Mac-1) expressed on leukocytes is often required to initiate inflammatory and immune responses (Simmons et al., 1988; Diamond et al., 1993; Sligh et al., 1993). The expression of ICAM-1 is induced by several pro-inflammatory cytokines (Dustin et al., 1986; Pober et al., 1986). However, ICAM-1 expression has also been shown to be upregulated by ionizing radiation in a p53-dependent manner (Hallahan et al., 1996; Gaugler et al., 1997; Hallahan & Virudachalam, 1997). Recently it was discovered that ICAM-1 expression correlates with senescence (see 4.1 and Gourgoulis et al., 2005).

4. The role of DDR in diseases

4.1 Senescence-associated secretory phenotype (SASP)

If low levels of DNA damage persist in cells, the DDR induces an irreversible cell cycle arrest called senescence. Recent data have shown *in vivo* accumulation of senescent cells with age (Herbig et al., 2006; Jeyapalan et al., 2007). Senescent cells secrete a broad spectrum of factors, including the cytokines IL-6, IL-8, transforming growth factor-b (TGF-β), plasminogen activator inhibitor 1 (PAI-1), and others, collectively often referred to as the senescence-associated secretory phenotype (SASP) (Kortlever & Bernards, 2006; Coppé et al., 2009; Rodier et al., 2009). There is good evidence that some of these factors contribute to senescence entry and maintenance. For instance, the autocrine secretion of IL-6 is required for the establishment of oncogene-induced senescence (Kuilman et al. 2008). Some IRFs, including IRF-1, IRF-5 and IRF-7, have been functionally linked to senescence (Li et al., 2008; Upreti et al., 2010). Some members of the SASP do not function exclusively in a cell-autonomous manner, but they also affect neighboring cells. Paradoxically, their paracrine effects sometimes promote tumorigenesis. IL-6 contributes to tumorigenesis by promoting angiogenesis (Wei et al., 2003; Fan et al., 2008). In addition, IL-6 secretion by HRasV12-transformed cancer cells has been reported to mediate tumour growth (Leslie 2010). Tumor-promoting effects have also been described for other SASP members, such as TGF-β (reviewed in Bierie & Moses, 2006), IL-1 (Dejana et al., 1988; Voronov et al., 2003) and IL-8 (Norgauer et al., 1996). These opposite effects may be explained by differences in cells type, stage of transformation or the mode of signaling (autocrine versus paracrine). It is possible that healthy, normal cells enter senescence in response to oncogene-induced DNA damage, and possibly due to the subsequent SASP, whereas the SASP can promote tumorigenesis in neighboring precancerous lesions harboring specific mutations. DNA damage-induced senescence may therefore have dual roles in preventing and promoting tumorigenesis, depending on the cellular context. Some characteristics of senescent cells, such as the ability of SASP members to modify the extracellular environment, may play a role in aging and age-related pathology (Chung et al., 2009). Of note many of DDR-induced ligands for activating immune receptors, such as NKG2D, DNAM-1 and LFA-1 are upregulated in senescent cells. It remains currently unclear if the underlying DDR in senescent cells is regulating the expression of these ligands or if the expression depends on senescence-specific pathways.

4.2 Cancer

As mentioned earlier, the DDR may represent a major barrier to tumorigenesis (Bartkova et al., 2005; Gorgoulis et al., 2005). Replication stress in response to oncogene activation results in the collapse of DNA replication forks. The resulting DNA breaks activate the DDR, leading to either senescence or cellular apoptosis. In addition to these largely cell-intrinsic barrier effects of the DDR, recent evidence suggests that cell-extrinsic barriers could exist, some of which may depend on the immune system. A link between the DDR and immune system was suggested by the upregulation of ligands for the activating immune receptors NKG2D, DNAM-1 and LFA-1 in tumor cells or in cells undergoing genotoxic stress. In addition the DDR also regulates the expression of the apoptosis-inducing death receptor 5 (DR5), a ligand for TRAIL (Wu et al., 1997). NKG2D, DNAM-1 and LFA-1 participate in 'induced self-recognition' of target cells by cytotoxic NK cells (Lakshmikanth et al., 2009). "Induced self-ligands" are absent or only poorly expressed by normal cells, but upregulated on diseased cells (Castriconi et al., 2004; Gasser et al., 2005; Gorgoulis et al., 2005). The activating receptors NKG2D, DNAM-1 and LFA-1 are mainly expressed by natural killer (NK) cells and T cells, which play an important role in the immunity against cancer (Shibuya et al., 1996; Barber et al., 2004; El-Sherbiny et al., 2007). The recognition of tumor cells by NK cells is governed by activating and inhibitory receptor-mediated signals (Gasser & Raulet, 2006). Many of the inhibitory receptors expressed by NK cells are specific for major histocompatibility complex (MHC) class I molecules. MHC class I molecules are expressed by normal cells but are often downregulated from tumour cells. Increased expression of activating ligands by tumor cells can override inhibitory receptor signaling, resulting in NK cell activation and NK cell-mediated lysis of tumor cells. NK cells also produce pro-inflammatory cytokines such as IFN-γ, which help to initiate an adaptive immune response (reviewed in Kos, 1998). In addition to their role in NK cells, NKG2D, DNAM-1 and LFA-1 provide signals that enhance the activation of specific T cell subsets, such as the cytotoxic CD8+ T cells (Shibuya et al., 1996; Barber et al., 2004; Gasser & Raulet, 2006). The qualitative and quantitative effector responses of NK and T cells are regulated by cytokines such as interleukin-2 (IL-2), IL-12, IL-15, IL-18, IL-21, TGF-β and the type I IFNs (Biron et al., 1999). Hence, in addition to the effects described above, the DDR-induced expression of type I interferons may also help in stimulating an immune response through the activation of NK and T cells.

4.3 Viral infections

The DDR is also triggered when cells are infected with certain viruses, including retroviruses such as the human immunodefiency virus 1 (HIV-1), adenoviruses, herpes simplex viruses 1 and 2 (HSV-1 and 2), cytomegalovirus (CMV), hepatitis B virus, Epstein-Barr virus (EBV) and the human papilloma virus type 16 and 18 (HPV-16 and 18) (Lilley et al., 2007). In many cases, the DDR is triggered in response to viral nucleic acid intermediates produced during the viral "life cycle" (Lilley et al., 2007). The importance of the DDR in preventing virus-induced tumorigenesis is evidenced by the fact that oncogenic viruses infect many cells but rarely lead to tumorigenesis. For example, infectious mononucleosis can be caused by the infection of EBV, but rarely leads to Burkitt's and Hodgkin's lymphoma (Lemon et al., 1977). The ATM-CHK2 pathway is triggered in B cells during a latent EBV infection, which is thought to supress EBV-induced transformation by inducing cell cycle arrest and apoptosis (Nikitin et al., 2010). Adenovirus infection results in the phosphorylation of ATM and H2AX, the stabilization of p53 and the downregulation of the anti-apoptotic protein myeloid cell leukemia 1 (MCL-1), thereby promoting the induction of apoptosis in virus-infected cells (Debbas & White, 1993; Lowe & Ruley, 1993a; Cuconati et al., 2003). In summary, the DDR is not restricted to controling tumorigenesis induced by the activation of host oncogenes, but also functions to control the activity of viral genes and may therefore participate in defending organisms from viral infections. In support of this idea, p53-deficient mice show higher viral titer and mortality after vesicular stomatitis virus infection (Takaoka et al., 2003). In another study, the knockdown of p53 in a liver cell line resulted in higher levels of hepatitis C virus replication (Dharel et al., 2008). In addition, p53 was shown to be activated in cells infected with the Newcastle disease virus, herpes simplex virus and influenza virus (Takaoka et al., 2003; Turpin et al., 2005).

Many viruses have developed means to interfere with the DDR, further supporting the idea that the DDR may restrict viral infection and proliferation of infected cells. The adenovirus core protein VII protects the viral genome from the DDR (Karen & Hearing, 2011). Tax, a protein encoded by HTLV-1 attenuates the ATM-mediated DDR by interacting with CHK1 and CHK2 (Park et al., 2004; Park et al., 2005). The activation of the DDR is disrupted by the human CMV through altering the localization of CHK2 by viral structural proteins (Gaspar & Shenk, 2005). During the EBV infection of B cells, the latent EBNA3C protein attenuates the DDR by modulating CHK2 and p53 activity (Nikita et al., 2010). Other proteins (E6 protein of the HPV-16, HPV-18, S40 large T antigen of simian virus etc.) of oncogenic viruses interfere with p53 functions in infected cells (Werness et al., 1990; Kessis et al., 1993).

Despite the potential antiviral properties of the DDR, many viruses have also evolved ways to activate at least part of the DDR for their own replication. In retroviral integration, for instance, the viral integrase cleaves the host DNA to facilitate the integration of the viral double-stranded cDNA, and as a consequence, leaves a dsDNA break that requires NHEJ repair (Skalka & Katz, 2005). Viral replication of HIV-1 was suppressed when cells were treated with an ATM-specific inhibitor (Lau et al., 2005). Furthermore, HIV-1 encodes a protein, Vpr, which activates the ATR-CHK1 pathway to arrest infected cells in the G2 phase of the cell cycle and to repair dsDNA breaks by homologous recombination (Goh et al., 1998; Roshal et al., 2003; Nakai-Murakami et al., 2006).

The activation of the DDR in response to viral infection renders cell sensitive to immune cell-mediated lysis by upregulating ligands for NKG2D, DNAM-1 and LFA-1. Two recent reports show that HIV-1 ATR-CHK1 activation by the HIV-1 Vpr upregulates the expression of ligands for the activating NKG2D receptor and promotes NK cell-mediated killing (Richard et al., 2009; Ward et al., 2009). EBV-transformed B-cell lines are relatively resistant to NK cell-mediated lysis possibly as a result of their attenuated DDR in addition to high expression of MHC class I molecules, which inhibit NK cells (Pappworth et al., 2007). However, the reactivation of EBV in transformed B cells renders them susceptible to NK-cell-mediated lysis, which was partially depends on NKG2D and DNAM-1 (Pappworth et al., 2007). NKG2D ligand expression is upregulated upon infection by a number of viruses, such as CMV, HBV, poxvirus and hepatitis C virus, although the role of the DDR in the regulation has yet to be explored in detail.

A number of viruses have developed means to interfere with the expression of ligands for activating receptors. This phenomenon is best characterized for the ligands of NKG2D. Nef (Negative factor) protein encoded by HIV-1 downregulates the expression of NKG2D ligands, HLA-A and HLA-B, to potentially evade recognition by NK cells and HLA-A-/HLA-B- restricted HIV-1-specific cytotoxic T cells (McMichael 1998; Cerboni et al., 2007). Hepatitis C virus impairs the NKG2D-dependent NK cell responses by downregulating NKG2D ligand and receptor expression (Wen et al., 2008). Both murine and human CMV have developed strategies to evade the NKG2D-dependent recognition. The murine CMV encodes the viral glycoproteins m138, m145 and m152 for evasion strategies. The m152 targets Rae1 for degradation (Lodoen et al., 2003), m145 and m138 prevent MULT1 expression (Krmpotic et al., 2005), while m138 cooperates with m155 to impair H60 expression (Lodoen et al., 2004; Lenac et al., 2006). The human CMV (HCMV)-encoded UL16 protein inhibits the expression of MICB, ULBP1, ULBP2 and RAET1G (Dunn et al., 2003; Rölle et al., 2003). The HCMV protein UL142 prevents the expression of some, but not all, alleles of MICA (Chalupny et al., 2006). Some alleles of MICA, such as the prevalent allele of MICA, MICA*008, are resistant to downregulation by HCMV because of a truncation of the cytoplasmic domain (Chalupny et al., 2006). These polymorphisms may reflect a counter-offensive of the host to evade viral protein-mediated inhibition of NKG2D ligand expression. Furthermore, it was recently discovered that a microRNA encoded by HCMV downregulates MICB expression by targeting a specific site in the *MICB* 3' untranslated region (Stern-Ginossar et al., 2007). Finally, the HCMV protein UL141 protein impedes the expression of DNAM-1 ligand CD155 (Tomasec et al., 2005). Interestingly, CD155 functions as a poliovirus receptor, but the role of NK cells or the DDR in poliovirus infection has not been studied in detail. Taken together, the DDR presents a challenge to many viruses as their replication critically depends on certain aspects of the DDR. At the same time, the DDR can induce apoptosis of infected cells or render infected cells sensitive to immune cell-mediated lysis (Figure 2). In response, viruses most likely target the specific effector molecules of the DDR that prevent their subsequent infection of new target cells, while leaving the part of the pathway required for their replication intact.

Host cell

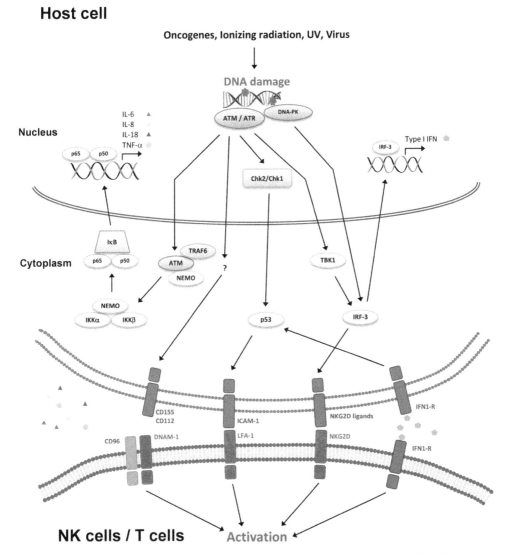

Fig. 2. Potential links between the DDR and the immune system. Activation of the DDR activates cytotoxic natural killer and T cells by inducing the expression of proinflammatory cytokines and ligands for activating immune receptors.

5. Conclusion

The DDR is activated in response to genotoxic stress caused by oncogene activation, viral infection or other environmental insults to the cell. The DDR initiates cell autonomous programmes to try to repair the damaged DNA, or to induce apoptosis if the damage is not repairable, in order to preserve the genome integrity and the survival of the organism.

Recent evidence links the DDR to innate and possibly, adaptive immunity. The activation of an immune response may contribute to the removal of these potentially harmful cells (Figure 2).

6. References

Abraham RT (2001) Cell cycle checkpoint signaling through the ATM and ATR kinases. *Genes & Development* 15: 2177 -2196

Achanta G, Pelicano H, Feng L, Plunkett W & Huang P (2001) Interaction of p53 and DNA-PK in Response to Nucleoside Analogues. *Cancer Research* 61: 8723 -8729

Akira S, Uematsu S & Takeuchi O (2006) Pathogen Recognition and Innate Immunity. *Cell* 124: 783-801

Annunziata CM, Davis RE, Demchenko Y, Bellamy W, Gabrea A, Zhan F, Lenz G, Hanamura I, Wright G & Xiao W (2007) Frequent Engagement of the Classical and Alternative NF-κB Pathways by Diverse Genetic Abnormalities in Multiple Myeloma. *Cancer Cell* 12: 115-130

Baeuerle PA & Henkel T (1994) Function and activation of NF-kappa B in the immune system. *Annu. Rev. Immunol* 12: 141-179

Banin S, Moyal L, Shieh S, Taya Y, Anderson C, Chessa L, Smorodinsky N, Prives C, Reiss Y & Shiloh Y (1998) Enhanced phosphorylation of p53 by ATM in response to DNA damage. *Science* 281: 1674

Barber DF, Faure M & Long EO (2004) LFA-1 Contributes an Early Signal for NK Cell Cytotoxicity. *The Journal of Immunology* 173: 3653 -3659

Barnes BJ, Kellum MJ, Pinder KE, Frisancho JA & Pitha PM (2003) Interferon Regulatory Factor 5, a Novel Mediator of Cell Cycle Arrest and Cell Death. *Cancer Research* 63: 6424 -6431

Barnes BJ, Moore PA & Pitha PM (2001) Virus-specific Activation of a Novel Interferon Regulatory Factor, IRF-5, Results in the Induction of Distinct Interferon alpha Genes. *J. Biol. Chem.* 276: 23382-23390

Bartek J, Falck J & Lukas J (2001) Chk2 kinase - a busy messenger. *Nat Rev Mol Cell Biol* 2: 877-886

Bartkova J, Horejsi Z, Koed K, Kramer A, Tort F, Zieger K, Guldberg P, Sehested M, Nesland JM, Lukas C, Orntoft T, Lukas J & Bartek J (2005) DNA damage response as a candidate anti-cancer barrier in early human tumorigenesis. *Nature* 434: 864-870

Basu S, Rosenzweig KR, Youmell M & Price BD (1998) The DNA-Dependent Protein Kinase Participates in the Activation of NF[kappa]B Following DNA Damage. *Biochemical and Biophysical Research Communications* 247: 79-83

Beg AA & Baltimore D (1996) An Essential Role for NF-κB in Preventing TNF-α-Induced Cell Death. *Science* 274: 782 -784

Bennett M, Macdonald K, Chan S, Luzio J, Simari R & Weissberg P (1998) Cell surface trafficking of Fas: a rapid mechanism of p53-mediated apoptosis. *Science* 282: 290

Bierie B & Moses HL (2006) TGF-b and cancer. *Cytokine & Growth Factor Reviews* 17: 29-40

Billadeau DD, Upshaw JL, Schoon RA, Dick CJ & Leibson PJ (2003) NKG2D-DAP10 triggers human NK cell-mediated killing via a Syk-independent regulatory pathway. *Nat Immunol* 4: 557-564

Biron CA, Nguyen KB, Pien GC, Cousens LP & Salazar-Mather TP (1999) NATURAL KILLER CELLS IN ANTIVIRAL DEFENSE: Function and Regulation by Innate Cytokines. *Annu. Rev. Immunol.* 17: 189-220

Bottino C, Castriconi R, Pende D, Rivera P, Nanni M, Carnemolla B, Cantoni C, Grassi J, Marcenaro S, Reymond N, Vitale M, Moretta L, Lopez M & Moretta A (2003) Identification of PVR (CD155) and Nectin-2 (CD112) as Cell Surface Ligands for the Human DNAM-1 (CD226) Activating Molecule. *The Journal of Experimental Medicine* 198: 557 -567

Brach MA, Hass R, Sherman ML, Gunji H, Weichselbaum R & Kufe D (1991) Ionizing radiation induces expression and binding activity of the nuclear factor kappa B. *J Clin Invest* 88: 691-695

Bredemeyer AL, Helmink BA, Innes CL, Calderon B, McGinnis LM, Mahowald GK, Gapud EJ, Walker LM, Collins JB, Weaver BK, Mandik-Nayak L, Schreiber RD, Allen PM, May MJ, Paules RS, Bassing CH & Sleckman BP (2008) DNA double-strand breaks activate a multi-functional genetic program in developing lymphocytes. *Nature* 456: 819-823

Brown EJ & Baltimore D (2000) ATR disruption leads to chromosomal fragmentation and early embryonic lethality. *Genes Dev* 14: 397-402

Cai Z, Chehab NH & Pavletich NP (2009) Structure and Activation Mechanism of the CHK2 DNA Damage Checkpoint Kinase. *Molecular Cell* 35: 818-829

Carlsten M, Björkström NK, Norell H, Bryceson Y, van Hall T, Baumann BC, Hanson M, Schedvins K, Kiessling R, Ljunggren H-G & Malmberg K-J (2007) DNAX Accessory Molecule-1 Mediated Recognition of Freshly Isolated Ovarian Carcinoma by Resting Natural Killer Cells. *Cancer Research* 67: 1317 -1325

Carter T, Vancurová I, Sun I, Lou W & DeLeon S (1990) A DNA-activated protein kinase from HeLa cell nuclei. *Mol Cell Biol* 10: 6460-6471

Carvalho G, Fabre C, Braun T, Grosjean J, Ades L, Agou F, Tasdemir E, Boehrer S, Israel A, Veron M, Fenaux P & Kroemer G (2007) Inhibition of NEMO, the regulatory subunit of the IKK complex, induces apoptosis in high-risk myelodysplastic syndrome and acute myeloid leukemia. *Oncogene* 26: 2299-2307

Castriconi R, Dondero A, Corrias MV, Lanino E, Pende D, Moretta L, Bottino C & Moretta A (2004) Natural Killer Cell-Mediated Killing of Freshly Isolated Neuroblastoma Cells. *Cancer Research* 64: 9180 -9184

Cerboni C, Neri F, Casartelli N, Zingoni A, Cosman D, Rossi P, Santoni A & Doria M (2007) Human immunodeficiency virus 1 Nef protein downmodulates the ligands of the activating receptor NKG2D and inhibits natural killer cell-mediated cytotoxicity. *J Gen Virol* 88: 242-250

Cerwenka A (2000) Retinoic Acid Early Inducible Genes Define a Ligand Family for the Activating NKG2D Receptor in Mice. *Immunity* 12: 721-727

Chalupny NJ, Rein-Weston A, Dosch S & Cosman D (2006) Down-regulation of the NKG2D ligand MICA by the human cytomegalovirus glycoprotein UL142. *Biochemical and Biophysical Research Communications* 346: 175-181

Chawla-Sarkar M, Lindner DJ, Liu Y-F, Williams BR, Sen GC, Silverman RH & Borden EC (2003) Apoptosis and interferons: role of interferon-stimulated genes as mediators of apoptosis. *Apoptosis* 8: 237-249

Chen X, Bargonetti J & Prives C (1995) p53, through p21 (WAF1/CIP1), Induces Cyclin D1 Synthesis. *Cancer Research* 55: 4257 -4263

Chipuk JE, Maurer U, Green DR & Schuler M (2003) Pharmacologic activation of p53 elicits Bax-dependent apoptosis in the absence of transcription. *Cancer Cell* 4: 371-381

Chung HY, Cesari M, Anton S, Marzetti E, Giovannini S, Seo AY, Carter C, Yu BP & Leeuwenburgh C (2009) Molecular inflammation: Underpinnings of aging and age-related diseases. *Ageing Research Reviews* 8: 18-30

Cogswell J, Godlevski M, Wisely G, Clay W, Leesnitzer L, Ways J & Gray J (1994) NF-kappa B regulates IL-1 beta transcription through a consensus NF- kappa B binding site and a nonconsensus CRE-like site. *The Journal of Immunology* 153: 712 -723

Coppé J-P, Patil CK, Rodier F, Sun Y, Muñoz DP, Goldstein J, Nelson PS, Desprez P-Y & Campisi J (2008) Senescence-Associated Secretory Phenotypes Reveal Cell-Nonautonomous Functions of Oncogenic RAS and the p53 Tumor Suppressor. *PLoS Biol* 6: e301

Cortez D, Guntuku S, Qin J & Elledge SJ (2001) ATR and ATRIP: Partners in Checkpoint Signaling. *Science* 294: 1713 -1716

Cosman D, Müllberg J, Sutherland CL, Chin W, Armitage R, Fanslow W, Kubin M & Chalupny NJ (2001) ULBPs, novel MHC class I-related molecules, bind to CMV glycoprotein UL16 and stimulate NK cytotoxicity through the NKG2D receptor. *Immunity* 14: 123-133

Creagh EM & O'Neill LAJ (2006) TLRs, NLRs and RLRs: a trinity of pathogen sensors that co-operate in innate immunity. *Trends in Immunology* 27: 352-357

Cuconati A, Mukherjee C, Perez D & White E (2003) DNA damage response and MCL-1 destruction initiate apoptosis in adenovirus-infected cells. *Genes Dev.* 17: 2922-2932

Debbas M & White E (1993) Wild-type p53 mediates apoptosis by E1A, which is inhibited by E1B. *Genes & Development* 7: 546 -554

Dejana E, Bertocchi F, Bortolami MC, Regonesi A, Tonta A, Breviario F & Giavazzi R (1988) Interleukin 1 promotes tumor cell adhesion to cultured human endothelial cells. *J. Clin. Invest.* 82: 1466-1470

deRojas-Walker T, Tamir S, Ji H, Wishnok JS & Tannenbaum SR (1995) Nitric oxide induces oxidative damage in addition to deamination in macrophage DNA. *Chem. Res. Toxicol* 8: 473-477

Das S, Boswell SA, Aaronson SA & Lee SW (2008) p53 promoter selection: Choosing between life and death. *cc* 7: 154-157

Dharel N, Kato N, Muroyama R, Taniguchi H, Otsuka M, Wang Y, Jazag A, Shao R, Chang J, Adler MK, Kawabe T & Omata M (2008) Potential contribution of tumor suppressor p53 in the host defense against hepatitis C virus. *Hepatology* 47: 1136-1149

Diamond MS, Garcia-Aguilar J, Bickford JK, Corbi AL & Springer TA (1993) The I domain is a major recognition site on the leukocyte integrin Mac-1 (CD11b/CD18) for four distinct adhesion ligands. *The Journal of Cell Biology* 120: 1031 -1043

Diefenbach A, Jamieson AM, Liu SD, Shastri N & Raulet DH (2000) Ligands for the murine NKG2D receptor: expression by tumor cells and activation of NK cells and macrophages. *Nat Immunol* 1: 119-126

Duguay D, Mercier F, Stagg J, Martineau D, Bramson J, Servant M, Lin R, Galipeau J & Hiscott J (2002) In Vivo Interferon Regulatory Factor 3 Tumor Suppressor Activity in B16 Melanoma Tumors. *Cancer Research* 62: 5148 -5152

Dujka ME, Puebla-Osorio N, Tavana O, Sang M & Zhu C (2009) ATM and p53 are essential in the cell-cycle containment of DNA breaks during V(D)J recombination in vivo. *Oncogene* 29: 957-965

Dumaz N & Meek DW (1999) Serine 15 phosphorylation stimulates p53 transactivation but does not directly influence interaction with HDM2. *EMBO J* 18: 7002-7010

Dunn C, Chalupny NJ, Sutherland CL, Dosch S, Sivakumar PV, Johnson DC & Cosman D (2003) Human Cytomegalovirus Glycoprotein UL16 Causes Intracellular Sequestration of NKG2D Ligands, Protecting Against Natural Killer Cell Cytotoxicity. *The Journal of Experimental Medicine* 197: 1427 -1439

Dustin ML, Rothlein R, Bhan AK, Dinarello CA & Springer TA (1986) Induction by IL 1 and interferon-gamma: tissue distribution, biochemistry, and function of a natural adherence molecule (ICAM-1). *J. Immunol* 137: 245-254

Dvorak HF (1986) Tumors: wounds that do not heal. Similarities between tumor stroma generation and wound healing. *N. Engl. J. Med* 315: 1650-1659

El-Sherbiny YM, Meade JL, Holmes TD, McGonagle D, Mackie SL, Morgan AW, Cook G, Feyler S, Richards SJ, Davies FE, Morgan GJ & Cook GP (2007) The Requirement for DNAM-1, NKG2D, and NKp46 in the Natural Killer Cell-Mediated Killing of Myeloma Cells. *Cancer Research* 67: 8444 -8449

Falck J, Mailand N, Syljuasen RG, Bartek J & Lukas J (2001) The ATM-Chk2-Cdc25A checkpoint pathway guards against radioresistant DNA synthesis. *Nature* 410: 842-847

Fan Y, Ye J, Shen F, Zhu Y, Yeghiazarians Y, Zhu W, Chen Y, Lawton MT, Young WL & Yang G-Y (2008) Interleukin-6 stimulates circulating blood-derived endothelial progenitor cell angiogenesis in vitro. *J Cereb Blood Flow Metab* 28: 90-98

Fitzgerald KA, McWhirter SM, Faia KL, Rowe DC, Latz E, Golenbock DT, Coyle AJ, Liao S-M & Maniatis T (2003) IKKε and TBK1 are essential components of the IRF3 signaling pathway. *Nat Immunol* 4: 491-496

Fuchs A, Cella M, Giurisato E, Shaw AS & Colonna M (2004) Cutting Edge: CD96 (Tactile) Promotes NK Cell-Target Cell Adhesion by Interacting with the Poliovirus Receptor (CD155). *The Journal of Immunology* 172: 3994 -3998

Gao J, Senthil M, Ren B, Yan J, Xing Q, Yu J, Zhang L & Yim J (2010) IRF-1 transcriptionally up-regulates PUMA which mediates the mitochondrial apoptotic pathway in IRF-1 induced apoptosis in cancer cells. *Cell Death Differ* 17: 699-709

Gatei M, Sloper K, Sörensen C, Syljuäsen R, Falck J, Hobson K, Savage K, Lukas J, Zhou B-B, Bartek J & Khanna KK (2003) Ataxia-telangiectasia-mutated (ATM) and NBS1-dependent Phosphorylation of Chk1 on Ser-317 in Response to Ionizing Radiation. *Journal of Biological Chemistry* 278: 14806 -14811

Gaspar M & Shenk T (2006) Human cytomegalovirus inhibits a DNA damage response by mislocalizing checkpoint proteins. *Proceedings of the National Academy of Sciences of the United States of America* 103: 2821 -2826

Gasser S (2007) DNA - damage response and development of targeted cancer treatments. *Annals of Medicine* 39: 457

Gasser S & Raulet DH (2006) Activation and self-tolerance of natural killer cells. *Immunological Reviews* 214: 130-142

Gasser S, Orsulic S, Brown EJ & Raulet DH (2005) The DNA damage pathway regulates innate immune system ligands of the NKG2D receptor. *Nature* 436: 1186-1190

Gaugler, C. Squiban, A. Van Der Mee M-H (1997) Late and persistent up-regulation of intercellular adhesion molecule-1 (ICAM-1) expression by ionizing radiation in human endothelial cells in vitro. *Int J Radiat Biol* 72: 201-209

Ghosh S & Karin M (2002) Missing Pieces in the NF-κB Puzzle. *Cell* 109: S81-S96

Ghosh S, May MJ & Kopp EB (1998) NF-κB AND REL PROTEINS: Evolutionarily Conserved Mediators of Immune Responses. *Annu. Rev. Immunol.* 16: 225-260

Goh WC, Rogel ME, Kinsey CM, Michael SF, Fultz PN, Nowak MA, Hahn BH & Emerman M (1998) HIV-1 Vpr increases viral expression by manipulation of the cell cycle: A mechanism for selection of Vpr in vivo. *Nat Med* 4: 65-71

Gorgoulis VG, Pratsinis H, Zacharatos P, Demoliou C, Sigala F, Asimacopoulos PJ, Papavassiliou AG & Kletsas D (2005) p53-Dependent ICAM-1 overexpression in senescent human cells identified in atherosclerotic lesions. *Lab Invest* 85: 502-511

Groh V, Rhinehart R, Secrist H, Bauer S, Grabstein KH & Spies T (1999) Broad tumor-associated expression and recognition by tumor-derived γδ T cells of MICA and MICB. *Proceedings of the National Academy of Sciences* 96: 6879 -6884

Grosjean-Raillard J, Tailler M, Ades L, Perfettini J-L, Fabre C, Braun T, De Botton S, Fenaux P & Kroemer G (2008) ATM mediates constitutive NF-[kappa]B activation in high-risk myelodysplastic syndrome and acute myeloid leukemia. *Oncogene* 28: 1099-1109

Halazonetis T, Gorgoulis V & Bartek J (2008) An oncogene-induced DNA damage model for cancer development. *Science* 319: 1352

Hallahan DE & Virudachalam S (1997) Ionizing Radiation Mediates Expression of Cell Adhesion Molecules in Distinct Histological Patterns within the Lung. *Cancer Research* 57: 2096 -2099

Hallahan D, Kuchibhotla J & Wyble C (1996) Cell Adhesion Molecules Mediate Radiation-induced Leukocyte Adhesion to the Vascular Endothelium. *Cancer Research* 56: 5150 -5155

Hanahan D & Weinberg RA (2000) The Hallmarks of Cancer. *Cell* 100: 57-70

Hayden MS & Ghosh S (2008) Shared Principles in NF-κB Signaling. *Cell* 132: 344-362

Herbig U, Ferreira M, Condel L, Carey D & Sedivy JM (2006) Cellular Senescence in Aging Primates. *Science* 311: 1257

Heylbroeck C, Balachandran S, Servant MJ, DeLuca C, Barber GN, Lin R & Hiscott J (2000) The IRF-3 transcription factor mediates Sendai virus-induced apoptosis. *J. Virol* 74: 3781-3792

Hinz M, Stilmann M, Arslan SÇ, Khanna KK, Dittmar G & Scheidereit C (2010) A Cytoplasmic ATM-TRAF6-cIAP1 Module Links Nuclear DNA Damage Signaling to Ubiquitin-Mediated NF-κB Activation. *Molecular Cell* 40: 63-74

Hirao A, Kong Y-Y, Matsuoka S, Wakeham A, Ruland J, Yoshida H, Liu D, Elledge SJ & Mak TW (2000) DNA Damage-Induced Activation of p53 by the Checkpoint Kinase Chk2. *Science* 287: 1824-1827

Honda K & Taniguchi T (2006) IRFs: master regulators of signalling by Toll-like receptors and cytosolic pattern-recognition receptors. *Nat Rev Immunol* 6: 644-658

Hu G, Mancl ME & Barnes BJ (2005) Signaling through IFN Regulatory Factor-5 Sensitizes p53-Deficient Tumors to DNA Damage-Induced Apoptosis and Cell Death. *Cancer Res* 65: 7403-7412

Huang TT, Feinberg SL, Suryanarayanan S & Miyamoto S (2002) The Zinc Finger Domain of NEMO Is Selectively Required for NF-κB Activation by UV Radiation and Topoisomerase Inhibitors. *Mol. Cell. Biol.* 22: 5813-5825

Huang TT, Wuerzberger-Davis SM, Seufzer BJ, Shumway SD, Kurama T, Boothman DA & Miyamoto S (2000) NF-κB Activation by Camptothecin. *Journal of Biological Chemistry* 275: 9501 -9509

Huang TT, Wuerzberger-Davis SM, Wu Z-H & Miyamoto S (2003) Sequential Modification of NEMO/IKKγ by SUMO-1 and Ubiquitin Mediates NF-κB Activation by Genotoxic Stress. *Cell* 115: 565-576

Iguchi-Manaka A, Kai H, Yamashita Y, Shibata K, Tahara-Hanaoka S, Honda S-ichiro, Yasui T, Kikutani H, Shibuya K & Shibuya A (2008) Accelerated tumor growth in mice deficient in DNAM-1 receptor. *The Journal of Experimental Medicine* 205: 2959 -2964

Jackson SP & Bartek J (2009) The DNA-damage response in human biology and disease. *Nature* 461: 1071-1078

Janssens S, Tinel A, Lippens S & Tschopp J (2005) PIDD Mediates NF-[kappa]B Activation in Response to DNA Damage. *Cell* 123: 1079-1092

Jeyapalan JC, Ferreira M, Sedivy JM & Herbig U (2007) Accumulation of senescent cells in mitotic tissue of aging primates. *Mechanisms of Ageing and Development* 128: 36-44

Kaneko YS, Watanabe N, Morisaki H, Akita H, Fujimoto A, Tominaga K, Terasawa M, Tachibana A, Ikeda K, Nakanishi M & Kaneko Y (1999) Cell-cycle-dependent and ATM-independent expression of human Chk1 kinase. *Oncogene* 18: 3673-3681

Kanneganti T-D, Lamkanfi M & Núñez G (2007) Intracellular NOD-like Receptors in Host Defense and Disease. *Immunity* 27: 549-559

Karen KA & Hearing P (2011) Adenovirus Core Protein VII Protects the Viral Genome from a DNA Damage Response at Early Times after Infection. *J. Virol.*: JVI.02540-10

Karpova AY, Trost M, Murray JM, Cantley LC & Howley PM (2002) Interferon regulatory factor-3 is an in vivo target of DNA-PK. *Proc Natl Acad Sci U S A.* 99: 2818–2823

Kastan M, Onyekwere O, Sidransky D, Vogelstein B & Craig R (1991) Participation of p53 protein in the cellular-response to DNA damage. *Cancer Research* 51: 6304-6311

Kawanishi S, Hiraku Y, Pinlaor S & Ma N (2006) Oxidative and nitrative DNA damage in animals and patients with inflammatory diseases in relation to inflammation-related carcinogenesis. *Biological Chemistry* 387: 365-372

Khanna. KK, Keating KE, Kozlov S, Scott S, Gatei M, Hobson K, Taya Y, Gabrielli B, Chan D, Lees-Miller SP & Lavin MF (1998) ATM associates with and phosphorylates p53: mapping the region of interaction. *Nat Genet* 20: 398-400

Kim TY, Lee K-H, Chang S, Chung C, Lee H-W, Yim J & Kim TK (2003) Oncogenic Potential of a Dominant Negative Mutant of Interferon Regulatory Factor 3. *Journal of Biological Chemistry* 278: 15272 -15278

Kim T, Kim TY, Song Y-H, Min IM, Yim J & Kim TK (1999) Activation of Interferon Regulatory Factor 3 in Response to DNA-damaging Agents. *J. Biol. Chem.* 274: 30686-30689

Kim T-K, Lee J-S, Jung J-E, Oh S-Y, Kwak S, Jin X, Lee S-Y, Lee J-B, Chung YG, Choi YK, You S & Kim H (2006) Interferon regulatory factor 3 activates p53-dependent cell growth inhibition. *Cancer Letters* 242: 215-221

Kirshner JR, Karpova AY, Kops M & Howley PM (2005) Identification of TRAIL as an Interferon Regulatory Factor 3 Transcriptional Target. *J. Virol.* 79: 9320-9324

Kessis TD, Slebos RJ, Nelson WG, Kastan MB, Plunkett BS, Han SM, Lorincz AT, Hedrick L & Cho KR (1993) Human papillomavirus 16 E6 expression disrupts the p53-mediated cellular response to DNA damage. *Proceedings of the National Academy of Sciences of the United States of America* 90: 3988 -3992

Kos FJ (1998) Regulation of adaptive immunity by natural killer cells. *Immunol Res* 17: 303-312

Kortlever RM & Bernards R (2006) Senescence, Wound Healing, and Cancer: the PAI-1 Connection. *cc* 5: 2697-2703

Krmpotic A, Hasan M, Loewendorf A, Saulig T, Halenius A, Lenac T, Polic B, Bubic I, Kriegeskorte A, Pernjak-Pugel E, Messerle M, Hengel H, Busch DH, Koszinowski UH & Jonjic S (2005) NK cell activation through the NKG2D ligand MULT-1 is selectively prevented by the glycoprotein encoded by mouse cytomegalovirus gene m145. *The Journal of Experimental Medicine* 201: 211 -220

Kuilman T, Michaloglou C, Vredeveld LCW, Douma S, Doorn R van, Desmet CJ, Aarden LA, Mooi WJ & Peeper DS (2008) Oncogene-Induced Senescence Relayed by an Interleukin-Dependent Inflammatory Network. *Cell* Vol 133: 1019-1031

Kumar KP, McBride KM, Weaver BK, Dingwall C & Reich NC (2000) Regulated Nuclear-Cytoplasmic Localization of Interferon Regulatory Factor 3, a Subunit of Double-Stranded RNA-Activated Factor 1. *Mol Cell Biol* 20: 4159-4168

Kunkel TA (2004) DNA Replication Fidelity. *Journal of Biological Chemistry* 279: 16895 -16898

Kunsch C, Lang R, Rosen C & Shannon M (1994) Synergistic transcriptional activation of the IL-8 gene by NF-kappa B p65 (RelA) and NF-IL-6. *The Journal of Immunology* 153: 153 -164

Kurimasa A, Kumano S, Boubnov NV, Story MD, Tung C-S, Peterson SR & Chen DJ (1999) Requirement for the Kinase Activity of Human DNA-Dependent Protein Kinase Catalytic Subunit in DNA Strand Break Rejoining. *Mol Cell Biol* 19: 3877-3884

Lakshmikanth T, Burke S, Ali TH, Kimpfler S, Ursini F, Ruggeri L, Capanni M, Umansky V, Paschen A, Sucker A, Pende D, Groh V, Biassoni R, Höglund P, Kato M, Shibuya K, Schadendorf D, Anichini A, Ferrone S, Velardi A, et al (2009) NCRs and DNAM-1 mediate NK cell recognition and lysis of human and mouse melanoma cell lines in vitro and in vivo. *J Clin Invest* 119: 1251-1263

Lau A, Swinbank KM, Ahmed PS, Taylor DL, Jackson SP, Smith GCM & O'Connor MJ (2005) Suppression of HIV-1 infection by a small molecule inhibitor of the ATM kinase. *Nat Cell Biol* 7: 493-500

Lemon SM, Hutt LM, Shaw JE, Li J-LH & Pagano JS (1977) Replication of EBV in epithelial cells during infectious mononucleosis. *Nature* 268: 268-270

Lenac T, Budt M, Arapovic J, Hasan M, Zimmermann A, Simic H, Krmpotic A, Messerle M, Ruzsics Z, Koszinowski UH, Hengel H & Jonjic S (2006) The herpesviral Fc receptor fcr-1 down-regulates the NKG2D ligands MULT-1 and H60. *The Journal of Experimental Medicine* 203: 1843 -1850

Leslie K, Gao S, Berishaj M, Podsypanina K, Ho H, Ivashkiv L & Bromberg J (2010) Differential interleukin-6/Stat3 signaling as a function of cellular context mediates Ras-induced transformation. *Breast Cancer Research* 12: R80

Li N, Banin S, Ouyang H, Li GC, Courtois G, Shiloh Y, Karin M & Rotman G (2001) ATM Is Required for IκB Kinase (IKK) Activation in Response to DNA Double Strand Breaks. *Journal of Biological Chemistry* 276: 8898-8903

Li Q, Tang L, Roberts PC, Kraniak JM, Fridman AL, Kulaeva OI, Tehrani OS & Tainsky MA (2008) Interferon Regulatory Factors IRF5 and IRF7 Inhibit Growth and Induce Senescence in Immortal Li-Fraumeni Fibroblasts. *Molecular Cancer Research* 6: 770 - 784

Libermann TA & Baltimore D (1990) Activation of interleukin-6 gene expression through the NF-kappa B transcription factor. *Mol. Cell. Biol.* 10: 2327-2334

Lilley CE, Schwartz RA & Weitzman MD (2007) Using or abusing: viruses and the cellular DNA damage response. *Trends in Microbiology* 15: 119-126

Lindahl T (1993) Instability and decay of the primary structure of DNA. *Nature* 362: 709-715

Liu Q, Guntuku S, Cui X-S, Matsuoka S, Cortez D, Tamai K, Luo G, Carattini-Rivera S, DeMayo F, Bradley A, Donehower LA & Elledge SJ (2000) Chk1 is an essential kinase that is regulated by Atr and required for the G2/M DNA damage checkpoint. *Genes & Development* 14: 1448 -1459

Lodoen M, Ogasawara K, Hamerman JA, Arase H, Houchins JP, Mocarski ES & Lanier LL (2003) NKG2D-mediated Natural Killer Cell Protection Against Cytomegalovirus Is Impaired by Viral gp40 Modulation of Retinoic Acid Early Inducible 1 Gene Molecules. *The Journal of Experimental Medicine* 197: 1245 -1253

Lodoen MB, Abenes G, Umamoto S, Houchins JP, Liu F & Lanier LL (2004) The Cytomegalovirus m155 Gene Product Subverts Natural Killer Cell Antiviral Protection by Disruption of H60–NKG2D Interactions. *The Journal of Experimental Medicine* 200: 1075 -1081

Lowe SW & Ruley HE (1993a) Stabilization of the p53 tumor suppressor is induced by adenovirus 5 E1A and accompanies apoptosis. *Genes & Development* 7: 535 -545

Lowe SW, Schmitt EM, Smith SW, Osborne BA & Jacks T (1993b) p53 is required for radiation-induced apoptosis in mouse thymocytes. *Nature* 362: 847-849

Lukas C, Bartkova J, Latella L, Falck J, Mailand N, Schroeder T, Sehested M, Lukas J & Bartek J (2001) DNA Damage-activated Kinase Chk2 Is Independent of Proliferation or Differentiation Yet Correlates with Tissue Biology. *Cancer Research* 61: 4990 -4993

Matsuoka S, Huang M & Elledge SJ (1998) Linkage of ATM to Cell Cycle Regulation by the Chk2 Protein Kinase. *Science* 282: 1893 -1897

Matsuoka S, Ballif BA, Smogorzewska A, McDonald ER, Hurov KE, Luo J, Bakalarski CE, Zhao Z, Solimini N, Lerenthal Y, Shiloh Y, Gygi SP & Elledge SJ (2007) ATM and

ATR Substrate Analysis Reveals Extensive Protein Networks Responsive to DNA Damage. *Science* 316: 1160-1166

McGowan CH (2002) Checking in on Cds1 (Chk2): A checkpoint kinase and tumor suppressor. *BioEssays* 24: 502-511

McMichael A (1998) T Cell Responses and Viral Escape. *Cell* 93: 673-676

Meylan E, Dooley AL, Feldser DM, Shen L, Turk E, Ouyang C & Jacks T (2009) Requirement for NF-κB signaling in a mouse model of lung adenocarcinoma. *Nature* 462: 104-107

Mihara M, Erster S, Zaika A, Petrenko O, Chittenden T, Pancoska P & Moll UM (2003) p53 has a direct apoptogenic role at the mitochondria. *Molecular Cell* 11: 577-590

Mori T, Anazawa Y, Iiizumi M, Fukuda S, Nakamura Y & Arakawa H (2002) Identification of the interferon regulatory factor 5 gene (IRF-5) as a direct target for p53. *Oncogene* 21: 2914-8

Nakai-Murakami C, Shimura M, Kinomoto M, Takizawa Y, Tokunaga K, Taguchi T, Hoshino S, Miyagawa K, Sata T, Kurumizaka H, Yuo A & Ishizaka Y (online) HIV-1 Vpr induces ATM-dependent cellular signal with enhanced homologous recombination. *Oncogene* 26: 477-486

Nikitin PA, Yan CM, Forte E, Bocedi A, Tourigny JP, White RE, Allday MJ, Patel A, Dave SS, Kim W, Hu K, Guo J, Tainter D, Rusyn E & Luftig MA (2010) An ATM/Chk2-Mediated DNA Damage-Responsive Signaling Pathway Suppresses Epstein-Barr Virus Transformation of Primary Human B Cells. *Cell Host & Microbe* 8: 510-522

Norgauer J, Metzner B & Schraufstatter I (1996) Expression and growth-promoting function of the IL-8 receptor beta in human melanoma cells. *The Journal of Immunology* 156: 1132 -1137

Nyberg KA, Michelson RJ, Putnam CW & Weinert TA (2002) Toward Maintaining the Genome: DNA Damage and Replication Checkpoints. *Annu. Rev. Genet.* 36: 617-656

Ou Y-H, Chung P-H, Sun T-P & Shieh S-Y (2005) p53 C-Terminal Phosphorylation by CHK1 and CHK2 Participates in the Regulation of DNA-Damage-induced C-Terminal Acetylation. *Mol Biol Cell* 16: 1684-1695

Pahl HL (1999) Activators and target genes of Rel/NF-kappaB transcription factors. *Oncogene* 18: 6853-6866

Pamment J, Ramsay E, Kelleher M, Dornan D & Ball KL (2002) Regulation of the IRF-1 tumour modifier during the response to genotoxic stress involves an ATM-dependent signalling pathway. *Oncogene* 21: 7776-85

Pappworth IY, Wang EC & Rowe M (2007) The Switch from Latent to Productive Infection in Epstein-Barr Virus-Infected B Cells Is Associated with Sensitization to NK Cell Killing. *J. Virol.* 81: 474-482

Park HU, Jeong S-J, Jeong J-H, Chung JH & Brady JN (2005) Human T-cell leukemia virus type 1 Tax attenuates γ-irradiation-induced apoptosis through physical interaction with Chk2. *Oncogene* 25: 438-447

Park HU, Jeong J-H, Chung JH & Brady JN (2004) Human T-cell leukemia virus type 1 Tax interacts with Chk1 and attenuates DNA-damage induced G2 arrest mediated by Chk1. *Oncogene* 23: 4966-4974

Parmar S & Platanias LC (2003) Interferons: mechanisms of action and clinical applications. *Curr Opin Oncol* 15: 431-439

Pende D, Rivera P, Marcenaro S, Chang C-C, Biassoni R, Conte R, Kubin M, Cosman D, Ferrone S, Moretta L & Moretta A (2002) Major Histocompatibility Complex Class I-related Chain A and UL16-Binding Protein Expression on Tumor Cell Lines of Different Histotypes. *Cancer Research* 62: 6178 -6186

Peraldi M-N, Berrou J, Dulphy N, Seidowsky A, Haas P, Boissel N, Metivier F, Randoux C, Kossari N, Guérin A, Geffroy S, Delavaud G, Marin-Esteban V, Glotz D, Charron D & Toubert A (2009) Oxidative Stress Mediates a Reduced Expression of the Activating Receptor NKG2D in NK Cells from End-Stage Renal Disease Patients. *The Journal of Immunology* 182: 1696 -1705

Perkins EJ, Nair A, Cowley DO, Van Dyke T, Chang Y & Ramsden DA (2002) Sensing of intermediates in V(D)J recombination by ATM. *Genes & Development* 16: 159 - 164

Pober JS, Gimbrone MA Jr, Lapierre LA, Mendrick DL, Fiers W, Rothlein R & Springer TA (1986) Overlapping patterns of activation of human endothelial cells by interleukin 1, tumor necrosis factor, and immune interferon. *J. Immunol* 137: 1893-1896

Raulet DH (2003) Roles of the NKG2D immunoreceptor and its ligands. *Nat Rev Immunol* 3: 781-790

Richard J, Sindhu S, Pham TNQ, Belzile J-P & Cohen ÉA (2010) HIV-1 Vpr up-regulates expression of ligands for the activating NKG2D receptor and promotes NK cell–mediated killing. *Blood* 115: 1354 -1363

Rodier F, Coppe J-P, Patil CK, Hoeijmakers WAM, Munoz DP, Raza SR, Freund A, Campeau E, Davalos AR & Campisi J (2009) Persistent DNA damage signalling triggers senescence-associated inflammatory cytokine secretion. *Nat Cell Biol* 11: 973-979

Rohner A, Langenkamp U, Siegler U, Kalberer CP & Wodnar-Filipowicz A (2007) Differentiation-promoting drugs up-regulate NKG2D ligand expression and enhance the susceptibility of acute myeloid leukemia cells to natural killer cell-mediated lysis. *Leukemia Research* 31: 1393-1402

Rölle A, Mousavi-Jazi M, Eriksson M, Odeberg J, Söderberg-Nauclér C, Cosman D, Kärre K & Cerboni C (2003) Effects of Human Cytomegalovirus Infection on Ligands for the Activating NKG2D Receptor of NK Cells: Up-Regulation of UL16-Binding Protein (ULBP)1 and ULBP2 Is Counteracted by the Viral UL16 Protein. *The Journal of Immunology* 171: 902 -908

Roshal M, Kim B, Zhu Y, Nghiem P & Planelles V (2003) Activation of the ATR-mediated DNA Damage Response by the HIV-1 Viral Protein R. *Journal of Biological Chemistry* 278: 25879 -25886

Rothlein R, Dustin M, Marlin S & Springer T (1986) A human intercellular adhesion molecule (ICAM-1) distinct from LFA-1. *The Journal of Immunology* 137: 1270 - 1274

Scheidereit C (2006) IκB kinase complexes: gateways to NF-κB activation and transcription. *Oncogene* 25: 6685-6705

Sen R & Baltimore D (1986) Inducibility of kappa immunoglobulin enhancer-binding protein Nf-kappa B by a posttranslational mechanism. *Cell* 47: 921-928

Shibuya A, Campbell D, Hannum C, Yssel H, Franz-Bacon K, McClanahan T, Kitamura T, Nicholl J, Sutherland GR, Lanier LL & Phillips JH (1996) DNAM-1, A Novel

Adhesion Molecule Involved in the Cytolytic Function of T Lymphocytes. *Immunity* 4: 573-581

Shieh S-Y, Ikeda M, Taya Y & Prives C (1997) DNA Damage-Induced Phosphorylation of p53 Alleviates Inhibition by MDM2. *Cell* 91: 325-334

Shieh S-Y, Ahn J, Tamai K, Taya Y & Prives C (2000) The human homologs of checkpoint kinases Chk1 and Cds1 (Chk2) phosphorylate p53 at multiple DNA damage-inducible sites. *Genes & Development* 14: 289 -300

Shiloh Y (2003) ATM and related protein kinases: safeguarding genome integrity. *Nat Rev Cancer* 3: 155-168

Simmons D, Makgoba MW & Seed B (1988) ICAM, an adhesion ligand of LFA-1, is homologous to the neural cell adhesion molecule NCAM. *Nature* 331: 624-627

Simon MM, Aragane Y, Schwarz A, Luger TA & Schwarz T (1994) UVB Light Induces Nuclear Factor κB (NFκB) Activity Independently from Chromosomal DNA Damage in Cell-Free Cytosolic Extracts. *J Investig Dermatol* 102: 422-427

Skalka AM & Katz RA (2005) Retroviral DNA integration and the DNA damage response. *Cell Death Differ* 12: 971-978

Sligh JE, Ballantyne CM, Rich SS, Hawkins HK, Smith CW, Bradley A & Beaudet AL (1993) Inflammatory and immune responses are impaired in mice deficient in intercellular adhesion molecule 1. *Proceedings of the National Academy of Sciences* 90: 8529 -8533

Sørensen CS, Syljuåsen RG, Falck J, Schroeder T, Rönnstrand L, Khanna KK, Zhou B-B, Bartek J & Lukas J (2003) Chk1 regulates the S phase checkpoint by coupling the physiological turnover and ionizing radiation-induced accelerated proteolysis of Cdc25A. *Cancer Cell* 3: 247-258

Soriani A, Zingoni A, Cerboni C, Iannitto ML, Ricciardi MR, Di Gialleonardo V, Cippitelli M, Fionda C, Petrucci MT, Guarini A, Foa R & Santoni A (2009) ATM-ATR-dependent up-regulation of DNAM-1 and NKG2D ligands on multiple myeloma cells by therapeutic agents results in enhanced NK-cell susceptibility and is associated with a senescent phenotype. *Blood* 113: 3503-3511

Stanietsky N, Simic H, Arapovic J, Toporik A, Levy O, Novik A, Levine Z, Beiman M, Dassa L, Achdout H, Stern-Ginossar N, Tsukerman P, Jonjic S & Mandelboim O (2009) The interaction of TIGIT with PVR and PVRL2 inhibits human NK cell cytotoxicity. *Proceedings of the National Academy of Sciences* 106: 17858 -17863

Stang MT, Armstrong MJ, Watson GA, Sung KY, Liu Y, Ren B & Yim JH (2007) Interferon regulatory factor-1-induced apoptosis mediated by a ligand-independent fas-associated death domain pathway in breast cancer cells. *Oncogene* 26: 6420-6430

Stern-Ginossar N, Elefant N, Zimmermann A, Wolf DG, Saleh N, Biton M, Horwitz E, Prokocimer Z, Prichard M, Hahn G, Goldman-Wohl D, Greenfield C, Yagel S, Hengel H, Altuvia Y, Margalit H & Mandelboim O (2007) Host Immune System Gene Targeting by a Viral miRNA. *Science* 317: 376 -381

Stiff T, O'Driscoll M, Rief N, Iwabuchi K, Löbrich M & Jeggo PA (2004) ATM and DNA-PK Function Redundantly to Phosphorylate H2AX after Exposure to Ionizing Radiation. *Cancer Research* 64: 2390 -2396

Swift LP, Rephaeli A, Nudelman A, Phillips DR & Cutts SM (2006) Doxorubicin-DNA Adducts Induce a Non-Topoisomerase II–Mediated Form of Cell Death. *Cancer Research* 66: 4863 -4871

Smyth MJ, Swann J, Cretney E, Zerafa N, Yokoyama WM & Hayakawa Y (2005) NKG2D function protects the host from tumor initiation. *J. Exp. Med* 202: 583-588

Takai H, Tominaga K, Motoyama N, Minamishima YA, Nagahama H, Tsukiyama T, Ikeda K, Nakayama K, Nakanishi M & Nakayama K-ichi (2000) Aberrant cell cycle checkpoint function and early embryonic death in Chk1 −/− mice. *Genes & Development* 14: 1439 -1447

Takai H, Naka K, Okada Y, Watanabe M, Harada N, Saito S, Anderson CW, Appella E, Nakanishi M, Suzuki H, Nagashima K, Sawa H, Ikeda K & Motoyama N (2002) Chk2-deficient mice exhibit radioresistance and defective p53-mediated transcription. *EMBO J* 21: 5195-5205

Takaoka A, Hayakawa S, Yanai H, Stoiber D, Negishi H, Kikuchi H, Sasaki S, Imai K, Shibue T, Honda K & Taniguchi T (2003) Integration of interferon-[alpha]/[beta] signalling to p53 responses in tumour suppression and antiviral defence. *Nature* 424: 516-523

Takaoka A, Yanai H, Kondo S, Duncan G, Negishi H, Mizutani T, Kano S-ichi, Honda K, Ohba Y, Mak TW & Taniguchi T (2005) Integral role of IRF-5 in the gene induction programme activated by Toll-like receptors. *Nature* 434: 243-249

Tamura T, Ishihara M, Lamphier MS, Tanaka N, Oishi I, Aizawa S, Matsuyama T, Mak TW, Taki S & Taniguchi T (1995) An IRF-1-dependent pathway of DNA damage-induced apoptosis in mitogen-activated T lymphocytes. *Nature* 376: 596-599

Tanaka N, Ishihara M, Kitagawa M, Harada H, Kimura T, Matsuyama T, Lamphier MS, Aizawa S, Mak TW & Taniguchi T (1994) Cellular commitment to oncogene-induced transformation or apoptosis is dependent on the transcription factor IRF-1. *Cell* 77: 829-839

Tanaka N, Sato M, Lamphier MS, Nozawa H, Oda E, Noguchi S, Schreiber RD, Tsujimoto Y & Taniguchi T (1998) Type I interferons are essential mediators of apoptotic death in virally infected cells. *Genes Cells* 3: 29-37

Tanaka N, Kawakami T & Taniguchi T (1993) Recognition DNA sequences of interferon regulatory factor 1 (IRF-1) and IRF-2, regulators of cell growth and the interferon system. *Mol Cell Biol.* 13: 4531–4538

Tanaka N, Ishihara M, Lamphier MS, Nozawa H, Matsuyama T, Mak TW, Aizawa S, Tokino T, Oren M & Taniguchi T (1996) Cooperation of the tumour suppressors IRF-1 and p53 in response to DNA damage. *Nature* 382: 816-818

Taniguchi T & Takaoka A (2002) The interferon-α/β system in antiviral responses: a multimodal machinery of gene regulation by the IRF family of transcription factors. *Current Opinion in Immunology* 14: 111-116

Taniguchi T, Ogasawara K, Takaoka A & Tanaka N (2001) IRF family of transcription factors as regulators of host defense. *Annu. Rev. Immunol.* 19: 623-655

Tibbetts RS, Brumbaugh KM, Williams JM, Sarkaria JN, Cliby WA, Shieh S-Y, Taya Y, Prives C & Abraham RT (1999) A role for ATR in the DNA damage-induced phosphorylation of p53. *Genes Dev* 13: 152-157

Tomasec P, Wang ECY, Davison AJ, Vojtesek B, Armstrong M, Griffin C, McSharry BP, Morris RJ, Llewellyn-Lacey S, Rickards C, Nomoto A, Sinzger C & Wilkinson GWG

(2005) Downregulation of natural killer cell-activating ligand CD155 by human cytomegalovirus UL141. *Nat Immunol* 6: 181-188

Turpin E, Luke K, Jones J, Tumpey T, Konan K & Schultz-Cherry S (2005) Influenza Virus Infection Increases p53 Activity: Role of p53 in Cell Death and Viral Replication. *J. Virol.* 79: 8802-8811

Upreti M, Koonce NA, Hennings L, Chambers TC & Griffin RJ (2010) Pegylated IFN-α sensitizes melanoma cells to chemotherapy and causes premature senescence in endothelial cells by IRF-1-mediated signaling. *Cell Death Dis* 1: e67

Upshaw JL, Arneson LN, Schoon RA, Dick CJ, Billadeau DD & Leibson PJ (2006) NKG2D-mediated signaling requires a DAP10-bound Grb2-Vav1 intermediate and phosphatidylinositol-3-kinase in human natural killer cells. *Nat Immunol* 7: 524-532

Unger T, Juven-Gershon T, Moallem E, Berger M, Vogt Sionov R, Lozano G, Oren M & Haupt Y (1999) Critical role for Ser20 of human p53 in the negative regulation of p53 by Mdm2. *EMBO J* 18: 1805-1814

Voronov E, Shouval DS, Krelin Y, Cagnano E, Benharroch D, Iwakura Y, Dinarello CA & Apte RN (2003) IL-1 is required for tumor invasiveness and angiogenesis. *Proceedings of the National Academy of Sciences of the United States of America* 100: 2645 -2650

Vousden KH & Lu X (2002) Live or let die: the cell's response to p53. *Nat Rev Cancer* 2: 594-604

Wade Harper J, Adami GR, Wei N, Keyomarsi K & Elledge SJ (1993) The p21 Cdk-interacting protein Cip1 is a potent inhibitor of G1 cyclin-dependent kinases. *Cell* 75: 805-816

Walker JR, Corpina RA & Goldberg J (2001) Structure of the Ku heterodimer bound to DNA and its implications for double-strand break repair. *Nature* 412: 607-614

Wang BX, Rahbar R & Fish EN (2011) Interferon: Current Status and Future Prospects in Cancer Therapy. *J Interferon Cytokine Res* ahead of print. doi:10.1089/jir.2010.0158.

Wang C-Y, Mayo MW & Baldwin AS (1996) TNF- and Cancer Therapy-Induced Apoptosis: Potentiation by Inhibition of NF-κB. *Science* 274: 784 -787

Wang C-Y, Mayo MW, Korneluk RG, Goeddel DV & Baldwin AS (1998) NF-kB Antiapoptosis: Induction of TRAF1 and TRAF2 and c-IAP1 and c-IAP2 to Suppress Caspase-8 Activation. *Science* 281: 1680-1683

Wang C-Y, Guttridge DC, Mayo MW & Baldwin AS (1999) NF-kappa B Induces Expression of the Bcl-2 Homologue A1/Bfl-1 To Preferentially Suppress Chemotherapy-Induced Apoptosis. *Mol. Cell. Biol.* 19: 5923-5929

Ward J, Davis Z, DeHart J, Zimmerman E, Bosque A, Brunetta E, Mavilio D, Planelles V & Barker E (2009) HIV-1 Vpr Triggers Natural Killer Cell–Mediated Lysis of Infected Cells through Activation of the ATR-Mediated DNA Damage Response. *PLoS Pathog* 5: e1000613

Weaver BK, Ando O, Kumar KP & Reich NC (2001) Apoptosis is promoted by the dsRNA-activated factor (DRAF1) during viral infection independent of the action of interferon or p53. *FASEB J* 15: 501-515

Weaver BK, Kumar KP & Reich NC (1998) Interferon Regulatory Factor 3 and CREB-Binding Protein/p300 Are Subunits of Double-Stranded RNA-Activated Transcription Factor DRAF1. *Mol. Cell. Biol.* 18: 1359-1368

Wei L-H, Kuo M-L, Chen C-A, Chou C-H, Lai K-B, Lee C-N & Hsieh C-Y (2003) Interleukin-6 promotes cervical tumor growth by VEGF-dependent angiogenesis via a STAT3 pathway. *Oncogene* 22: 1517-1527

Wen C, He X, Ma H, Hou N, Wei C, Song T, Zhang Y, Sun L, Ma Q & Zhong H (2008) Hepatitis C Virus Infection Downregulates the Ligands of the Activating Receptor NKG2D. *Cell Mol Immunol* 5: 475-478

Werness B, Levine A & Howley P (1990) Association of human papillomavirus types 16 and 18 E6 proteins with p53. *Science* 248: 76 -79

Wold MS (1997) Replication protein A: a heterotrimeric, single-stranded DNA-binding protein required for eukaryotic DNA metabolism. *Annu. Rev. Biochem* 66: 61-92

Wu GS, Burns TF, McDonald ER, Jiang W, Meng R, Krantz ID, Kao G, Gan D-D, Zhou J-Y, Muschel R, Hamilton SR, Spinner NB, Markowitz S, Wu G & El-Deiry WS (1997) KILLER/DR5 is a DNA damage-inducible p53-regulated death receptor gene. *Nat Genet* 17: 141-143

Wu Z-H, Shi Y, Tibbetts RS & Miyamoto S (2006) Molecular Linkage Between the Kinase ATM and NF-{kappa}B Signaling in Response to Genotoxic Stimuli. *Science* 311: 1141-1146

Wu Z-H, Wong ET, Shi Y, Niu J, Chen Z, Miyamoto S & Tergaonkar V (2010) ATM- and NEMO-Dependent ELKS Ubiquitination Coordinates TAK1-Mediated IKK Activation in Response to Genotoxic Stress. *Molecular Cell* 40: 75-86

Yajima H, Lee K-J & Chen BPC (2006) ATR-Dependent Phosphorylation of DNA-Dependent Protein Kinase Catalytic Subunit in Response to UV-Induced Replication Stress. *Mol Cell Biol* 26: 7520-7528

Yang J, Yu Y, Hamrick HE & Duerksen-Hughes PJ (2003) ATM, ATR and DNA-PK: initiators of the cellular genotoxic stress responses. *Carcinogenesis* 24: 1571 -1580

Yanai H, Chen H-min, Inuzuka T, Kondo S, Mak TW, Takaoka A, Honda K & Taniguchi T (2007) Role of IFN regulatory factor 5 transcription factor in antiviral immunity and tumor suppression. *Proc Natl Acad Sci U S A.* 104: 3402–3407

Yoneyama M & Fujita T (2007) Function of RIG-I-like Receptors in Antiviral Innate Immunity. *J. Biol. Chem.* 282: 15315-15318

Yu X, Harden K, C Gonzalez L, Francesco M, Chiang E, Irving B, Tom I, Ivelja S, Refino CJ, Clark H, Eaton D & Grogan JL (2009) The surface protein TIGIT suppresses T cell activation by promoting the generation of mature immunoregulatory dendritic cells. *Nat Immunol* 10: 48-57

Yuan X-wei, Zhu X-feng, Huang X-fang, Sheng P-yi, He A-shan, Yang Z-bo, Deng R, Feng G-kan & Liao W-ming (2007) Interferon-[alpha] enhances sensitivity of human osteosarcoma U2OS cells to doxorubicin by p53-dependent apoptosis. *Acta Pharmacol Sin* 28: 1835-1841

Zhao H & Piwnica-Worms H (2001) ATR-Mediated Checkpoint Pathways Regulate Phosphorylation and Activation of Human Chk1. *Mol. Cell. Biol.* 21: 4129-4139

Zhao H, Watkins JL & Piwnica-Worms H (2002) Disruption of the checkpoint kinase 1/cell division cycle 25A pathway abrogates ionizing radiation-induced S and G2 checkpoints. *Proceedings of the National Academy of Sciences* 99: 14795 -14800

Zhou B-BS & Elledge SJ (2000) The DNA damage response: putting checkpoints in perspective. *Nature* 408: 433-439

Zou L & Elledge SJ (2003) Sensing DNA damage through ATRIP recognition of RPA-ssDNA
    complexes. *Science* 300: 1542-1548

8

Inhibition of DNA Polymerase λ, a DNA Repair Enzyme, and Anti-Inflammation: Chemical Knockout Analysis for DNA Polymerase λ Using Curcumin Derivatives

Yoshiyuki Mizushina[1,2], Masayuki Nishida[3],
Takeshi Azuma[3] and Masaru Yoshida[3,4,5]
[1]*Laboratory of Food & Nutritional Sciences*
Department of Nutritional Science, Kobe-Gakuin University
[2]*Cooperative Research Center of Life Sciences*
Kobe-Gakuin University
[3]*Division of Gastroenterology, Department of Internal Medicine*
Kobe University Graduate School of Medicine
[4]*The Integrated Center for Mass Spectrometry*
Kobe University Graduate School of Medicine
[5]*Division of Metabolomics Research*
Kobe University Graduate School of Medicine
Japan

1. Introduction

DNA polymerase (i.e., DNA-dependent DNA polymerase [pol], E.C. 2.7.7.7) catalyzes the polymerization of deoxyribonucleotides alongside a DNA strand, which it "reads" and uses as a template (Kornberg & Baker, 1992). The newly polymerized molecule is complementary to the template strand and identical to the template's partner strand. Pol can add free nucleotides only to the 3′ end of the newly formed strand, meaning that elongation of the new strand occurs in a 5′ to 3′ direction.

The human genome encodes at least 14 pols that conduct cellular DNA synthesis (Bebenek & Kunkel, 2004; Hubscher et al., 2002). Eukaryotic cells contain 3 DNA replicative pols (α, δ and ε), 1 mitochondrial pol (γ), and at least 10 DNA repair and/or recombination-related pols (β, ζ, η, θ, ι, κ, λ, μ and ν, and REV1) (Friedberg et al., 2000; Takata et al., 2006). Pols have a highly conserved structure, which means that their overall catalytic subunits show little variance among species. Enzymes with conserved structures usually perform important cellular functions, the maintenance of which provides evolutionary advantages. On the basis of sequence homology, eukaryotic pols can be divided into 4 main families, termed A, B, X and Y (Friedberg et al., 2000). Family A includes mitochondrial pol γ, as well as pols θ and ν. Family B includes 3 DNA replicative pols (α, δ and ε) and pol ζ. Family X comprises pols β, λ and μ; and lastly, family Y includes pols η, ι and κ, in addition to REV1.

We have been screening for selective inhibitors of each pol derived from natural products including food materials and nutrients for more than 15 years (Mizushina, 2009; Sakaguchi et al., 2002). In our studies of pol inhibitors, we have found that selective inhibitors of pol λ, which is a DNA repair-related pol, have anti-inflammatory activity against 12-O-tetradecanoylphorbol-13-acetate (TPA)-induced inflammation (Mizushina et al., 2003; Mizushina, 2009). Although tumor promoters such as TPA are classified as compounds that promote tumor formation (Hecker, 1978), they also cause inflammation and are commonly used as artificial inducers of inflammation in order to screen for anti-inflammatory agents (Fujiki & Sugimura, 1987). Tumor promoter-induced inflammation can be distinguished from acute inflammation, which is exudative and accompanied by fibroblast proliferation and granulation. The tumor promoter TPA is frequently used to search for new types of anti-inflammatory compound. TPA not only causes inflammation, but also influences mammalian cell growth (Nakamura et al., 1995), suggesting that the molecular basis of the inflammation stems from pol reactions related to cell proliferation. This relationship, however, needs to be investigated more closely.

In this review, we examine the relationship between pol λ inhibition and anti-inflammation using pol λ-specific inhibitors, such as chemically synthesized curcumin derivatives. On the basis of these results, the pol λ-inhibitory mechanism and anti-inflammation effects of monoacetyl-curcumin, which was the strongest pol λ inhibitor among the compounds tested, is discussed.

2. Effect of curcumin derivatives on the activities of mammalian pols

2.1 Pol assay for inhibitor screening

A pol activity assay to detect pol inhibitors was established by Mizushina et al. (1996a; 1996b; 1997). Purified mammalian pols α, β, γ, δ, ε, η, ι, κ and λ, which have high activity, were kind gifts from pol researchers around the world. As shown in Fig. 1, poly(dA)/oligo(dT)$_{18}$ (A/T = 2/1) and 2'-deoxythymidine 5'-triphosphate (dTTP) were used as the DNA template-primer and nucleotide (dNTP, 2'-deoxynucleotide 5'-triphosphate) substrate, respectively. The candidate inhibitors, which were low molecular weight organic compounds, were dissolved in distilled dimethyl sulfoxide (DMSO) at various concentrations and sonicated for 30 s. Aliquots (4 μL) of the sonicated samples were mixed with 16 μl of each enzyme (final amount 0.05 units) in 50 mM Tris–HCl (pH 7.5) containing 1 mM dithiothreitol, 50% glycerol and 0.1 mM EDTA, and pre-incubated at 0 °C for 10 min. These inhibitor–enzyme mixtures (8 μL) were then added to 16 μl of each of the enzyme standard reaction mixtures, and incubation was carried out at 37 °C for 60 min, except for *Taq* pol, which was incubated at 74 °C for 60 min. Activity without the inhibitor was considered 100%, and the remaining activity at each concentration of the inhibitor was determined relative to this value. One unit of pol activity was defined as the amount of enzyme that catalyzed the incorporation of 1 nmol of dNTP (i.e., dTTP) into synthetic DNA template–primers in 60 min at 37 °C under the normal reaction conditions for each enzyme (Mizushina et al., 1996b; 1997).

2.2 Mammalian pol inhibitory effect of curcumin derivatives

As described above, we are searching for natural inhibitors specific to each of the mammalian pols. A phenolic compound produced from a higher plant, a Japanese vegetable

Inhibition of DNA Polymerase λ, a DNA Repair Enzyme, and Anti-Inflammation: Chemical Knockout Analysis
for DNA Polymerase λ Using Curcumin Derivatives

167

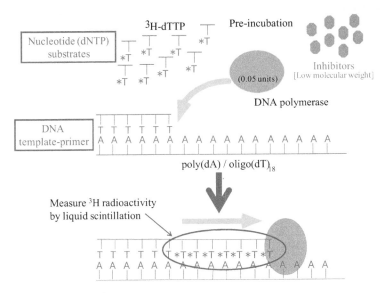

Fig. 1. Pol inhibitor assay scheme

(*Petasites japonicus*) collected from Akita prefecture, Japan, was found to inhibit pol λ activity selectively (Mizushina et al., 2002). The compound was purified and its chemical structure was analyzed, and it was identified as petasiphenol (compound **1** in Fig. 2) (Iriye et al., 1992). The three-dimensional relationship between pol inhibitors and the pol structure was investigated, which suggested that some phenolic compounds might be pol inhibitors. It was therefore tested whether commercial or easily obtainable phenolic compounds might also be pol λ-specific inhibitors. As a result, curcumin (diferuloylmethane, compound **2** in Fig. 2), which is the same type of phenolic compound as petasiphenol, and 13 chemically synthesized derivatives of curcumin (compounds **3–15** in Fig. 2) were prepared, and then tested for their inhibitory effects on mammalian pols.

The inhibition of four mammalian pols, namely calf pol α, human pol γ, human pol κ and human pol λ, by each compound at 10 μM was investigated. Pols α, γ, κ and λ were used as representatives of the B, A, Y and X families of pols, respectively (Bebenek & Kunkel, 2004; Hubscher et al., 2002; Takata et al., 2006). As shown in Fig. 3, petasiphenol (**1**) and curcumin (**2**) inhibited human pol λ activity. The inhibitory effect on pol λ of compounds **4, 5, 13** and **14** was stronger than that of curcumin (**2**). Compounds **6** to **11**, which do not have any enone moieties, did not affect pol λ activity; thus, the enone moiety, which is present in petasiphenol, might be important or essential for pol λ inhibition. As mentioned above, compounds **4, 5** and **13**, which have one or more acetoxy moieties, strongly inhibited the activity of pol λ, and compound **13** (monoacetyl-curcumin) was the strongest inhibitor among the compounds tested. The one acetoxy moiety at position C4" in monoacetyl-curcumin (13) might stimulate the inhibitory effect on pol λ. On the other hand, at 10 μM, none of the compounds inhibited the activity of calf pol α, human pol γ or human pol κ.

On the basis of these results, we concentrated on curcumin (**2**), which is a major food component, and monoacetyl-curcumin (**13**), which was the strongest inhibitor of pol λ among the curcumin derivatives tested, in the next part of this study.

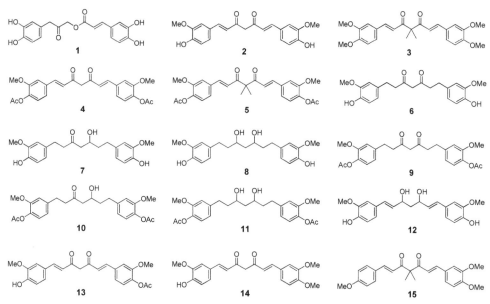

Fig. 2. Structure of curcumin derivatives. Compound **1**: petasiphenol; compound **2**: curcumin (diferuloylmethane); compound **3**: (1E,6E)-1,7-bis(3′,4′-dimethoxyphenyl)-4,4-dimethyl-1,6-heptadien-3,5-dione; compound **4**: (1E,4Z,6E)-1,7-bis(4′-acetoxy-3′-methoxyphenyl)-5-hydroxy-1,4,6-heptatrien-3-one (diacetyl-curcumin); compound **5**: (1E,6E)-1,7-bis(4′-acetoxy-3′-methoxyphenyl)-4,4-dimethyl-1,6-heptadien-3,5-dione; compound **6**: 1,7-bis4-hydroxy-3-methoxyphenyl-3,5-heptadione; compound **7**: 1,7-bis4-hydroxy-3-methoxyphenyl-5-hydroxy-3-heptanone; compound **8**: 1,7-bis4-hydroxy-3-methoxyphenyl-3,5-heptadiol; compound **9**: 1,7-bis4-acetoxy-3-methoxyphenyl-3,5-heptadione; compound **10**: 1,7-bis4-acetoxy-3-methoxyphenyl-5-hydroxy-3-heptanone; compound **11**: 1E,6E-1,7-bis4-acetoxy-3-methoxyphenyl-3,5-dihydroxyheptane; compound **12**: 1E,6E-1,7-bis4-hydroxy-3-methoxyphenyl-3,5-dihydroxy-1,6-heptadiene; compound **13**: (1E,4Z,6E)-7-(4″-acetoxy-3″-methoxyphenyl)-5-hydroxy-1-(4′-hydroxy-3′-methoxyphenyl)hepta-1,4,6-trien-3-one (monoacetyl-curcumin); compound **14**: (1E,4Z,6E)-1-(3′,4′-dimethoxyphenyl)-5-hydroxy-7-[4″-hydroxy-3″-methoxypheny]hepta-1,4,6-trien-3-one (monometyl-curcumin); compound **15**: 1E,6E-1-3,4-dimethoxyphenyl-4,4-dimethyl-7-4-methoxyphenylhepta-1,6-dien-3,5-diol.

3. Effect of curcumin (2) and monoacetyl-curcumin (13) on the activities of pols and other DNA metabolic enzymes

Curcumin (**2**) and monoacetyl-curcumin (**13**) were effective at inhibiting human pol λ activity, and the inhibition was dose-dependent with 50% inhibition observed at a concentration of 7.0 and 3.9 μM, respectively (Table 1). These compounds had no influence on the activities of not only DNA replicative pols such as calf pol α, human pol δ and human pol ε, or mitochondrial DNA replicative pols such as human pol γ, but also DNA repair-related pols such as rat pol β, human pols η, ι and κ. It is interesting that these compounds had no affect on the activity of pol β, because pols β and λ both belong to the

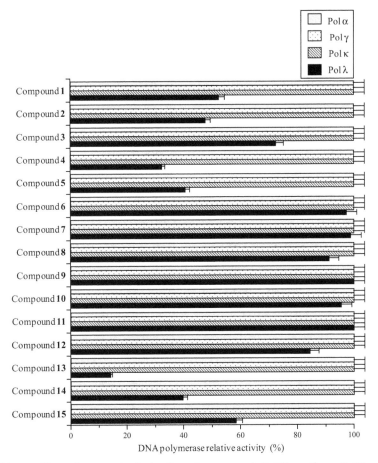

Fig. 3. Inhibitory effect of curcumin derivatives (compounds **1–15**) on the activities of mammalian pols. Each compound (10 μM) was incubated with calf pol α (B-family pol), human pol γ (A-family pol), human pol κ (Y-family pol) and human pol λ (X-family pol) (0.05 units each). Pol activity in the absence of the compound was taken as 100%, and the relative activity is shown. Data are shown as the mean ± SE (n=3).

X-family of pols, and the three-dimensional structure of pol β is thought to be highly similar to pol λ (Garcia-Diaz et al., 2004).

Curcumin (**2**) and monoacetyl-curcumin (**13**) also had no inhibitory effect on cherry salmon (fish) pols α and δ, cauliflower (higher plant) pol α, prokaryotic pols such as the Klenow fragment of *E. coli* pol I, *Taq* pol and T4 pol, and other DNA metabolic enzymes such as calf DNA primase of pol α, human immunodeficiency virus type-1 (HIV-1) reverse transcriptase, T7 RNA polymerase, T4 polynucleotide kinase and bovine deoxyribonuclease I. Therefore, these phenolic compounds were specific inhibitors of human pol λ among the pols and DNA metabolic enzymes tested. Petasiphenol (**1**) also selectively inhibited the activity of eukaryotic pol λ such as curcumin (**2**) and monoacetyl-curcumin (**13**) (Mizushina et al., 2002).

Enzyme	IC$_{50}$ value (μM)	
	Curcumin (2)	Monoacetyl-curcumin (13)
– Mammalian DNA polymerases –		
Calf DNA polymerase α	>100	>100
Rat DNA polymerase β	>100	>100
Human DNA polymerase γ	>100	>100
Human DNA polymerase δ	>100	>100
Human DNA polymerase ϵ	>100	>100
Human DNA polymerase η	>100	>100
Human DNA polymerase ι	>100	>100
Human DNA polymerase κ	>100	>100
Human DNA polymerase λ	7.0 $\pm$ 0.39	3.9 $\pm$ 0.25
– Fish DNA polymerases –		
Cherry salmon DNA polymerase α	>100	>100
Cherry salmon DNA polymerase δ	>100	>100
– Plant DNA polymerases –		
Cauliflower DNA polymerase α	>100	>100
– Prokaryotic DNA polymerases –		
E. coli DNA polymerase I	>100	>100
Taq DNA polymerase	>100	>100
T4 DNA polymerase	>100	>100
– Other DNA metabolic enzymes –		
Calf primase of DNA polymerase α	>100	>100
HIV-1 reverse transcriptase	>100	>100
T7 RNA polymerase	>100	>100
T4 polynucleotide kinase	>100	>100
Bovine deoxyribonuclease I	>100	>100

Table 1. IC$_{50}$ values of curcumin (2) and monoacetyl-curcumin (13) for various pols and other DNA metabolic enzymes. The compounds were incubated with each enzyme (0.05 units). Enzyme activity in the absence of the compound was taken as 100%. Data are shown as the mean $\pm$ SE (n=3).

When activated DNA (i.e., bovine deoxyribonuclease I-treated DNA) and dNTP were used as the DNA template-primer and nucleotide substrate instead of synthesized DNA [poly(dA)/oligo(dT)$_{18}$ (A/T = 2/1)] and dTTP, respectively, the inhibitory effects of these compounds did not change.

4. Effect of curcumin derivatives on TPA-induced anti-inflammatory activity

As mentioned in the Introduction, TPA is known to cause inflammation and is commonly used in screens for anti-inflammatory agents (Fujiki & Sugimura, 1987). Curcumin (2) is known as an anti-TPA-induced inflammatory compound (Ammon & Wahl, 1991), but the other agents (compounds 1 and 3–15) had not previously been tested for anti-TPA-induced inflammatory activity.

Inhibition of DNA Polymerase λ, a DNA Repair Enzyme, and Anti-Inflammation: Chemical Knockout Analysis
for DNA Polymerase λ Using Curcumin Derivatives

171

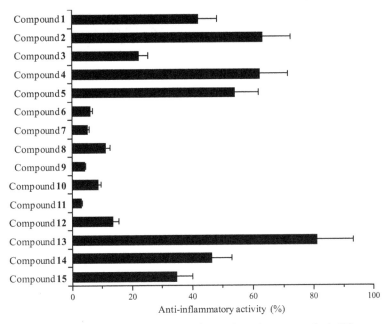

Fig. 4. Anti-inflammatory activity of curcumin derivatives (compounds **1–15**) toward TPA-induced edema on mouse ear. Each compound (250 μg) was applied to one of the mouse ears and, after 30 min, TPA (0.5 μg) was applied to both ears. Edema was evaluated after 7 h. The anti-inflammatory activity (%) is expressed as the percentage reduction in edema as compared with the non-treated ear. Data are shown as the mean ± SE (n=5).

Using an inflammation test in mice, the anti-inflammatory activity of these compounds was examined. The application of TPA (0.5 μg) to a mouse ear induced edema with a 241% increase in the weight of the ear disk at 7 h after application. As expected, curcumin (**2**) inhibited this inflammation at an applied dose of at least 250 μg (inhibitory effect (IE) = 63%) (Fig. 4). Petasiphenol (**1**), which was purified from Japanese vegetable (*Petasites japonicus*), was also an anti-inflammatory agent, although its effect was a third weaker than that of curcumin (**2**). Thus, both petasiphenol (**1**) and curcumin (**2**) could be potent inhibitors of inflammation caused by TPA. Interestingly, other curcumin derivatives also caused a marked reduction in TPA-induced inflammation: notably, the anti-inflammatory effect of monoacetyl-curcumin (**13**) was stronger than that of curcumin (**2**) with an IE of 81%, indicating that this compound possesses strong anti-inflammatory activity.

5. Structure–activity relationship of curcumin derivatives

Pol λ inhibition had a significant correlation (correlation coefficient = 0.9608) with anti-inflammatory activity, as shown by Fig. 3 and Fig. 4, which led us to speculate that TPA-induced inflammation may involve a process requiring pol λ, which is a DNA repair-related pol. Thus, to confirm whether there is a relationship between pol λ inhibition and anti-inflammation, the inhibitory effects of the curcumin derivatives (compounds **1–15**) on the two bio-activities were compared.

Among the fifteen curcumin derivatives tested, including curcumin (**2**) itself (Fig. 1), monoacetyl-curcumin (**13**) was the strongest inhibitor of both pol λ and anti-inflammation. Considering the structure of monoacetyl-curcumin (**13**) (Fig. 5), the essential moieties of the structure for these activities might be: <1> two enone moieties, <2> one hydroxyl group at position C4′, and <3> one acetoxy group at position C4″. These moieties are specific to monoacetyl-curcumin (**13**); therefore, these moieties are likely to be involved in the activities of both pol λ inhibition and anti-inflammation.

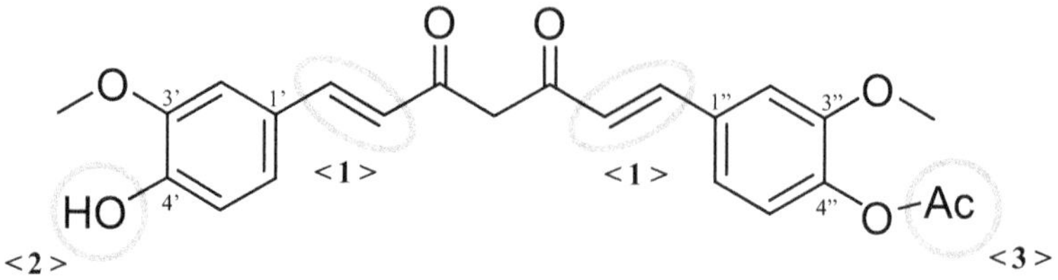

Fig. 5. Chemical structure of monoacetyl-curcumin (**13**). The functional groups likely to be essential for both pol λ inhibitory activity and anti-inflammatory activity in the curcumin derivatives are shown (<1> to <3>).

6. Inhibitory activity of curcumin (2) and monoacetyl-curcumin (13) against inflammatory responses in cultured cells

Next, because curcumin (**2**) and monoacetyl-curcumin (**13**) might be chemical knockout agents for DNA repair-related pol λ activity (Table 1), we used these compounds to investigate the anti-inflammatory mechanism of pol λ specific inhibitors in the murine macrophage cell line RAW264.7 treated with lipopolysaccharide (LPS or endotoxin), which stimulates macrophages to release inflammatory cytokines, interleukins (ILs) and tumor necrosis factor (TNF) (Hsu & Wen, 2002).

RAW264.7 cells were seeded on a 12-well plate at 1×10^5 cells/well and incubated for 24 h. The cells were pre-treated with 10 or 50 μM curcumin (**2**) or monoacetyl-curcumin (**13**) for 30 min and then stimulated with 100 ng/mL of LPS. After 30 min or 24 h, the cell culture medium was collected to measure the levels of inflammatory cytokines, such as tumor necrosis factor-α (TNF-α), nuclear factor-κB (NF-κB) and IκB. In RAW264.7 cells, cytotoxicity of these compounds at 50 μM was not observed (data not shown).

As shown in Fig. 6A, at 50 μM, curcumin (**2**) and monoacetyl-curcumin (**13**) both significantly suppressed LPS-stimulated production of TNF-α, and monoacetyl-curcumin (**13**) showed greater inhibition than curcumin (**2**). At 10 μM, monoacetyl-curcumin (**13**) still showed suppression of TNF-α production, although curcumin (**2**) at 10 μM did not significantly inhibit TNF-α production.

Next, the effect of monoacetyl-curcumin (**13**) on the expression level of pol λ protein in LPS-treated RAW264.7 cells was investigated. Fig. 6B shows that these macrophages underwent a more than 3-fold increase in the expression of pol λ after LPS stimulation, but this increase was suppressed by 50 μM monoacetyl-curcumin (**13**). These results suggest that there is the positive correlation between inflammatory induction by LPS and pol λ expression; thus, not only the DNA polymerization activity but also the protein expression of DNA repair-related pol λ is likely to be important in inflammation.

Inhibition of DNA Polymerase λ, a DNA Repair Enzyme, and Anti-Inflammation: Chemical Knockout Analysis
for DNA Polymerase λ Using Curcumin Derivatives

173

NF-κB is known to be the rate-controlling factor in inflammatory responses. Therefore, the inhibitory effects of curcumin (2) and monoacetyl-curcumin (13) on the LPS-induced nuclear translocation of NF-κB were examined in RAW264.7 cells. At 50 μM, curcumin (2) and monoacetyl-curcumin (13) both inhibited NF-κB nuclear translocation stimulated by 100 ng/mL of LPS, and the effect of monoacetyl-curcumin (13) was stronger than that of curcumin (2) (Fig. 6C). Stimulation with LPS results in activation of Toll-like receptor 4 and the downstream IκB kinases (IKKs), which in turn phosphorylate IκB, leading to degradation of IκB and translocation of NF-κB into the nucleus (Hashimoto et al., 2002). Therefore, the suppressive effects of curcumin (2) and monoacetyl-curcumin (13) on the LPS-induced phosphorylation of IκB were examined in RAW264.7 cells. By Western blot analysis, it was revealed that, at 50 μM, both curcumin (2) and monoacetyl-curcumin (13) significantly inhibited the LPS-induced phosphorylation of IκB (Fig. 6D). These results demonstrate that monoacetyl-curcumin (13), as well as curcumin (2), suppresses NF-κB nuclear translocation by inhibiting the phosphorylation of IκB.

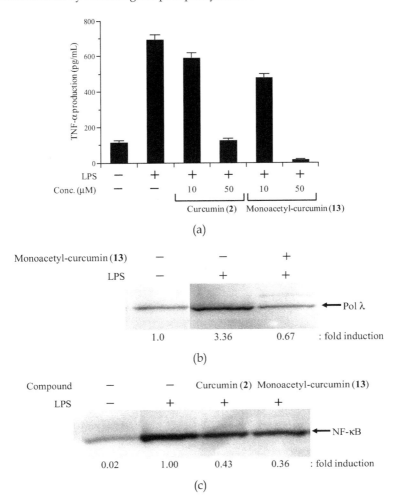

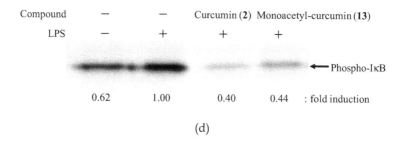

(d)

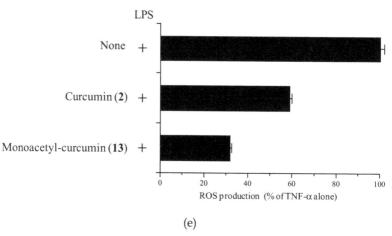

(e)

Fig. 6. Inhibitory activities of curcumin (2) and monoacetyl-curcumin (13) against inflammatory responses in the cultured murine macrophage cell line RAW264.7. (a) RAW264.7 cells were pre-treated with 10 or 50 μM curcumin (2) or monoacetyl-curcumin (13) for 30 min and then incubated with 100 ng/mL of LPS for 24 h. The TNF-α level in the culture medium was measured by ELISA. Data are shown as the mean ± SE (n=4). (b) RAW264.7 cells were pre-treated with 50 μM monoacetyl-curcumin (13), and then incubated with 100 ng/mL of LPS for 30 min. The expression level of pol λ was evaluated by Western blot analysis. The intensity of each band was analyzed, and the values relative to non-treatment with LPS are represented at the lower edge of the image. (c and d) RAW264.7 cells were pre-treated with 50 μM curcumin (2) or monoacetyl-curcumin (13), and then incubated with 100 ng/mL of LPS for 30 min. Nuclear translocation of NF-κB p65 (c) and the phosphorylation of IκB (d) were evaluated by Western blot analysis. The intensity of each band was analyzed, and the values relative to treatment with LPS alone are represented at the lower edge of the image. (e) RAW264.7 cells were pre-treated with 50 μM curcumin (2) or monoacetyl-curcumin (13) for 30 min, and then treated with 50 ng/mL of TNF-α and 4 μM DCFH-DA for 30 min. The fluorescent intensity of DCF, which indicates ROS production, was measured as described in a previous report (Corda et al., 2001). Data are shown as the mean ± SE (n=4).

Inhibition of DNA Polymerase λ, a DNA Repair Enzyme, and Anti-Inflammation: Chemical Knockout Analysis for DNA Polymerase λ Using Curcumin Derivatives

175

Anti-oxidative activity has been reported to be linked to anti-inflammatory activity (Rahman et al., 2006). We therefore investigated the anti-oxidative activity of curcumin (2) and monoacetyl-curcumin (13) against the production of reactive oxygen species (ROS) induced by TNF-α. Measurement of intracellular ROS was performed according to the method of a previous report (Corda et al., 2001). In RAW264.7 cells, at 50 μM, the two compounds decreased the production of ROS by 50 ng/mL of TNF-α to 59.5% and 32.1%, respectively (Fig. 6E). These results suggest that both compounds possess anti-oxidative activity, but that monoacetyl-curcumin (13) has stronger activity than curcumin (2).

7. Inhibitory activity of curcumin (2) and monoacetyl-curcumin (13) against LPS-induced inflammation *in vivo*

To assess their anti-inflammatory effects *in vivo*, the inhibitory activity of curcumin (2) and monoacetyl-curcumin (13) against LPS-induced acute inflammation was investigated in mice (Fig. 7). As shown in Fig. 7A, treatment with 250 μg/kg (body weight, BW) of LPS increased the serum TNF-α level, and an oral injection of 100 mg/kg (BW) of monoacetyl-curcumin (13) significantly decreased the LPS-induced production of TNF-α to 36%. By contrast, curcumin (2) had no effect. Next, the inhibitory effects of these compounds on nuclear translocation of NF-κB in the liver were examined. Fig. 7B shows that LPS caused translocation of NF-κB into the nucleus, and monoacetyl-curcumin (13) blocked this nuclear translocation. Notably, curcumin (2) also inhibited nuclear translocation of NF-κB even though it did not block TNF-α production.

The serum levels of curcumin (2) and monoacetyl-curcumin (13) 2 h after oral administration were measured in the mice by liquid-chromatography mass spectrometry. The serum concentrations were below the detection limit and, thus, were less than 0.3 nM for both curcumin (2) and monoacetyl-curcumin (13) (data not shown). It has been reported that curcumin (2) is poorly absorbed in the body (Anand et al., 2007). Thus, a lower concentration of monoacetyl-curcumin (13) than of curcumin (2) might be able to decrease the serum TNF-α level in mice treated with LPS.

8. Discussion

Inflammatory mediators, such as TPA and LPS, quickly stimulate ROS (Hsu & Wen, 2002), and ROS are known to mediate oxidative DNA damage. As shown in Fig. 8, DNA repair pols such as pol λ induce protein expression and increase DNA polymerization activity to repair the damaged DNA. Furthermore, we consider that pol λ might have a great effect on inflammatory responses, such as TNF-α production, NF-κB activation, secretion of cytokines [e.g. interferons (IFNs) and interleukins (ILs) etc], tissue damage and cell death. The results summarized in this review suggest that inhibition of DNA repair by pol λ is related to anti-inflammatory pathways, and that pol λ-specific inhibitors such as monoacetyl-curcumin (13) might be chemotherapeutic drugs for inflammatory diseases. The detailed molecular mechanism underlying the correlation between DNA repair inhibition by pol λ and anti-inflammatory responses is not yet known; therefore, experiments with small interfering RNA (siRNA) targeting pol λ would help in further analyses.

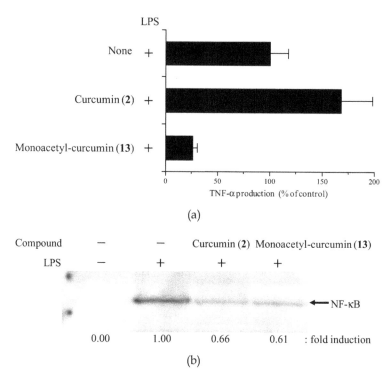

Fig. 7. The inhibitory activity of curcumin (2) and monoacetyl-curcumin (13) against LPS-induced inflammation *in vivo*. Male 8-week-old C57BL/6 mice were given an oral dose of 100 mg/kg (BW) of curcumin (2) or monoacetyl-curcumin (13) dissolved in corn oil or 200 μL of corn oil as a vehicle control. After 2 h, the mice were intraperitoneally injected with 250 μg/kg (BW) of LPS dissolved in phosphate-buffered saline (PBS) or 200 μL of PBS as a vehicle control. After 1 h, the mice were killed. (a) The TNF-α level in serum was measured by ELISA. Data are shown as the mean ± SE (n=4). The treatment with corn oil and LPS (positive control) was taken as 100% (TNF-α level, 728 pg/mL) and that with corn oil and saline (negative control) as taken as 0% (TNF-α level, 32 pg/mL). (b) NF-κB p65 in the nuclei of mouse liver cells was detected by Western blotting. The intensity of each band was analyzed, and the values relative to treatment with LPS alone are represented at the lower edge of the image.

As mentioned above, eukaryotic cells reportedly contain 14 pol species belonging to four families (Friedberg et al., 2000; Takata et al., 2006). Among the X family of pols, pol λ has an unclear biochemical function, although it seems to work in a similar way to pol β (Garcia-Diaz et al., 2002). Pol β is involved in the short-patch base excision repair (BER) pathway (Matsumoto & Kim, 1995; Singhal & Wilson, 1993; Sobol et al., 1996), as well as playing an essential role in neural development (Sugo et al., 2000). Recently, pol λ was found to possess 5'-deoxyribose-5-phosphate (dRP) lyase activity, but not apurinic/apyrimidinic (AP) lyase activity (Garcia-Diaz et al., 2001). Pol λ is able to substitute for pol β during *in vitro* BER, suggesting that pol λ also participates in BER. Northern blot analysis indicated that transcripts of pol β are abundantly expressed in the

Inhibition of DNA Polymerase λ, a DNA Repair Enzyme, and Anti-Inflammation: Chemical Knockout Analysis
for DNA Polymerase λ Using Curcumin Derivatives

177

testis, thymus and brain in rats (Hirose et al., 1989), whereas pol λ is efficiently transcribed mostly in the testis (Garcia-Diaz et al., 2000). Bertocci et al. reported that mice in which pol λ expression is knocked down are not only viable and fertile, but also display a normal hyper-mutation pattern (Bertocci et al., 2002).

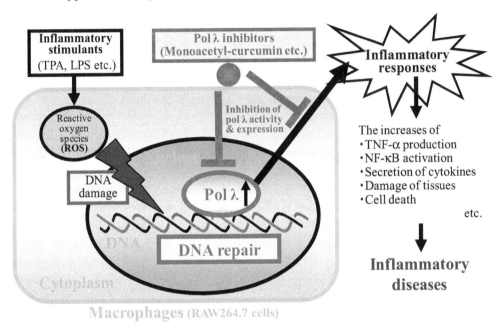

Fig. 8. The relationship between DNA repair by pol λ and inflammation

As well as causing inflammation, TPA influences cell proliferation and has physiological effects on cells because it has tumor promoter activity (Nakamura et al., 1995). Therefore, anti-inflammatory agents are expected to suppress DNA replication/repair/recombination in nuclei in relation to the action of TPA. Because pol λ is a DNA repair-related pol (Garcia-Diaz et al., 2002), our finding – that the molecular target of curcumin derivatives as monoacetyl-curcumin (13) is pol λ – is in good agreement with this expected mechanism of anti-inflammatory agents. As a result, any inhibitor of DNA repair-related pol λ might also be an inflammatory suppressor.

9. Conclusion

This review summarizes data showing that a major anti-inflammatory food compound, curcumin (2), selectively inhibits the activity of pol λ among 9 species of mammalian pols tested. Monoacetyl-curcumin (13) was the strongest inhibitor of pol λ among the 13 chemically synthesized derivatives of curcumin (2), suggesting that monoacetyl-curcumin (13) is a potent candidate for a functional compound. In addition, the inhibitory effects of monoacetyl-curcumin (13) on inflammatory responses in comparison to those of curcumin (2) *in vitro* and *in vivo* were investigated. Monoacetyl-curcumin (13) suppressed NF-κB activation induced by LPS and TNF-α in RAW264.7 murine macrophages. Moreover, monoacetyl-curcumin (**13**) exerted inhibitory effects on TNF-α production and NF-κB activation in an animal model of LPS-induced acute inflammation. These results of the chemical knock out of pol λ by monoacetyl-curcumin (**13**) suggest that the inhibition of pol λ, which is a DNA repair-related pol, is related to anti-inflammatory processes.

10. Acknowledgment

We are grateful for the donations of calf pol α by Dr. M. Takemura of Tokyo University of Science (Tokyo, Japan); rat pol β and human pol δ by Dr. K. Sakaguchi of Tokyo University of Science (Chiba, Japan); human pol γ by Dr. M. Suzuki of Nagoya University School of Medicine (Nagoya, Japan); human pol ε by Dr. S. Linn of University of California, Berkeley (CA, USA); human pols η and ι by Dr. F. Hanaoka and Dr. C. Masutani of Osaka University (Osaka, Japan); human pol κ by Dr. H. Ohmori of Kyoto University (Kyoto, Japan); and human pol λ by Dr. O. Koiwai of Tokyo University of Science (Chiba, Japan).
This work was supported in part by the Global COE Program "Global Center of Excellence for Education and Research on Signal Transduction Medicine in the Coming Generation" from MEXT (Ministry of Education, Culture, Sports, Science and Technology of Japan) (T.A and M.Y.), Young Researchers Training Program for Promoting Innovation of the Special Coordination Fund for Promoting Science and Technology from MEXT (T.A.).

11. References

Anand, P.; Kunnumakkara, A.B.; Newman, R.A. & Aggarwal, B.B. (2007). Bioavailability of curcumin: problems and promises. *Molecular Pharmacology*, Vol.4, No.6, pp. 807-818, ISSN 0026-895X

Ammon, H.P. & Wahl, M.A. (1991). Pharmacology of Curcuma longa. *Planta Medica*, Vol.57, No.1, pp. 1-7, ISSN 0032-0943

Bebenek, K. & Kunkel, T.A. (2004). DNA Repair and Replication. In: *Advances in Protein Chemistry*, W. Yang (Ed.), Vol. 69, pp. 137-165, Elsevier: San Diego, CA, USA

Bertocci, B.; De Smet, A.; Flatter, E.; Dahan, A.; Bories, J.C.; Landreau, C.; Weill, J.C. & Reynaud, C.A. (2002). Cutting edge: DNA polymerases μ and λ are dispensable for Ig gene hypermutation. *The Journal of Immunology*, Vol.168, No.8, pp. 3702-3706, ISSN 0022-1767

Corda, S.; Laplace, C.; Vicaut, E. & Duranteau, J. (2001). Rapid reactive oxygen species production by mitochondria in endothelial cells exposed to tumor necrosis factor-alpha is mediated by ceramide. *The American Journal of Respiratory Cell and Molecular Biology*, Vol.24, No.6, pp. 762-768, ISSN 1044-1549

Friedberg, E.C.; Feaver, W.J. & Gerlach, V.L. (2000). The many faces of DNA polymerases: strategies for mutagenesis and for mutational avoidance. *Proceedings of the National Academy of Sciences USA*, Vol.97, No.11, pp. 5681-5683, ISSN 0027-8424

Fujiki, H. & Sugimura, T. (1987). *Advances in Cancer Research*, Academic Press Inc., pp. 223-264, London, UK

Garcia-Diaz, M.; Dominguez, O.; Lopez-Fernandez, L.A.; De Lera, L.T.; Saniger, M.L.; Ruiz, J.F.; Parraga, M.; Garcia-Ortiz, M.J.; Kirchhoff, T.; Del Mazo, J.; Bernad, A. & Blanco, L. (2000). DNA polymerase λ, a novel DNA repair enzyme in human cells. *Journal of Molecular Biology*, Vol.301, No.4, pp. 851–867, ISSN 0022-2836

Inhibition of DNA Polymerase λ, a DNA Repair Enzyme, and Anti-Inflammation: Chemical Knockout Analysis
for DNA Polymerase λ Using Curcumin Derivatives

179

Garcia-Diaz, M.; Bebenek, K.; Kunkel, T.A. & Blanco, L. (2001). Identification of an intrinsic 5'-deoxyribose-5-phosphate lyase activity in human DNA polymerase λ: a possible role in base excision repair. *The Journal of Biological Chemistry*, Vol.276, No.37, pp. 34659-34663, ISSN 0021-9258

Garcia-Diaz, M.; Bebenek, K.; Sabariegos, R.; Dominguez, O.; Rodriguez, J.; Kirchhoff, T.; Garcia-Palomero, E.; Picher, A.J.; Juarez, R.; Ruiz, J.F.; Kunkel, T.A. & Blanco, L. (2002). DNA polymerase λ, a novel DNA repair enzyme in human cells. *The Journal of Biological Chemistry*, Vol.277, No.15, pp. 13184-13191, ISSN 0021-9258

Garcia-Diaz, M.; Bebenek, K.; Krahn, J.M.; Blanco, L.; Kunkel, T.A. & Pedersen, L.C. (2004). A structural solution for the DNA polymerase λ-dependent repair of DNA gaps with minimal homology. *Molecular Cell*, Vol.13, No.4, pp. 561-572, ISSN 1097-2765

Hashimoto, T.; Nonaka, Y.; Minato, K.; Kawakami, S.; Mizuno, M.; Fukuda, I.; Kanazawa, K. & Ashida, H. (2002). Suppressive effect of polysaccharides from the edible and medicinal mushrooms, *Lentinus edodes* and *Agaricus blazei*, on the expression of cytochrome P450s in mice. *Bioscience, Biotechnology, and Biochemistry*, Vol.66, No.7, pp. 1610-1614, ISSN 0916-8451

Hecker, E. (1978). *Carcinogenesis*, Raben Press, pp. 11-48, NY, USA

Hirose, F.; Hotta, Y.; Yamaguchi, M. & Matsukage, A. (1989). Difference in the expression level of DNA polymerase β among mouse tissues: high expression in the pachytene spermatocyte. *Experimental Cell Research*, Vol.181, No.1, pp. 169-180, ISSN 0014-4827

Hsu, H.Y. & Wen, M.H. (2002). Lipopolysaccharide-mediated reactive oxygen species and signal transduction in the regulation of interleukin-1 gene expression. *The Journal of Biological Chemistry*, Vol.277, No.25, pp. 22131-22139, ISSN 0021-9258

Hubscher, U.; Maga, G. & Spadari, S. (2002). Eukaryotic DNA polymerases. *The Annual Review of Biochemistry*, Vol.71, pp.133-163, ISSN 0066-4154

Iriye, R.; Furukawa, K.; Nishida, R.; Kim, C. & Fukami, H. (1992). Isolation and synthesis of a new bio-antimutagen, petasiphenol, from scapes of *Petasites japonicum. Bioscience, Biotechnology, and Biochemistry*, Vol.56, No.11, pp. 1773-1775, ISSN 0916-8451

Kornberg, A. & Baker, T.A. (1992). Eukaryotic DNA polymerase, In: *DNA replication, Second Edition*, W.D. Freeman & Co. (Ed), Chapter 6, pp. 197-225, New York, USA, ISBN 1-891389-44-0

Matsumoto, Y. & Kim, K. (1995). Excision of deoxyribose phosphate residues by DNA polymerase β during DNA repair. *Science*, Vol.269, No.5224, pp. 699-702, ISSN 0036-8075

Mizushina, Y.; Tanaka, N.; Yagi, H.; Kurosawa, T.; Onoue, M.; Seto, H.; Horie, T.; Aoyagi, N.; Yamaoka, M.; Matsukage, A.; Yoshida, S. & Sakaguchi, K. (1996a). Fatty acids selectively inhibit eukaryotic DNA polymerase activities in vitro. *Biochimica et Biophysica Acta*, Vol.1308, No.3, pp. 256-262, ISSN 0304-4165

Mizushina, Y.; Yagi, H.; Tanaka, N.; Kurosawa, T.; Seto, H.; Katsumi, K.; Onoue, M.; Ishida, H.; Iseki, A.; Nara, T.; Morohashi, K.; Horie, T.; Onomura, Y.; Narusawa, M.; Aoyagi, N.; Takami, K.; Yamaoka, M.; Inoue, Y.; Matsukage, A.; Yoshida, S. & Sakaguchi, K. (1996b). Screening of inhibitor of eukaryotic DNA polymerases produced by microorganisms. *The Journal of Antibiotics*, Vol.49, No.5, pp. 491-492, ISSN 0021-8820

Mizushina, Y.; Yoshida, S.; Matsukage, A. & Sakaguchi, K. (1997). The inhibitory action of fatty acids on DNA polymerase β. *Biochimica et Biophysica Acta*, Vol.1336, No.3, pp. 509-521, ISSN 0304-4165

Mizushina, Y.; Kamisuki, S.; Kasai, N.; Ishidoh, T.; Shimazaki, N.; Takemura, M.; Asahara, H.; Linn, S.; Yoshida, S.; Koiwai, O.; Sugawara, F.; Yoshida, H. & Sakaguchi, K. (2002). Petasiphenol: a DNA polymerase λ inhibitor. *Biochemistry*, Vol.41, No.49, pp. 14463-14471, ISSN 0006-2960

Mizushina, Y.; Hirota, M.; Murakami, C.; Ishidoh, T.; Kamisuki, S.; Shimazaki, N.; Takemura, M.; Perpelescu, M.; Suzuki, M.; Yoshida, H.; Sugawara, F.; Koiwai, O. & Sakaguchi, K. (2003). Some anti-chronic inflammatory compounds are DNA polymerase λ-specific inhibitors. *Biochemical Pharmacology*, Vol.66, No.10, pp. 1935-1944, ISSN 0006-2952

Mizushina, Y. (2009). Specific inhibitors of mammalian DNA polymerase species. *Bioscience, Biotechnology, and Biochemistry*, Vol.73, No.6, pp. 1239-1251, ISSN 0916-8451

Nakamura, Y.; Murakami, A.; Ohto, Y.; Torikai, K.; Tanaka, T. & Ohigashi, H. (1998). Suppression of tumor promoter-induced oxidative stress and inflammatory responses in mouse skin by a superoxide generation inhibitor 1'-acetoxychavicol acetate. *Cancer Research*, Vol.58, No.21, pp. 4832–4839, ISSN 0008-5472

Rahman, I.; Biswas, S.K. & Kirkham, P.A. (2006). Regulation of inflammation and redox signaling by dietary polyphenols. *Biochemical Pharmacology*, Vol.72, No.11, pp. 1439-1452, ISSN 0006-2952

Ramadan, K.; Shevelev, I.V.; Maga, G. & Hubscher, U. (2002). DNA polymerase λ from calf thymus preferentially replicates damaged DNA. *The Journal of Biological Chemistry*, Vol.277, No.21, pp. 18454-18458, ISSN 0021-9258

Sakaguchi, K.; Sugawara, F. & Mizushina, Y. (2002). Inhibitors of eukaryotic DNA polymerases. *Seikagaku*, Vol.74, No.3, pp. 244-251

Singhal, R.K. & Wilson, S.H. (1993). Short gap-filling synthesis by DNA polymerase β is processive. *The Journal of Biological Chemistry*, Vol.268, No.21, pp. 15906-15911, ISSN 0021-9258

Sobol, R.W.; Horton, J.K.; Kuhn, R.; Gu, H.; Singhal, R.K.; Prasad, R.; Rajewsky, K. & Wilson, S.H. (1996). Requirement of mammalian DNA polymerase-β in base-excision repair. *Nature*, Vol.379, No.6561, pp. 183-186, ISSN 0028-0836

Sugo, N.; Aratani, Y.; Nagashima, Y.; Kubota, Y. & Koyama, H. (2000). Neonatal lethality with abnormal neurogenesis in mice deficient in DNA polymerase β. *The EMBO Journal*, Vol.19, No.6, pp. 1397-1404, ISSN 0261-4189

Takata, K.; Shimizu, T.; Iwai, S. & Wood, R.D. (2006). Human DNA polymerase N (POLN) is a low fidelity enzyme capable of error-free bypass of 5S-thymine glycol. *The Journal of Biological Chemistry*, Vol.281, No.33, pp. 23445-23455, ISSN 0021-9258

Permissions

The contributors of this book come from diverse backgrounds, making this book a truly international effort. This book will bring forth new frontiers with its revolutionizing research information and detailed analysis of the nascent developments around the world.

We would like to thank Dr. Sonya Vengrova, for lending her expertise to make the book truly unique. She has played a crucial role in the development of this book. Without her invaluable contribution this book wouldn't have been possible. She has made vital efforts to compile up to date information on the varied aspects of this subject to make this book a valuable addition to the collection of many professionals and students.

This book was conceptualized with the vision of imparting up-to-date information and advanced data in this field. To ensure the same, a matchless editorial board was set up. Every individual on the board went through rigorous rounds of assessment to prove their worth. After which they invested a large part of their time researching and compiling the most relevant data for our readers. Conferences and sessions were held from time to time between the editorial board and the contributing authors to present the data in the most comprehensible form. The editorial team has worked tirelessly to provide valuable and valid information to help people across the globe.

Every chapter published in this book has been scrutinized by our experts. Their significance has been extensively debated. The topics covered herein carry significant findings which will fuel the growth of the discipline. They may even be implemented as practical applications or may be referred to as a beginning point for another development. Chapters in this book were first published by InTech; hereby published with permission under the Creative Commons Attribution License or equivalent.

The editorial board has been involved in producing this book since its inception. They have spent rigorous hours researching and exploring the diverse topics which have resulted in the successful publishing of this book. They have passed on their knowledge of decades through this book. To expedite this challenging task, the publisher supported the team at every step. A small team of assistant editors was also appointed to further simplify the editing procedure and attain best results for the readers.

Our editorial team has been hand-picked from every corner of the world. Their multi-ethnicity adds dynamic inputs to the discussions which result in innovative outcomes. These outcomes are then further discussed with the researchers and contributors who give their valuable feedback and opinion regarding the same. The feedback is then collaborated with the researches and they are edited in a comprehensive manner to aid the understanding of the subject.

Apart from the editorial board, the designing team has also invested a significant amount of their time in understanding the subject and creating the most relevant covers. They scrutinized every image to scout for the most suitable representation of the subject and create an appropriate cover for the book.

The publishing team has been involved in this book since its early stages. They were actively engaged in every process, be it collecting the data, connecting with the contributors or procuring relevant information. The team has been an ardent support to the editorial, designing and production team. Their endless efforts to recruit the best for this project, has resulted in the accomplishment of this book. They are a veteran in the field of academics and their pool of knowledge is as vast as their experience in printing. Their expertise and guidance has proved useful at every step. Their uncompromising quality standards have made this book an exceptional effort. Their encouragement from time to time has been an inspiration for everyone.

The publisher and the editorial board hope that this book will prove to be a valuable piece of knowledge for researchers, students, practitioners and scholars across the globe.

List of Contributors

Robin Assfalg and Sebastian Iben
Department of Dermatology and Allergic Diseases, University of Ulm, Germany

Chunmei Wang, Erxu Pi, Qinglei Zhan and Sai-ming Ngai
School of Life Sciences, State Key laboratory of Agrobiotechnology, The Chinese University of Hong Kong, China

Sarah Vose and James Mitchell
Harvard School of Public Health, Department of Genetics and Complex Diseases, Boston, MA
USA

Kyungmi Min and Susan E. Ebeler
Department of Viticulture & Enology, University of California, Davis, USA

Kei Adachi and Hiroyuki Nakai
Department of Microbiology and Molecular Genetics, University of Pittsburgh School of Medicine, USA
Department of Molecular & Medical Genetics, Oregon Health & Science University School of Medicine, USA

Harpreet K. Dibra, Chris J. Perry and Iain D. Nicholl
University of Wolverhampton, UK

Gordon M. Xiong and Stephan Gasser
Department of Microbiology, National University of Singapore, Singapore

Yoshiyuki Mizushina
Laboratory of Food & Nutritional Sciences, Department of Nutritional Science, Kobe-Gakuin University, Japan

Yoshiyuki Mizushina
Cooperative Research Center of Life Sciences, Kobe-Gakuin University, Japan

Masayuki Nishida, Takeshi Azuma and Masaru Yoshida
Division of Gastroenterology, Department of Internal Medicine, Kobe University Graduate School of Medicine, Japan

Masaru Yoshida
The Integrated Center for Mass Spectrometry, Kobe University Graduate School of Medicine, Japan
Division of Metabolomics Research, Kobe University Graduate School of Medicine, Japan

Printed in the USA
CPSIA information can be obtained
at www.ICGtesting.com
JSHW011354221024
72173JS00003B/277